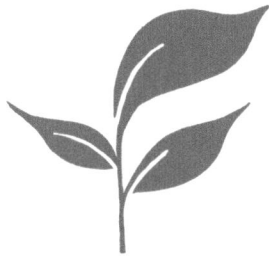

WHOLESOME
WORLD

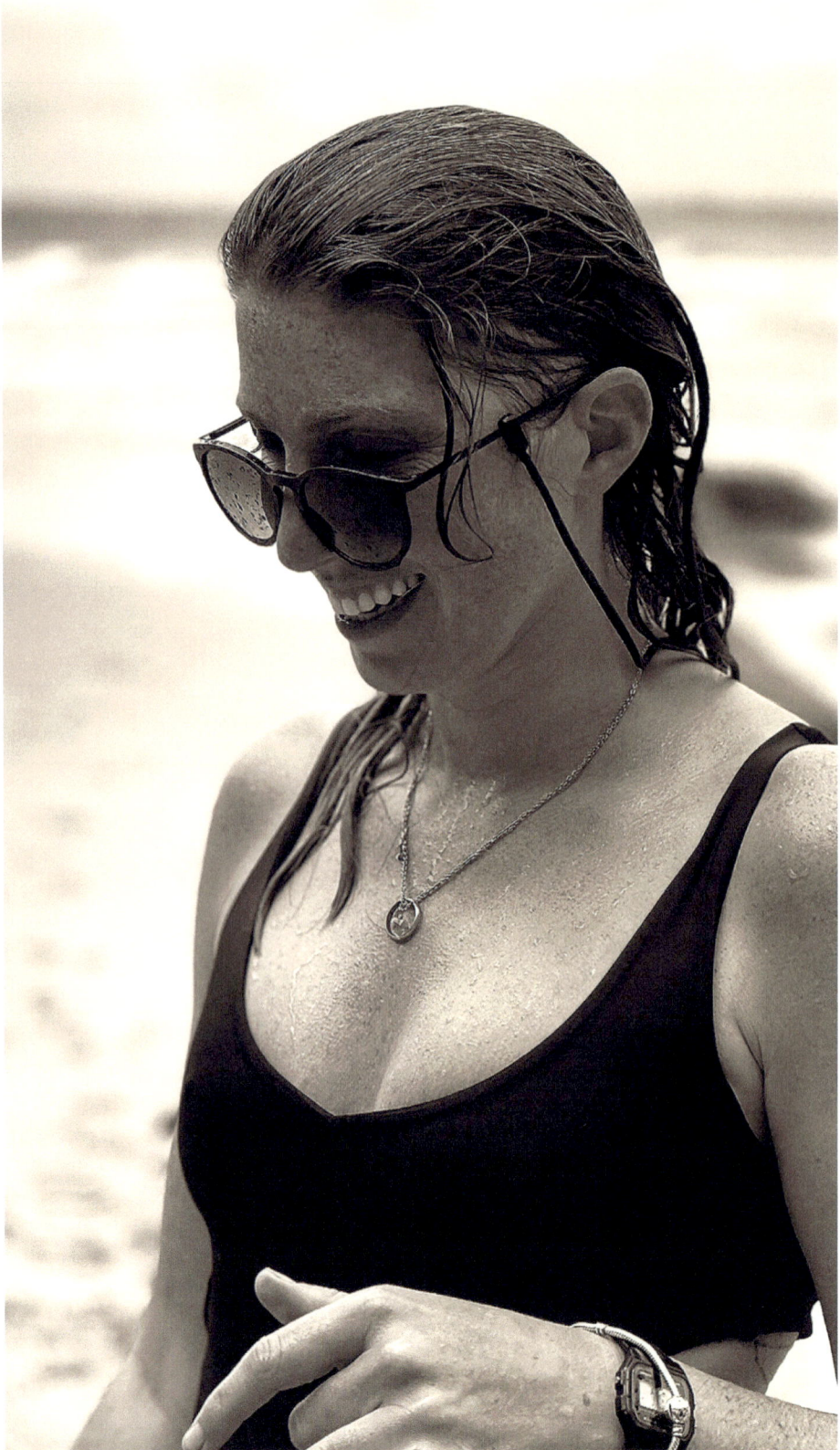

WELCOME TO MY WHOLESOME WORLD

Welcome to my life and book.

Let me tell you a bit about myself, show you who I am and the life hits that I have had to deal with, and how I managed to create a healthy, happy world.

My wholesome book can help you to learn how to set a new path towards improving your health from all different aspects of your life. I want to share life science insights through optimising nutritional, physical and mental health platforms.

I will satiate you with more than 100 delicious recipes from simple to quirky, where you will fall into my Wholesome World.

Full of my love from start to finish.

-

Freyja x

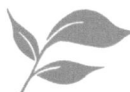

WHOLESOME WORLD COOKBOOK & LIFE

ISBN 978-1-3999-4974-3

Printed and bound in Great Britain by TJ Books Limited, Padstow.

WHOLESOME WORLD

A healthy diet & healthy life

"The important thing is not to stop questioning. Curiosity has its own reason for existing."

Albert Einstein

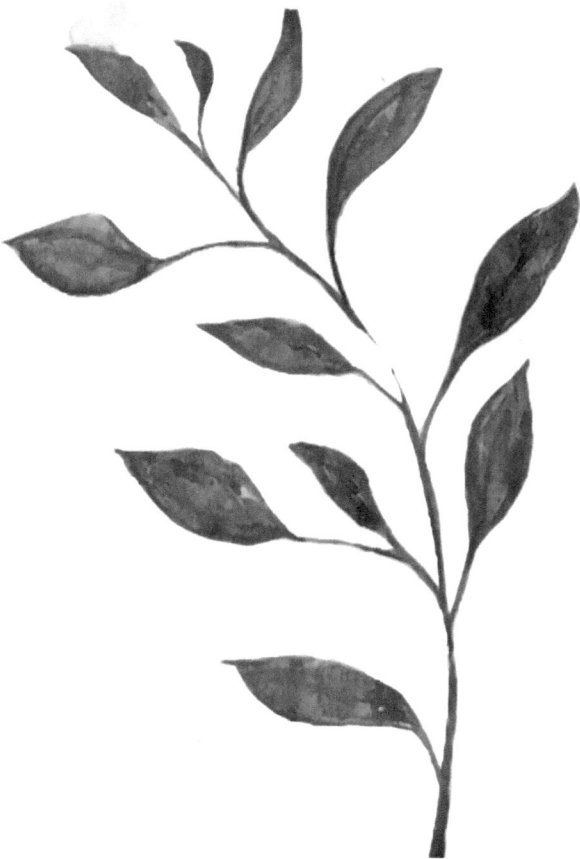

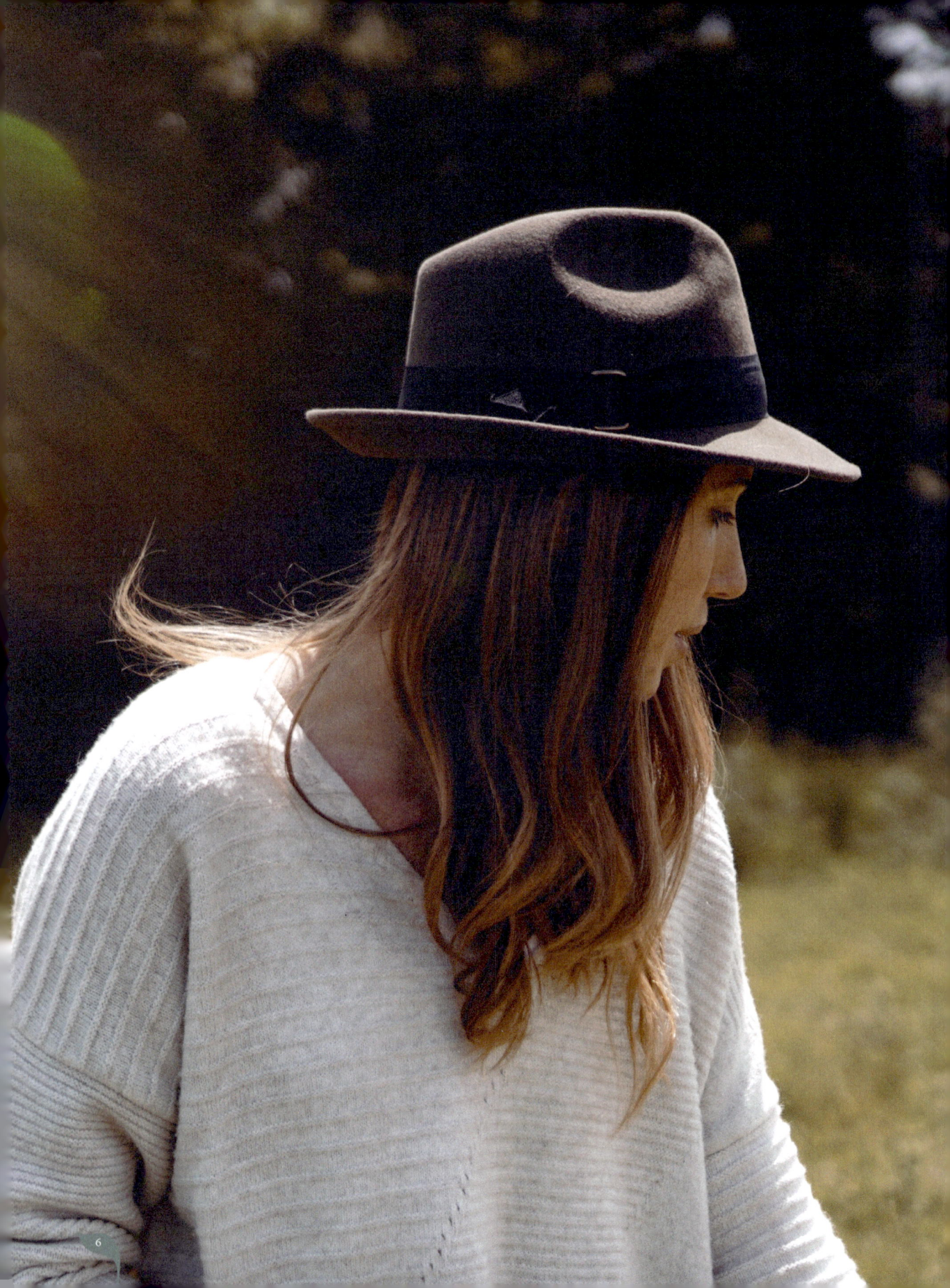

FREYJA'S LIFE

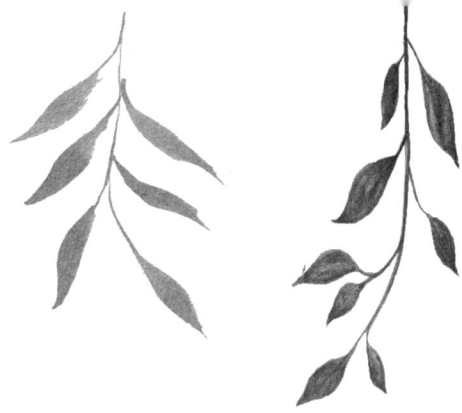

Ten years ago, I was 24, returning from working in Australia via Indonesia and enjoying the freedom to travel. I met an amazing man in the islands, and simply fell in love – which diverted my plans to a completely different journey.

Within the first year, he was hit with a rare type of cancer; treatment for the disease restricted us to living in Europe.

In the following years, coping with my partner's recurring cancer was a learning curve for us both; we were determined to find out everything we could about his illness and try whatever diet, medical practice and philosophy that might help.

As a remarkably strong man he cooked, meditated, medicated and had repeated rounds of chemo. He researched and surfed, climbed a mountain with me and so much more. He wanted to try every path that could be health positive. We wanted to share our discoveries and practical experience with other people searching for a way to maximise their health. Lars made notes about whatever he found useful and even started writing a book.

> *"My husband Lars died from cancer when we were 27.*
>
> *Ten months later I was diagnosed with a grade III/IV cancerous brain tumour."*

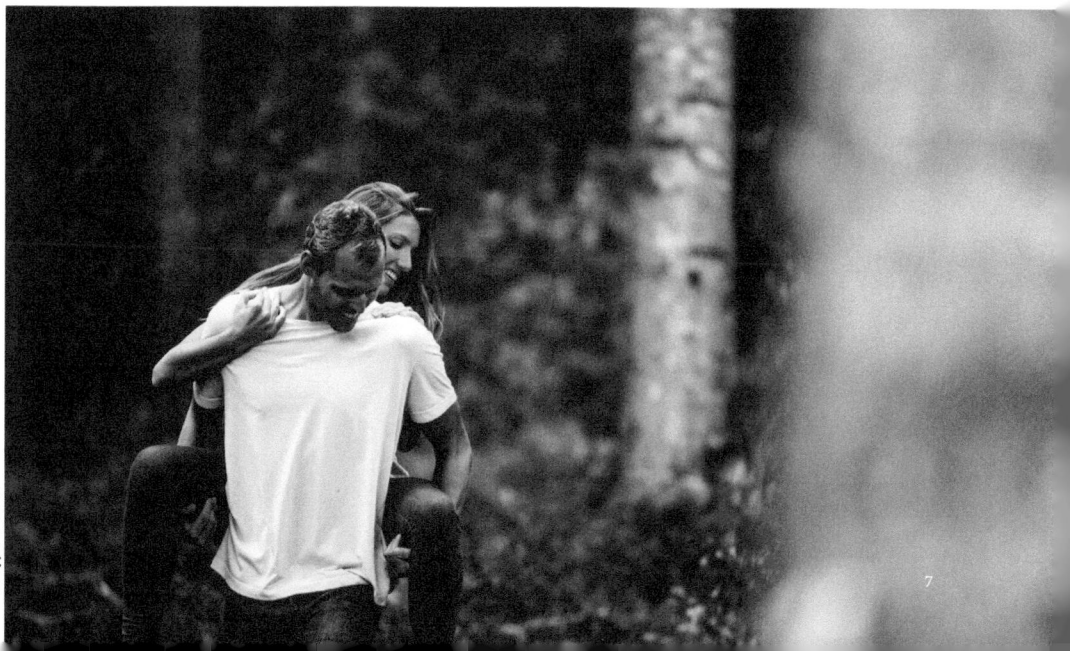

Freyja & Lars

After months of clumsiness and head rushes (my name for 'petit mal' epileptic seizures) and having to push for tests and scans because I knew something was wrong, getting a diagnosis was a relief. And it might sound odd, but I felt lucky. I had spent 2 years with Lars when he had cancer, so I had learnt alongside him about being as fit as possible: physically, nutritionally, mentally, everything. I'd also seen the importance of doing the things that make you happy to improve your chances of survival; how getting in the sea boosted Lars' mood and energy to battle what life was throwing at him.

Because Lars was gone, I had the courage to make bold decisions. If something went wrong maybe I'd find him on the other side, if there is one. But I knew he would be really pissed off with me if I hadn't put up a fight. One bold decision I made was to have aggressive surgery to try and get rid of the whole tumour. But that came with potential risks to my cognitive function and, at worst, my life.

This descision was made a fraction easier with advice from Dr Ian Sabin, my neurosurgeon. He gifted me with the understanding and confidence to open my mind to this potentially life-threatening surgery. Having the knowledge to make such poignant choices, continues to motivate me to share Wholesome World to this day.

My extra bit of luck was that my brother had just finished his PhD in neuroscience. His knowledge meant that, as I struggled with all of the information and the anticipated change to my brain function, he had insight into the science in a way that the average cancer patient did not.

I went through the serious, deep operation, radiotherapy and chemotherapy with his support, and that of some amazing souls within the NHS. Brain surgery on my temporal lobe was absurd — you lose your mental health, not just your physical. It isn't visible, but it is so much more.

Life Now...

Since my operation and treatment was completed in early 2016, my scans remain clear. Though I am still being tested every 6 months through an MRI, magnetic resonance imaging (sounds quite beautiful), which I weirdly see as a calming 'tick-off' life moment due to the severity of the original brain tumour; a plum sized oligodendroglioma cytoma.

Finding the way back to appreciating my life has been a journey, living by the sea, creating good food, travelling again to see good friends when possible and re-educating my brain to new challenges after the heavy surgery; my healing continues. My language still stumbles, my memory is limited... this is my world now.

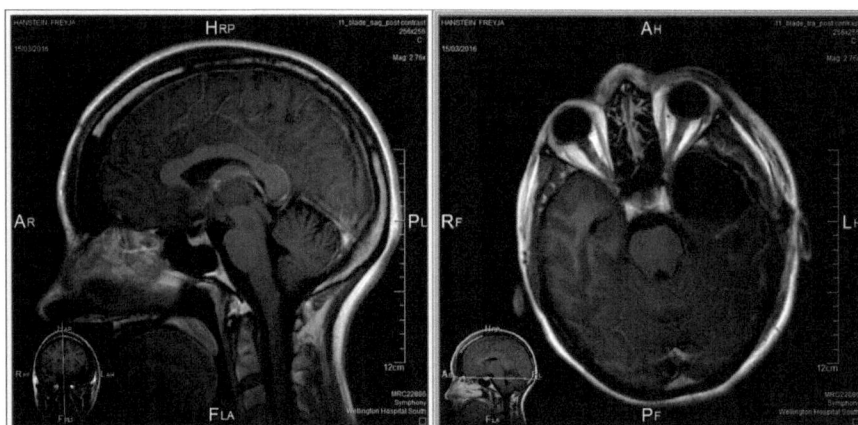

Freyja Hanstein MRI Brain Scan | 03.2016

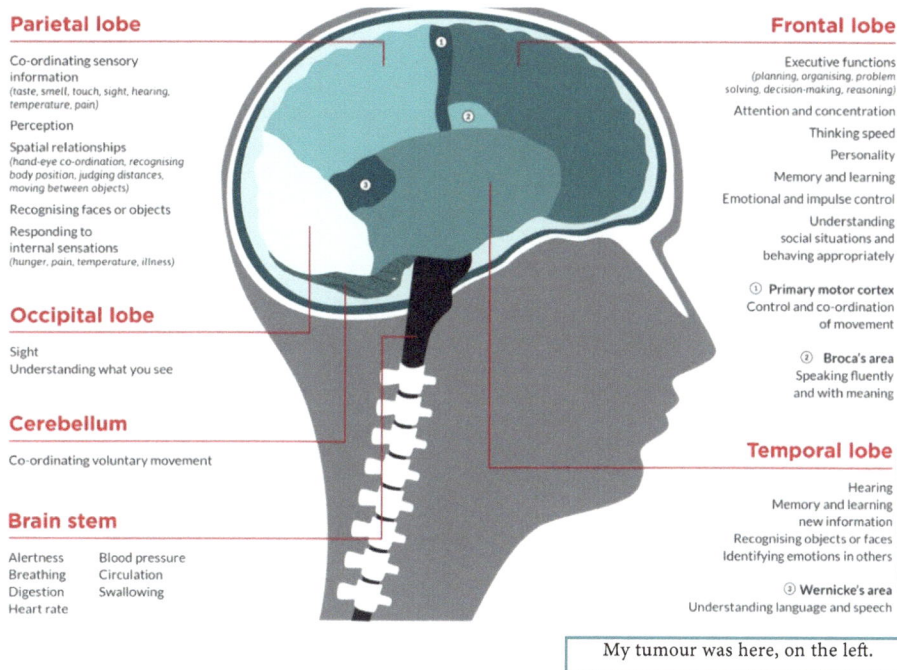

Parietal lobe

Co-ordinating sensory information
(taste, smell, touch, sight, hearing, temperature, pain)

Perception

Spatial relationships
(hand-eye co-ordination, recognising body position, judging distances, moving between objects)

Recognising faces or objects

Responding to internal sensations
(hunger, pain, temperature, illness)

Occipital lobe

Sight
Understanding what you see

Cerebellum

Co-ordinating voluntary movement

Brain stem

Alertness   Blood pressure
Breathing   Circulation
Digestion   Swallowing
Heart rate

Frontal lobe

Executive functions
(planning, organising, problem solving, decision-making, reasoning)

Attention and concentration

Thinking speed

Personality

Memory and learning

Emotional and impulse control

Understanding social situations and behaving appropriately

① Primary motor cortex
Control and co-ordination of movement

② Broca's area
Speaking fluently and with meaning

Temporal lobe

Hearing
Memory and learning new information
Recognising objects or faces
Identifying emotions in others

③ Wernicke's area
Understanding language and speech

My tumour was here, on the left.

Life Glitches...

After the operation I was left with the weirdest, unamendable version of myself. I lost the ability to decipher what my body wanted... was I hungry, tired or did I need the toilet (front or back!)?

My concentration and memory suffered; I lost all nouns, including obvious and basic names, even those of my parents. Language was a mystery. Sentences were impossible to get out of my head to talk to others or simply, how to order a cup of tea. Today, searching for what I want to say is still hard.

The temporal lobe is strongly implicated in language and semantics. I couldn't even memorise the sentences as they built paragraphs in a book, and the same with tv and the stories or news that was on. It was just tea, music, mini exhausted walks, and staring at a satiating homemade fire.

On top of that, due to my seizures, I lost my driving licence for 3 years. I lost my freedom and felt imprisoned. Particularly as I lived in such a small village with strongly limited public transport. Even going for a little surf beyond my local break was out of the question.

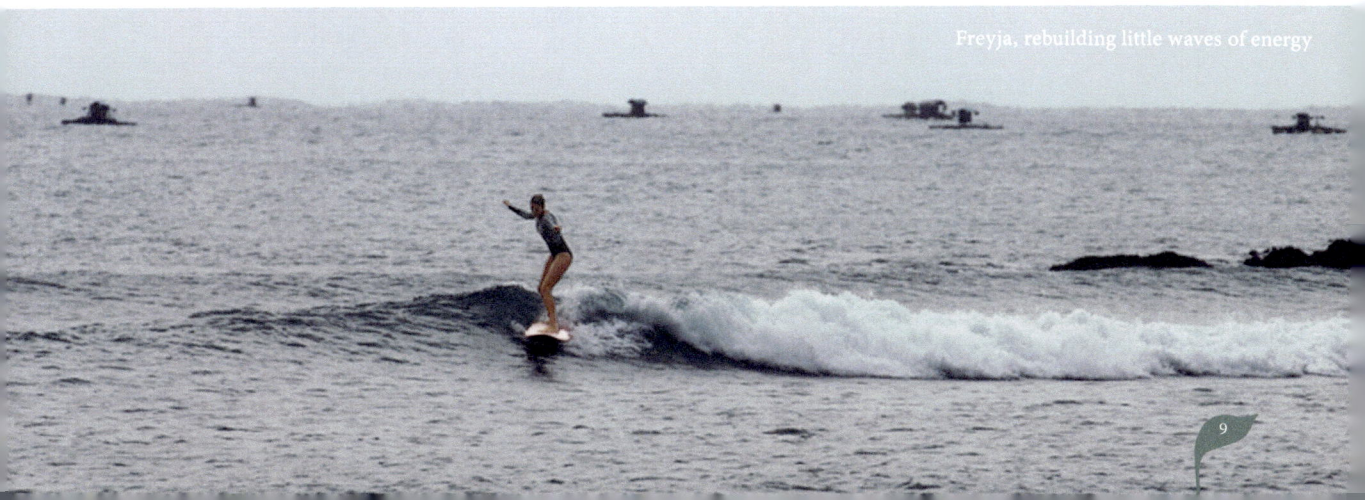

Freyja, rebuilding little waves of energy

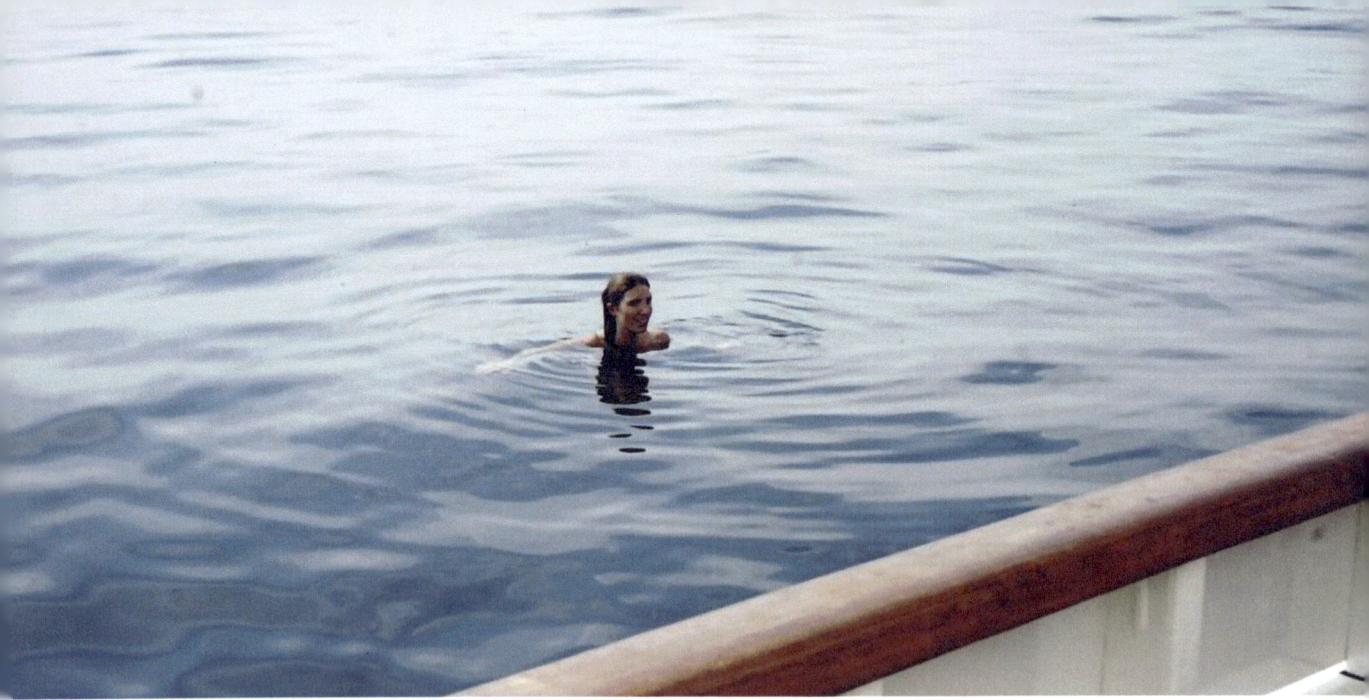

Life Hacks...

My great friend Ryan had the idea to create a Top Trumps-style card game using photos of friends and family with their names and characters to help me re-learn, in a non boring way who my friends were, and re-establish the basic facts about them and our most memorable moments. Other friends were amazingly supportive, such as my friend Snowy moving in with me in London during the radiotherapy treatment wave.

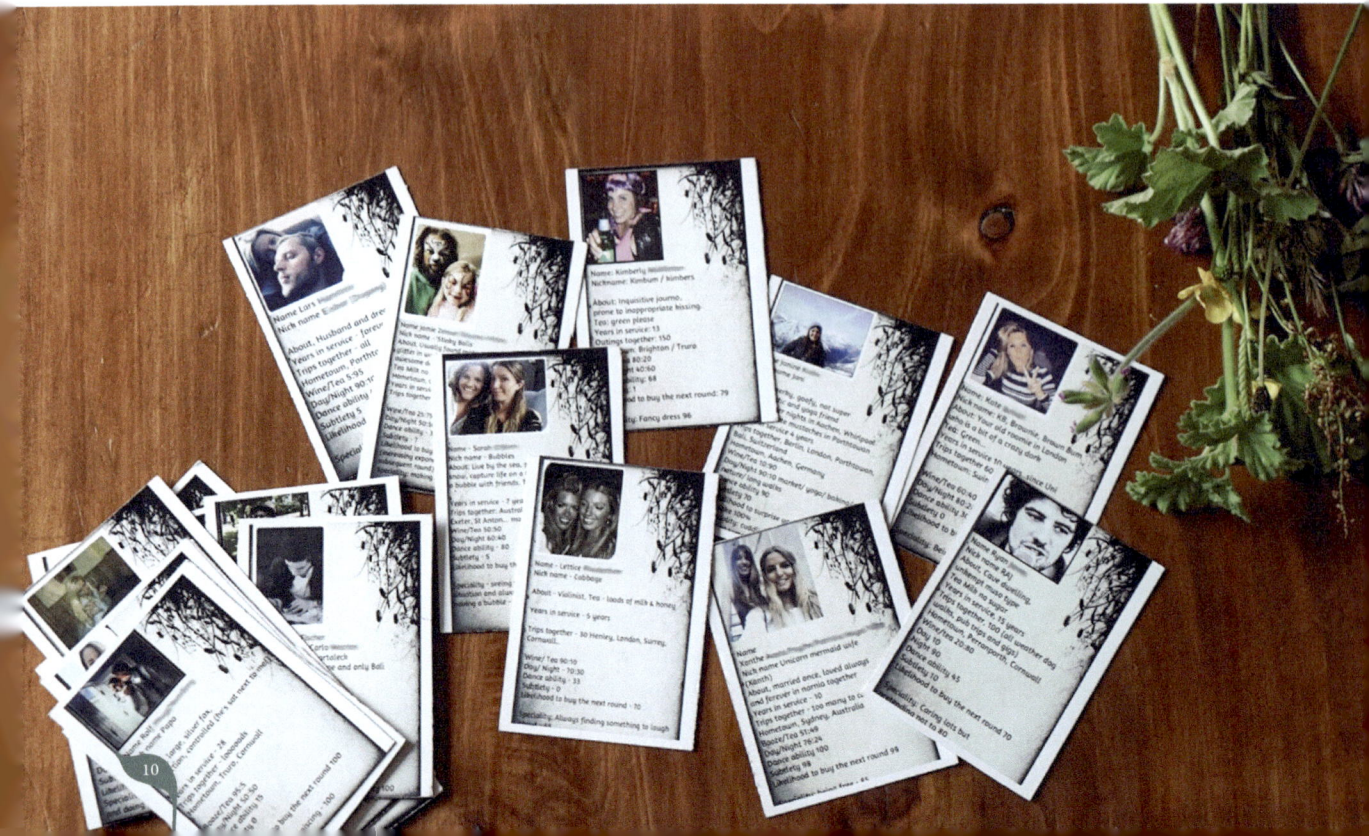

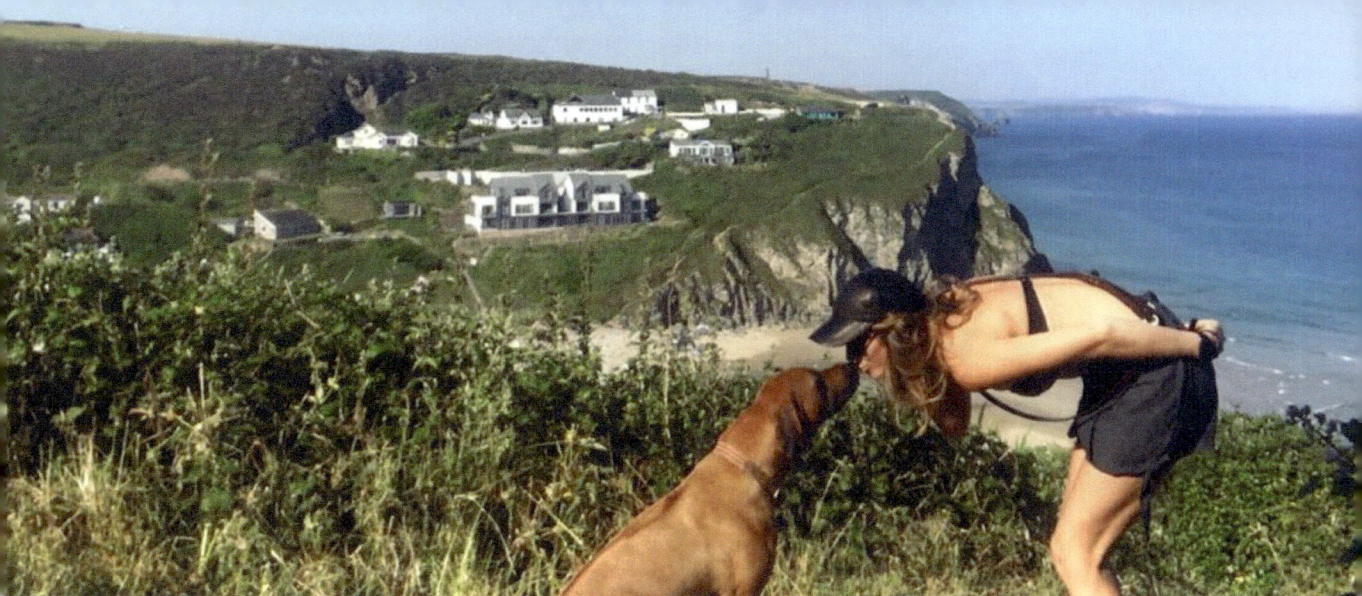

Freyja & Nalu (woof) — out for a little walk

There aren't many better memories from the days of treatment than the company of my dreamboat Ridgeback beast. Meet Nalu, she simply fills my soul with love. Science tells us that pets can aid the reduction of stress, anxiety and depression, whilst encouraging exercise, rest and recuperation. Nalu joined me and Lars near the end of our time together. This connection between us is unconditional, she is a consistent soul that dealt with my emotion whenever I chose. Meaning, I didn't even need to make the effort and describe what I was going through to my friends and family, who wanted to be there for me. This aided me, as I didn't have the energy to open a mental door and rehash the life story with a broken brain and communication skills. She is an everlasting link and I'm forever grateful and thankful to her.

On top of so many other waves I had to deal with, there were hits and hurdles that flew in and out of my life. For instance, my little house flooded, whilst sneaking up to London for my birthday back in 2017. The was just after the brain surgery and repairs took over a year to refurb the floor and more. Even more stressful as the London trip was strongly involved with the intense terrorist attack in Borough Market.

I couldn't have travelled without having a phone. The new-age techno vessels became my memory. This benefit of digital platforms being available to hand – mobile, was key to my mini-freedoms. To be on the safe side, I took extra battery chargers x2 for my trip to Australia for Dec 2016.

I also stumbled upon brain cancer groups, and two weird therapists, luckily followed by a normal dreamboat one. Strong paths for my confusion and stress relief.

I hope to share my desire and the need for good food with you through this book which could enhance your health.

I still feel unbelievably lucky for the foundation of knowledge and expertise that I had around me which allowed me to take an active role in my cancer treatment. Wholesome World started as an app, which is constantly growing and evolving due to new scientific discoveries and extra recipes being added every month. I want to share that foundation with others – not only people with cancer, but anyone who wants to nourish their body and soul.

Realising what makes you happy and strong is one of the most vital parts of living.

High grade/anaplastic oligodendroglioma:
About 30 to 38% of people with this type of tumour will survive for 5 years or more after they are diagnosed.[4]

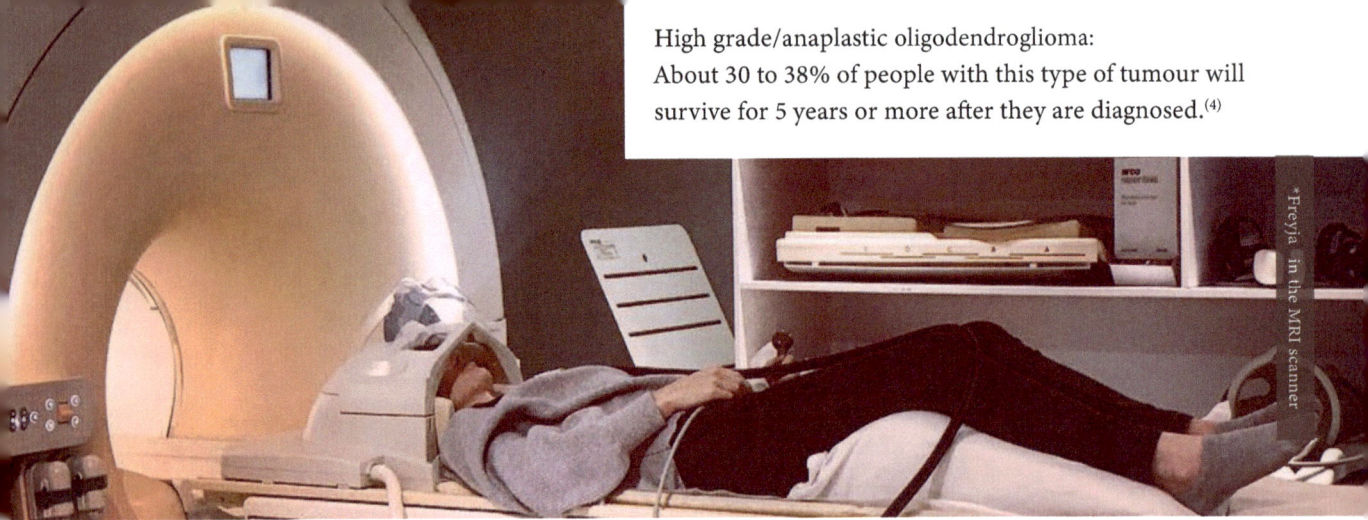

*Freyja in the MRI scanner

"In 2019 we met Freyja and Wholesome World to share her personal story and creation of the original app, as a source of inspiration to so many others going through similar experiences.

It is important to realise that adults report that their brain tumour affects their emotional and mental health[1] as Brain tumours reduce life expectancy by an average of 20 years, the highest of any cancer[2]. The Brain Tumour Charity provides support for everyone affected so that they can live as full a life as possible.

We fund pioneering research to find new treatments, improve understanding, increase survival rates and bring us closer to a cure, and are the UK's largest dedicated brain tumour charity, committed to fighting brain tumours on all fronts." [3]

Piers Townley The Brain Tumour Charity

The figures listed above are given in 1, 2, 5 and 10 year intervals simply because doctors use these intervals for research/measuring purposes – they are not meant to represent how long a person will live past those intervals.

For example, a patient who is a 5 year survivor might live as long as any other healthy person, depending on their circumstances.

It is important to remember that statistics and averages cannot tell you what will happen to you specifically.

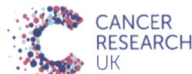

Find connections to charities here

There are so many charities that helped me through my health hit making me understand the technical tasks to push both my governmental tick lists off and understand what was available in our NHS health system.

The Brain Tumour Charity, gave me the awareness and understanding of what is now a 'normal' world.

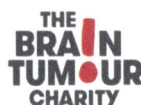

Progress in research into brain tumours has been slow - since 1971 there has been an overall increase in survival of less than 10% for people with a high grade brain tumour, one of the poorest improvements across all cancers. This highlights the need for investment in this field of research.[4]

Such a heavy wave to hear about the current research in this field, but just recently seeing the speed that research can develop and approach heavy medicinal defence, in hits like COVID, shows what secret doors there are to be found, not just for brain tumour research, but so many health related aspects.

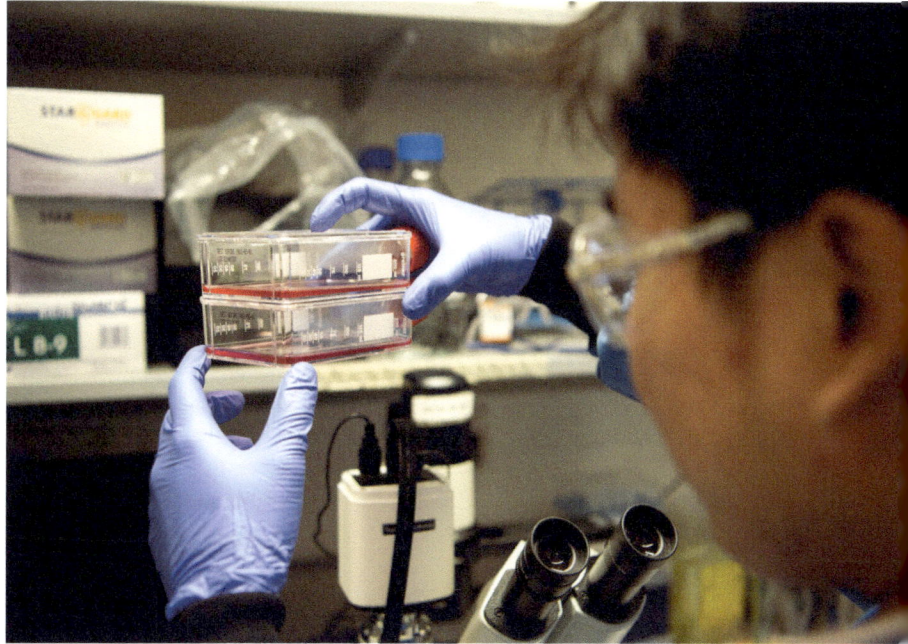

Publicly funded research bodies such as the National Institute for Health Research (NIHR) and the Research Councils are open to applications from researchers working on any condition and judged in open competition. However, the priorities of institutions and researchers can be determined by the perception of Government priorities.

Prof Richard Gilbertson:

"These great minds are now working together to solve the problem of cancer and are defining a new roadmap for cancer science in Cambridge for the next five years."

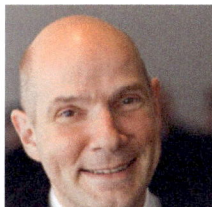

Professor
Martin Taphoorn

Patient Reported Outcome (PRO) measures used in neuro-oncology

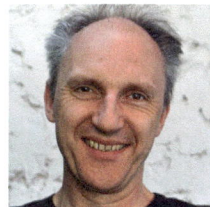

Professor
Sebastian Brandner

Nanoparticle Couriers for GBM treatments

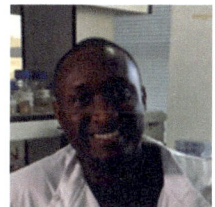

Dr Ola Rominiyi

3D models to understand invading GBM cells

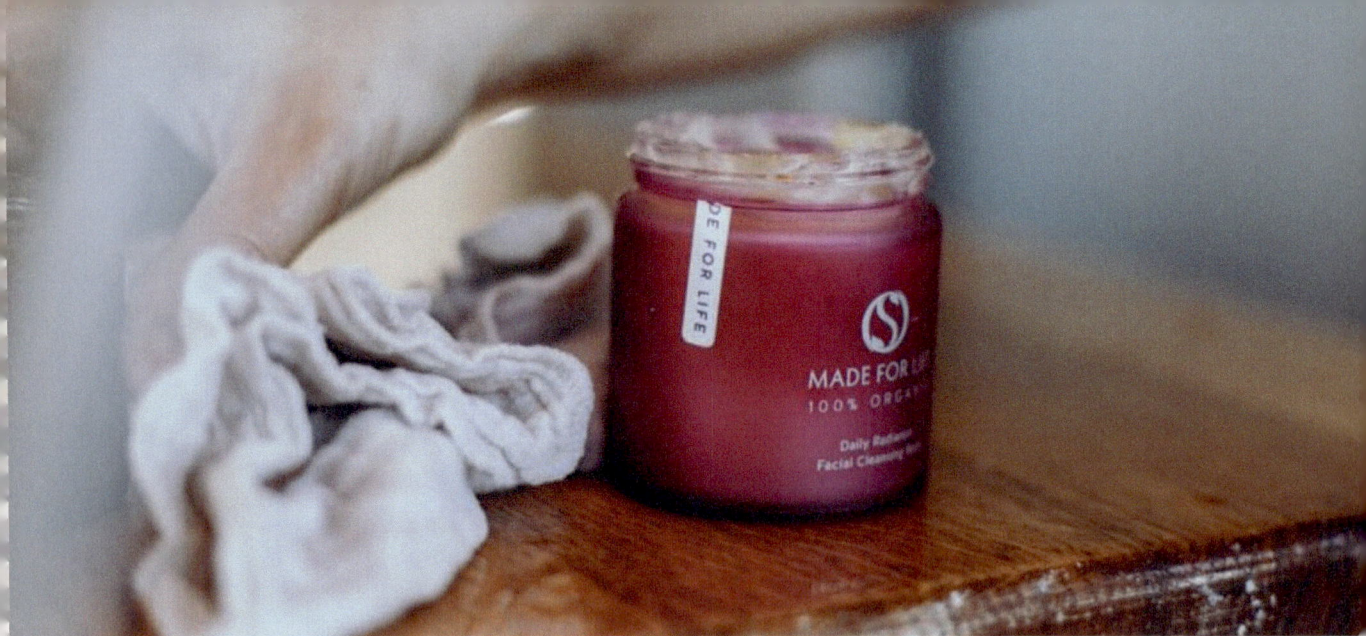

Made for Life is a beautiful 100% organic skincare range, which I stumbled across and worked with years ago. I still feel so enriched, that I have to throw the word out.

The range is both organic, raw and toxin free which nourishes you from tip to toe. It's even for those with sensitive skin as it can delightfully and safely nurture our skin through cancer treatments. One of those secret benefits of going through cancer maybe...

Another surprising benefit is that this skincare is edible! For instance, I remember using the beautiful flavours of the products to improve the taste of my thrown together pistachio and rose macaroons using their facial oil.

This is a cancer researched, 100% organic skincare company that I am an ambassador for, and just simply love through and through. One of the most solid ranges — for every soul on this planet.

The team there also have conducted scientific research to increase the availability of massage, and support and widen its priority, particularly for those with cancer.

My Top 3 that I can't live without are:

Skin Solve A calendula based body balm which soothes during the healing process.
Facial Oil I love the ease of use and benefits from this one, laden with rose and vanilla to benefit both the scent and skin.
Restorative Body Balm Their rose geranium is one of my favourite scents and is great for easing stress too.

The skin absorbs what you put on it, in a similar fashion to what your body consumes, but a lower amount. So it's much more important to invest in that which will enter your body, than just your facade.

My advice is to nourish yourself before others. Your skincare is a strong part of this too.

The highlighted benefits from the research showed that Touch Therapy massage will lower cortisol and boost serotonin levels without any side effects. It's great to 'catch the breath' and boost your immune system. Additional research showed the positive benefits of using some essential oils (at low level) and botanicals as an aromatherapy treat.

It's also great to soothe the soul, mind and body. You can find these across not just the UK but the world, in beautiful places like The Browns Hotel in London.

MADE FOR LIFE
ORGANICS
CORNWALL

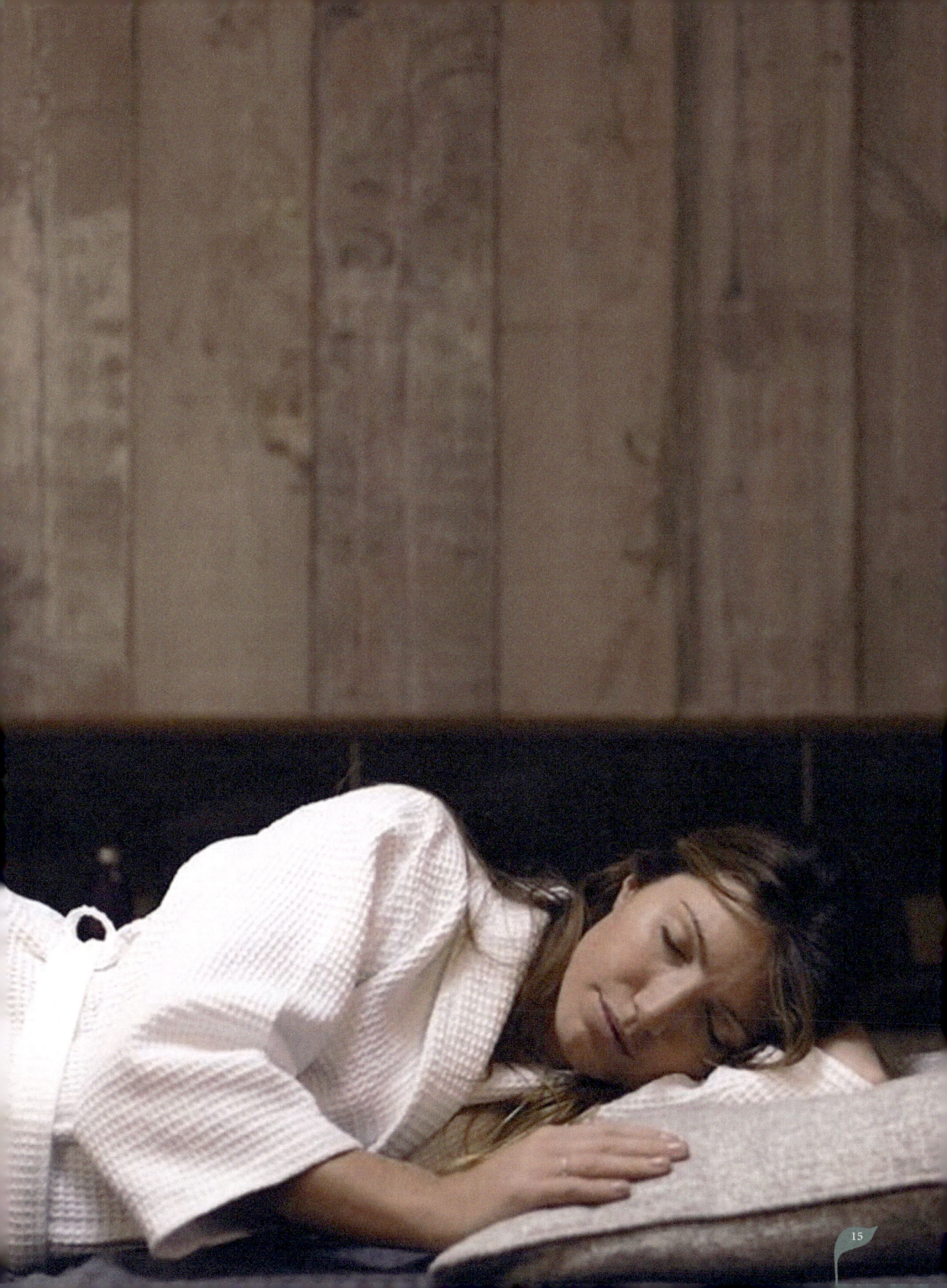

FOOD FOR THE BRAIN

"All disease begins in the gut"
- Hippocrates -

One of the aspects I found really interesting was how you can support your brain through nutrition...

Not many of us think about the importance of good nutrition on our brains, and yet the brain and the gut communicate continuously. In fact **the gut is often referred to as the second brain.** Chemicals, known as neurotransmitters, are made in the gut and communicate with the brain via the vagus nerve. Serotonin, known as the 'happy hormone' is one such neurotransmitter but there are many which can have a profound effect on our mood and wellbeing.

The gut microbiome is key to brain health, too as it also influences communication between the gut and the brain. In fact it works both ways as the brain can equally influence the health of the microbiome. This is why stress can be so detrimental to the gut.

To feed our microbiome and keep it healthy we need to eat a varied diet, rich in plant fibre, fermented foods (such as yoghurt, miso, sauerkraut), healthy fats and reduce unhealthy sugars and starches which feed our 'non-beneficial' microbiota. The health of the microbiome and the gut is also key to a healthy immune system as 70% of our immune system is housed in the gut.

The brain weighs just 1.5kg but utilises around 25% of the body's energy. The type of fuel the brain uses can be key to its performance. The brain is extremely glucose hungry but large amounts or unregulated amounts can have detrimental, toxic effects. Therefore, eating foods that maintain a healthy blood sugar balance is very important. This means not only avoiding refined carbohydrates which raise our blood sugar levels significantly but keeping the amount of carbohydrate we eat in check.

Refined carbohydrate-rich meals, such as those with white pasta, rice, bread and cereals are not good for the brain, due to the rapid release of a large amount of glucose into the bloodstream.

Add in healthy fats and protein to offset the effects, have small portions of carbohydrates, and skip a sugary dessert to maintain glucose balance.

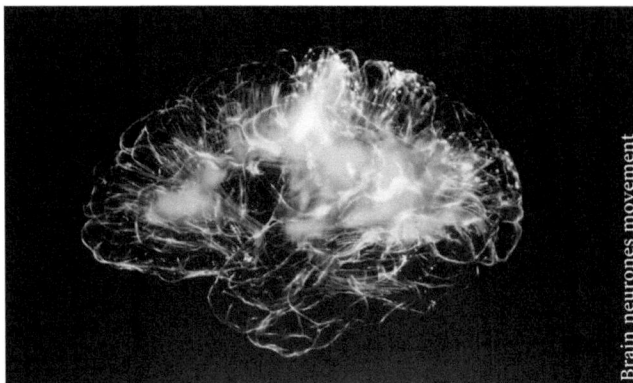

Brain neurones movement

Heathy fats such as Omega 3, 6 and 9 are vital for the body and particularly the functioning of the brain which is made of around 60% fat. These fats are found in oily fish, nuts, seeds, green veg, oils, grass fed meat and dairy. Omega 9 is mainly found in Olive Oil, but can be produced in the body, making it 'non essential'.

Omega 3 and 6 are essential fatty acids (ESF) as we cannot make them in our bodies. They are known to have opposite effects; omega-6s are pro-inflammatory, while omega-3s are anti-inflammatory[1], for which the speed of new age diet change over the last century has weighted the intake of the Omega 6 through processed food.

Ketogenic Diet
-
A low carb, high fat way of eating which switches the fuel in the body from glucose to ketones.

Research into the ketogenic diet which is a low carb, high fat diet has particularly looked at the effects on the brain and those with brain tumours.

Biochemical research that has been done is very positive. As yet we do not have sufficient evidence for the 'keto' diet to recommend this way of eating but there are enough studies and patient experience data to show that reducing carbs,[2] managing blood sugar levels and potentially switching the body's fuel source to fats can greatly increase some people's energy levels and cognitive clarity. It is also being effectively used in many weight management programmes.

Food is not all about providing energy, it has also been shown to have an effect on neuroplasticity. This is the ability of the brain to change and reorganise its response to injury and our learning experiences. Knowledge in this area is gaining momentum and this should be influencing our dietary behaviour, as neurological disease is becoming an epidemic of the 21st century.

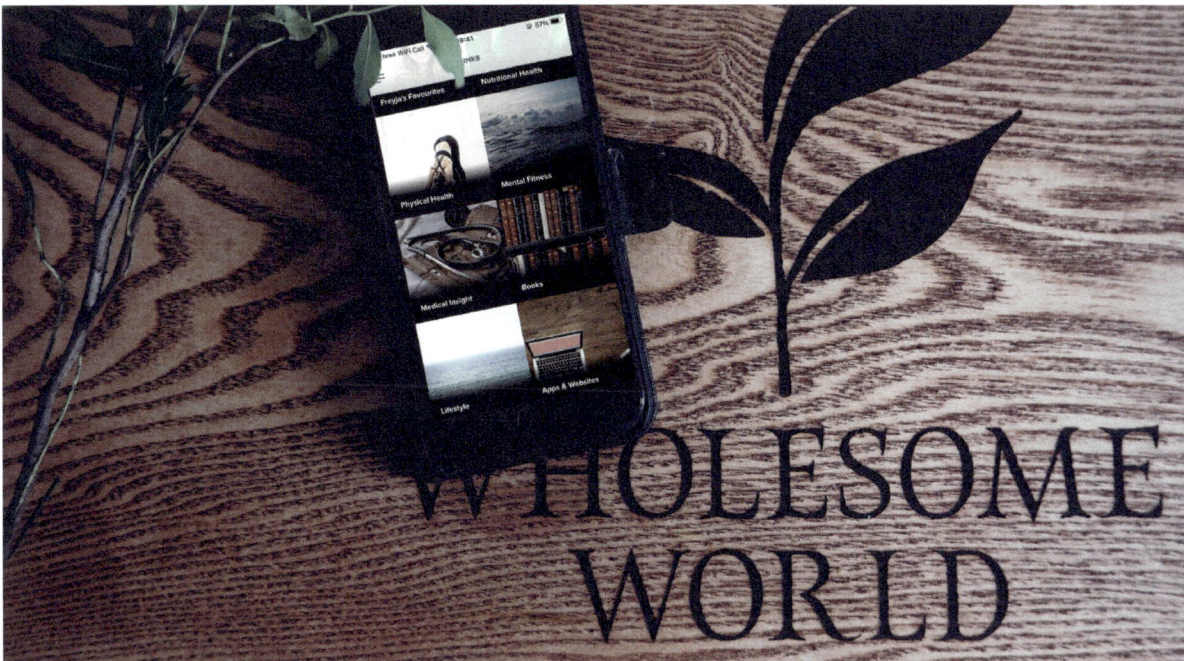

LIFE SCIENCE

sources

There are 3 aspects to life science and home health;

Mental Health | Physical Health | Nutrition

This ethos comes from David Servan-Schreiber, a French physician, neuroscientist, physchiatrist and author who incorporated a great deal of scientific health research into his recommended lifestyle. For which all are significantly important and can be interlaced with each other. It strengthens my life management, and enforces the importance of realising that general health relies on all 3 of these life elements.

His book, Anticancer: A New Way of Life, is a great reference for data to understand health issue prevention, causes, and for self-help if you get cancer, and applies to other types of illness both for prevention and treatment.

Good solid, authorised data sources are so important to affirm and satisfy the steps you take.

PubMed is top of my list to help find and understand medicinal research. It gives you a step to understanding medicinal health and support your queries and questions that you are looking to ask your doctor or health team. It is simply public medicinal papers that you can forage through for the latest research through abstracts, or as deep as you like.

TEDtalks are the next step for me as you can avoid reading, and be interacted with by scientists, or the general public. They simply talk to the world, and recognise that everyone is different, easing the understanding to so many topics. When I was just about to have my brain surgery, I watched snippets of souls that had been through what I was undertaking, scientists confirming my choice in undertaking it, and sometimes distracting me to new worlds that take my mind away from my problems.

*See p270 for some of my favourite TED Talks.

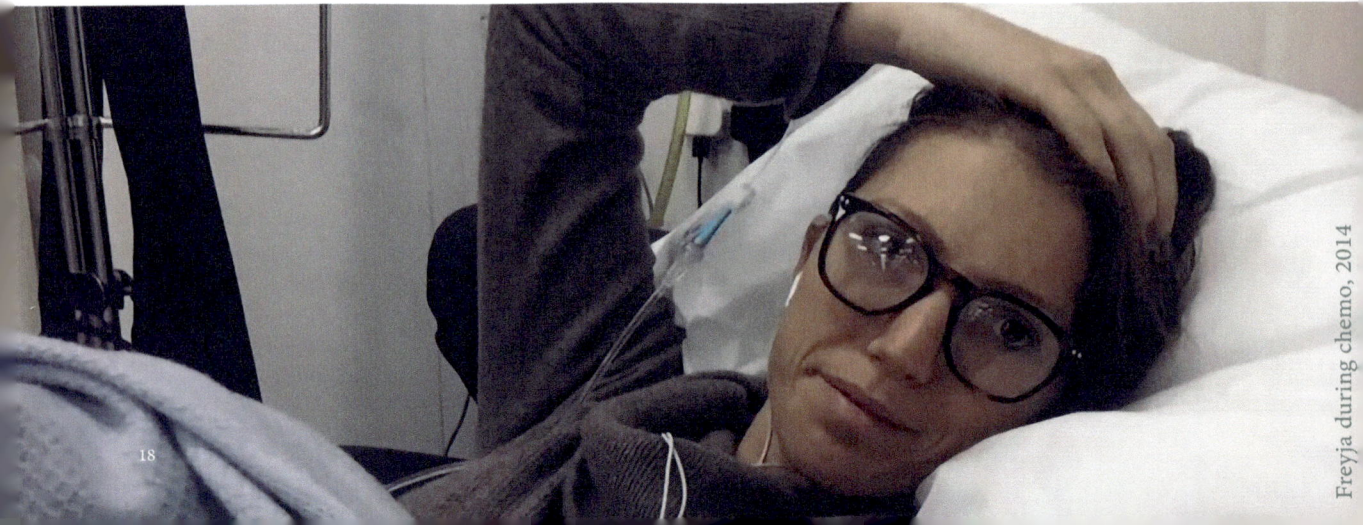

Freyja during chemo, 2014

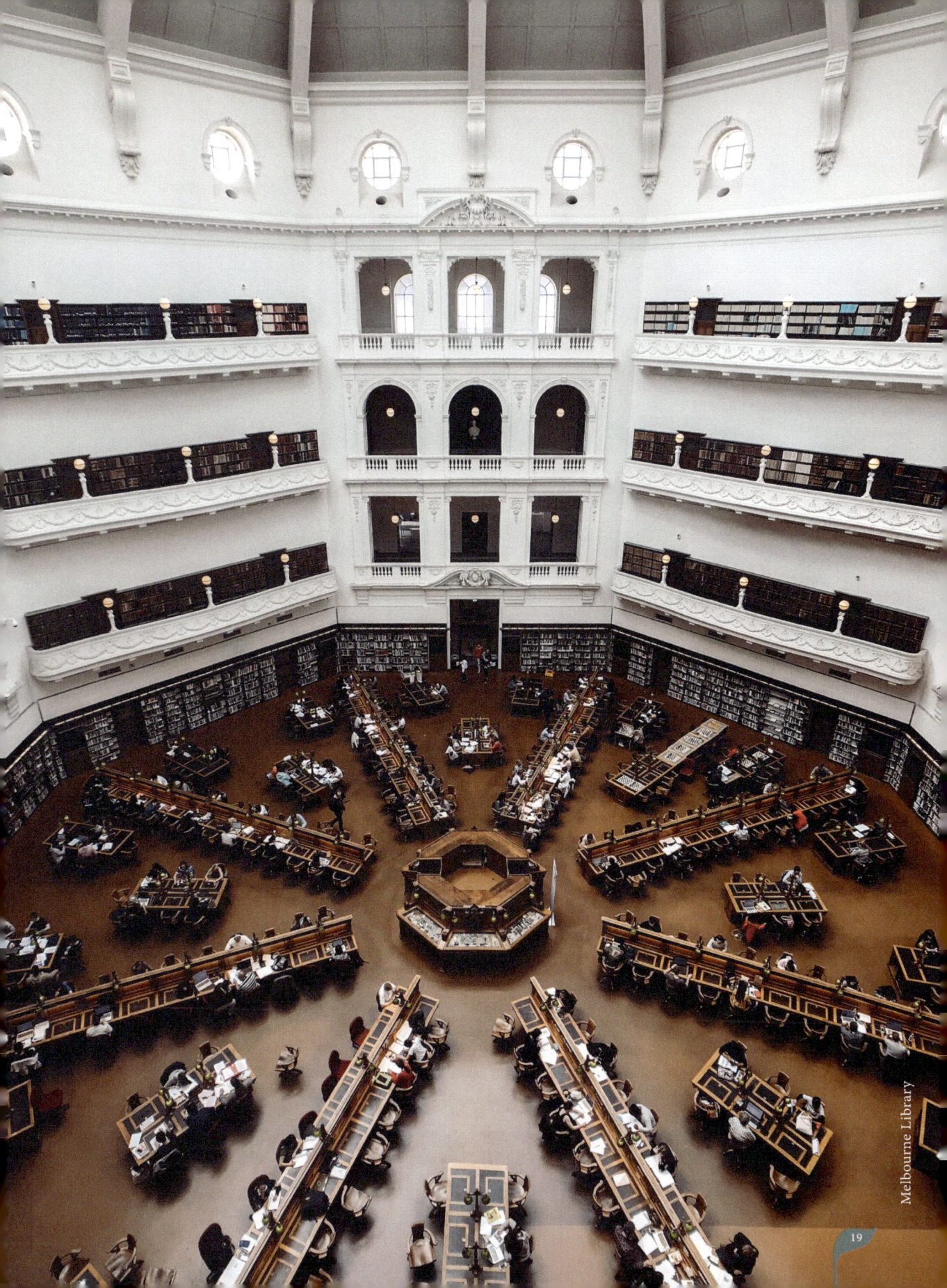

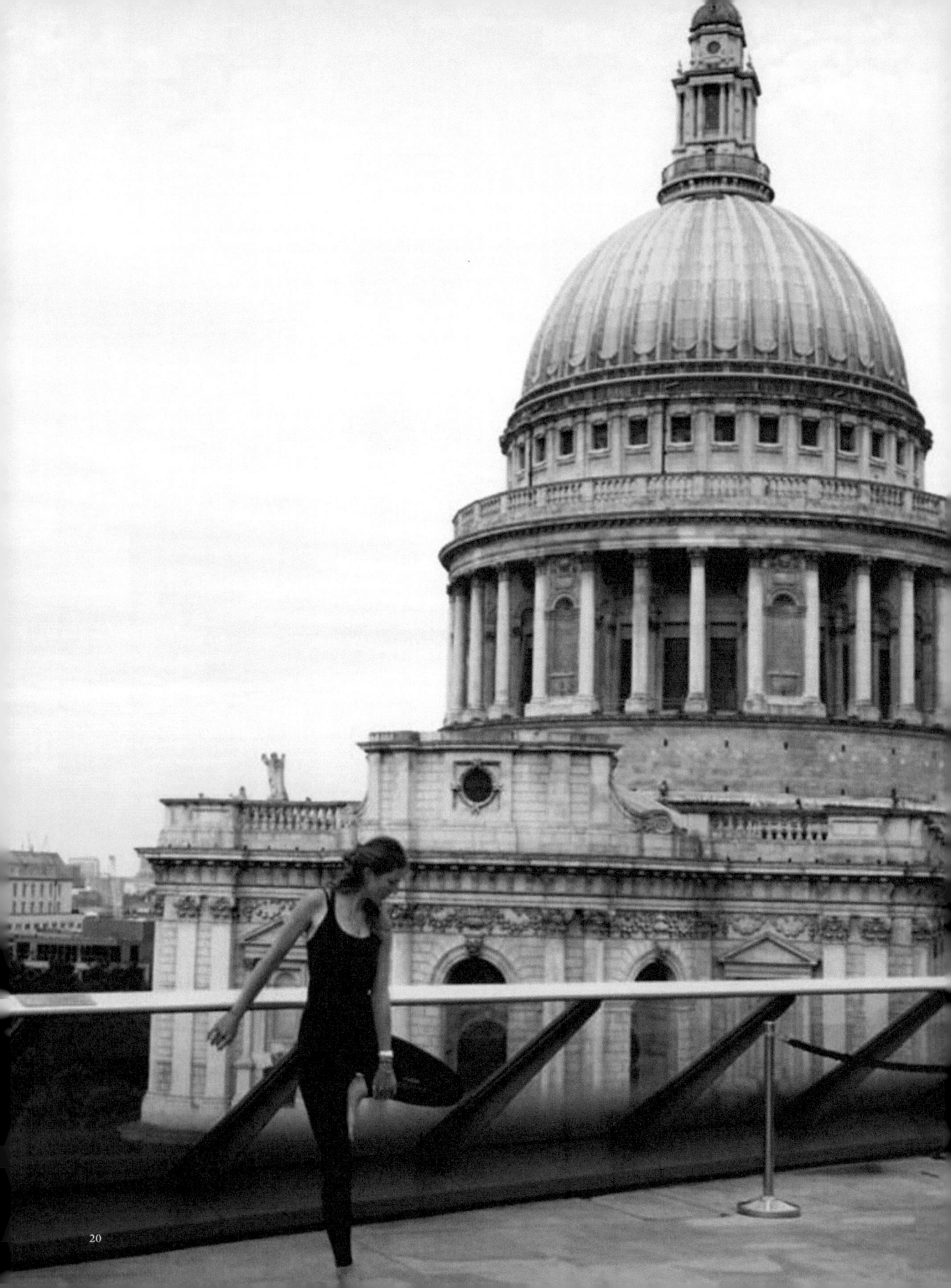

HEALTHY LIVING

for everyone

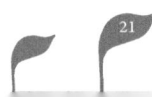

Freyja post op
& during radiotherapy

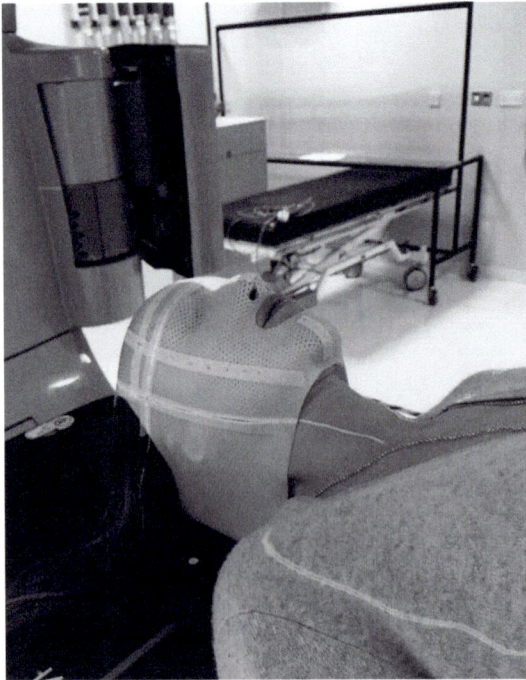

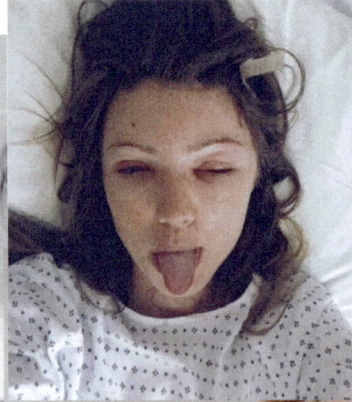

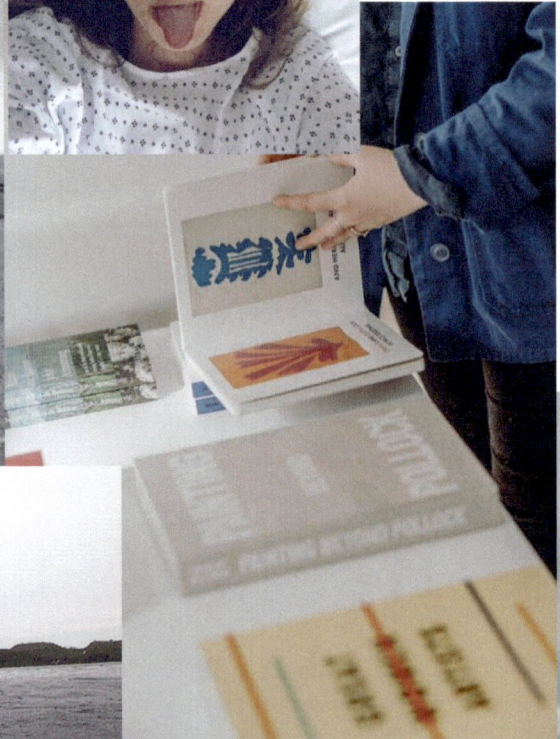

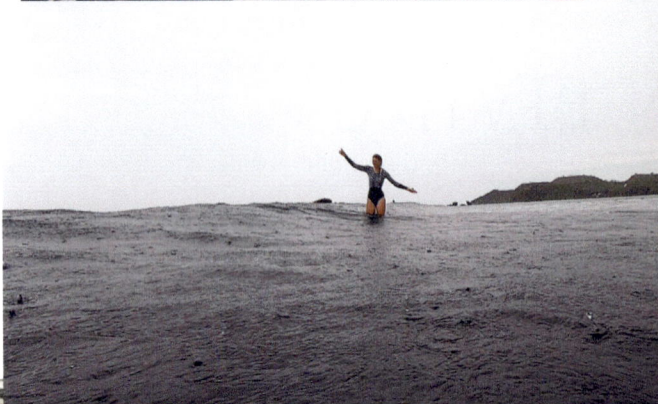

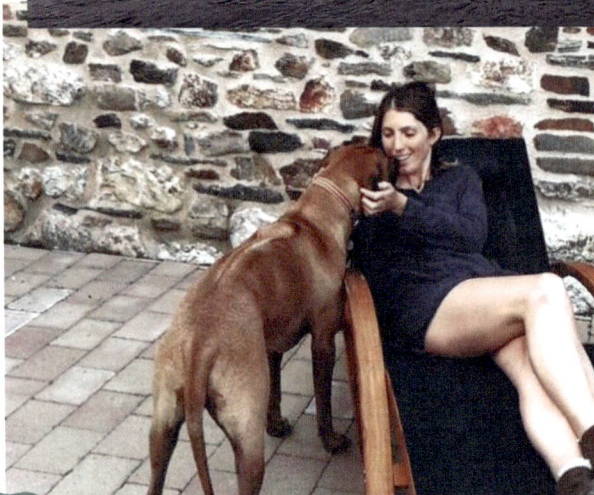

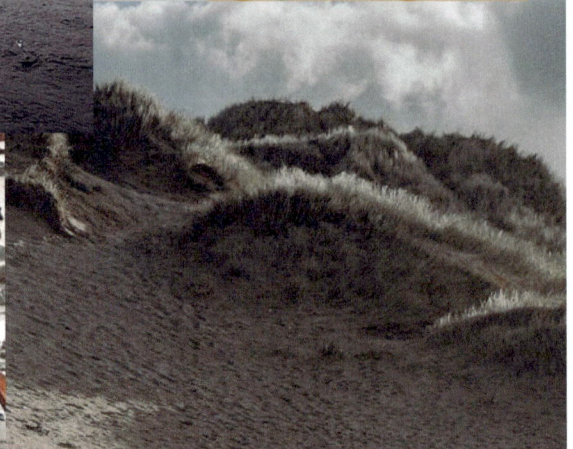

"Nutrition is one of the most under-utilised medications of the 21st century, for our physical and mental health"

Katy Griffin,
NHS Mental Health Nurse
& founder of Thera-Sea

HEALTHY LIVING

Taking control of your health, is a big step towards improving your body and mind's viability.

You need to get back to the basics. I would like to encourage you to modify your eating, move your body a little bit further and keep to a simple path to enhance your wellbeing.

Wholesome definition, Cambridge Dictionary:
'good for you, and likely to improve your life either physically, morally, or emotionally'

For me the aspects of life, health and satisfaction break down into 3 elements.

Mental, physical and nutritional. These aspects are are all important to your wellbeing, and each are improved or masked through medical treatment. The aim of this book is to help you integrate these 3 elements and enforce your life balance and strength. They interact, and improving each one, improves all.

A healthy life doesn't limit itself to your nutrition or exercise, it includes your home, environment and friends.

Throughout my life I have pushed my lifestyle to include physical activity. After my initial cancer treatment it was Nalu, my Ridgeback, who inspired me to maintain consistent physical activity even when I could only manage a few steps per day. Taking her out, meant opening the door to both physical satisfaction and my mental positivity too. Each factor interlaces, though food I find is the simplest starter step, opening the door to the other, harder parts of my world.

So let's look at these 3 elements:

Mental Health
Ayurveda, is one of the world's oldest whole-body healing systems, to maintain wellbeing. However, I am amazed how Western medicine can rescue you from severe disease that can impact your life.
I appreciated both sides and needed to understand each to improve my health and remove stress as much as possible.
It's essential to understand that everyone is different. Our minds and bodies are different and it takes time for changes to take effect.

Physical Health
An easy starting step is to do a light, ten minute walk, morning and evening, this will energise your body and change your mental perspective. My walks are inspired by my dog, Nalu. She is a strong positive reinforcement for my mindset and fuels my energy wave to start the day. Another simple aspect is, if possible, having strong deep sleep.

Nutritional Health
In terms of diet, I have flexed between paleo, pescatarian, vegetarian and vegan and finally taken elements from all of these for maximum benefit in my life. You should be wary of the short term energy boost provided by the intake of refined sugar and carbohydrates.

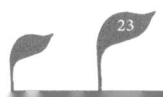

MENTAL HEALTH

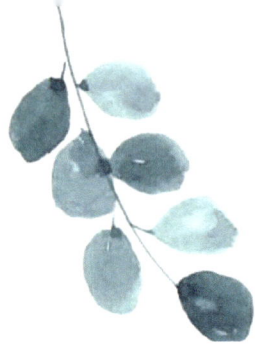

What is mental health?

The World Health Organisation (WHO) defines mental health as 'a state of wellbeing in which the individual realises his or her abilities, can cope with the normal stresses of life, work productively and fruitfully, and is able to make a contribution to his or her community'.

A healthy mind is protective against physical illness, social inequalities and unhealthy lifestyles. It helps us manage stress. High levels of stress and anxiety can lead to serious mental illness, such as depression.

When you are stressed, you feel threatened and your nervous system responds by releasing a flood of stress hormones, including adrenaline and cortisol, which rouse the body for emergency action. Your heart pounds faster, muscles tighten, blood pressure rises, breath quickens, and your senses become sharper.

The elevated levels of cortisol may actually suppress your immune system. You could be more susceptible to colds and contagious illnesses. Your risk of cancer and autoimmune diseases increases and you may develop food allergies and digestive problems.

When my man, Lars, passed away, I initially felt it as the heaviest weight in my world. So, I closed the door to my 'pandora's box' and let it swell and grow and drag me down into depression and a life swamp.

How can we cope when we are dragged down by emotional distress or physical limitations? How do we convert these 'rocks' pulling us under into happy bouyant balloons lifting us into a state of wellbeing, from glass half empty to glass half full? I think the hit of cancer that I went through though pushed me into the realisation that I could move forward, that I could benefit through having witnessed his strength and use it to help me see the reality of the body's capacity to recover if you pushed it as strongly as he had shown me.

WHAT do you do when you fall back into glass half empty? Why is it no longer half full?
What are the balloon floaters to pull you back up?

For me those balloons included using gratitude journals, mindfulness, meditation, a brain cancer charity, group therapy and a number of cognitive pursuits, good sleep, music and food.

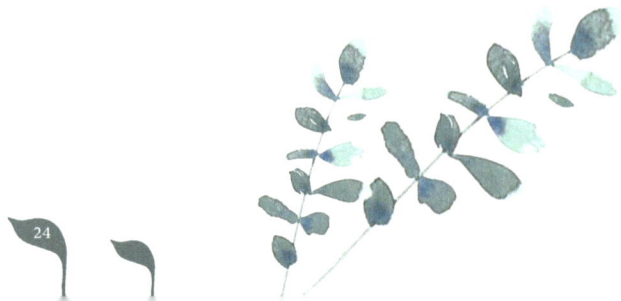

> "Every thought that we have creates a cascade of chemical reactions in the human body."
> - Dr Anna du Cauze De Nazelle

Gratitude journals

Gratitude Journals involve writing down three things at the end of the day that you are thankful for. Many people find this rewarding and beneficial to do as it rewires our neuroplastic brains to consciously remove our negative biases or the things that didn't go well that day and instead focus on the positive things that did go well; I find that it's simple and easy to download an app on your phone these days to prompt you to perform your daily gratitude.

Mindfulness and Meditation

Mindfulness can be defined as a mental state achieved by focusing one's awareness on the present moment, while calmly acknowledging and accepting one's feelings, thoughts, and bodily sensations.

Mindfulness can be used to help us channel our thoughts and again the more we practice, like many things, the better we get. Apps such as Calm or Headspace can help you with this practice. It helps us focus the mind on the present moment rather than worrying about the future or ruminating about the past. For some cancer patients, meditation has been shown to help relieve anxiety, stress, fatigue, and improve sleep and mood, when used along with standard medical treatment.

Surfing Waves = Mind Waves

Talking therapies such as CBT

If you need extra help and support, it is worth booking an appointment with your GP who can refer you to services such as 'health in mind' where trained therapists can confidentially provide talking therapy such as cognitive-behavioral therapy (CBT). You can also access these talking therapies online. According to Health In Mind UK, CBT is seen as effective as medication.

Cognitive Pursuits

Games and activities that stimulate the mind such as Lego, puzzles, card games, crosswords, sudoku, playing pool, snooker and so many others, are helpful. They occupy your time and focus your attention, when maybe too much is in your life. It can build your life satisfaction by being able to complete a task.

Sleep

Sleep is very important for us. Sleep hygiene practices can help to increase the amount of sleep we get and the quality of the sleep we get. Getting up and going to sleep at the same time, exercising, establishing a night-time routine such as getting a bath before bedtime, limiting caffeine, turning off electronics one hour before going to bed to reduce screen time and turning off the blue lights on your electronic devices[1] all help. Add the sleep mode automatically to your mobile, or keep it out of the bedroom, as creating a healthy sleep environment helps to maximize your chances of good night's sleep and rest.

Exposure to room light before bedtime, surpresses melatonin onset and shortens melatonin duration.[2] It basically delays getting to sleep and affects both quality and length of sleep too. As humans, we are designed to get up in the morning when the sun rises, and to go to sleep as it sets. However we need to be conscious to realise this process, and avoid the effects of artificial, electric and blue lights.

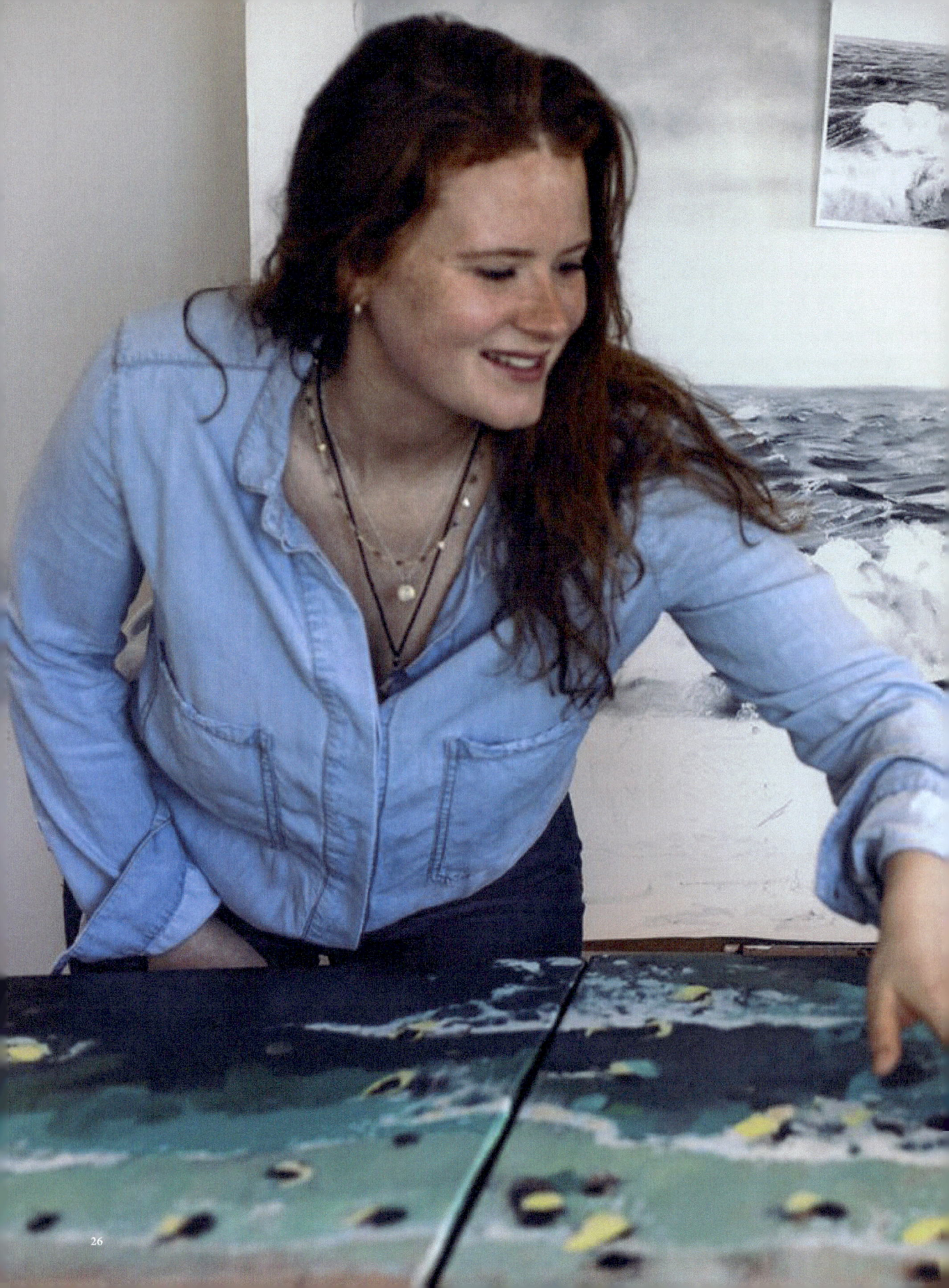

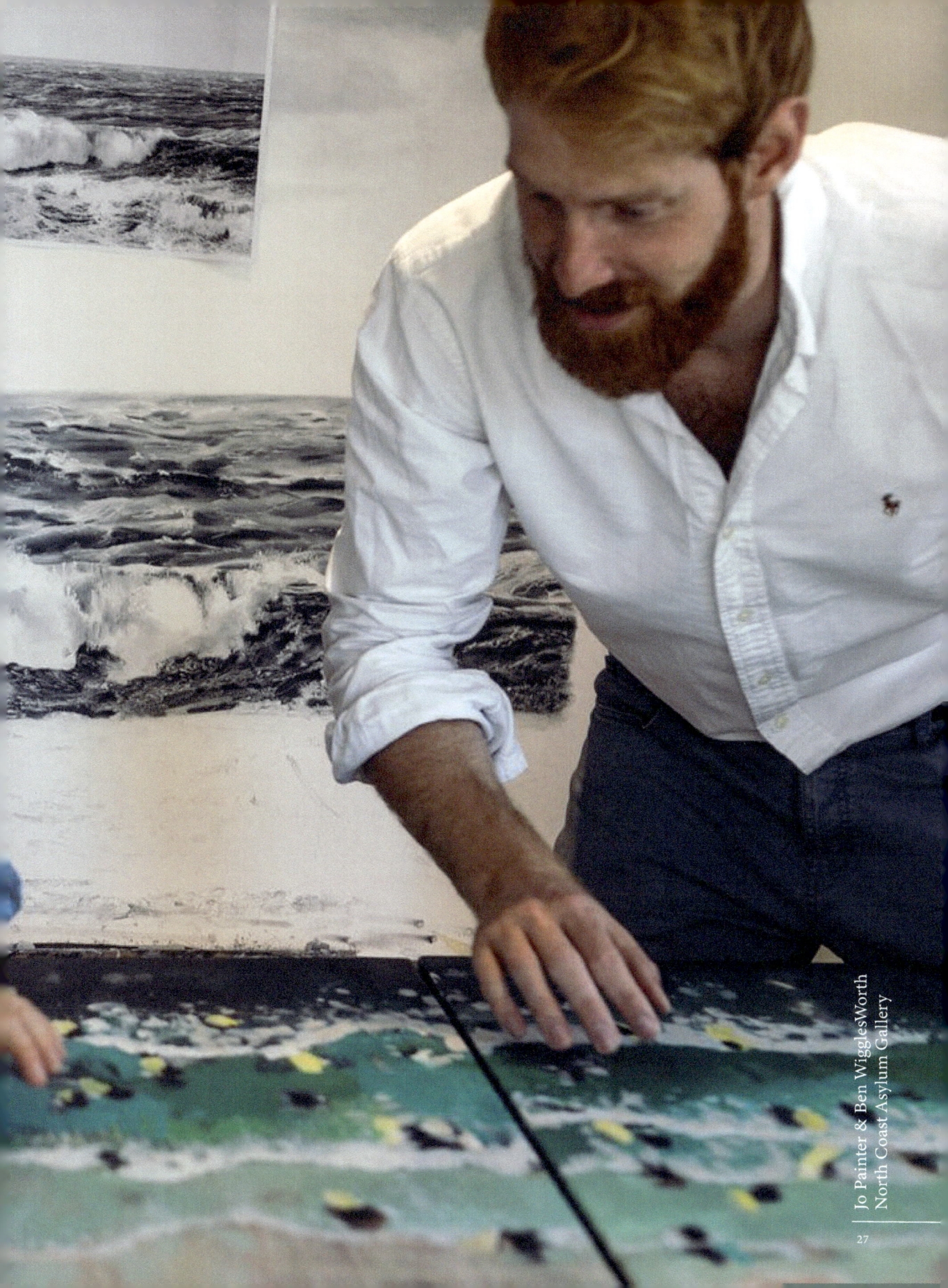

Jo Painter & Ben WigglesWorth
North Coast Asylum Gallery

How can we stay well?

A really helpful tool is to write yourself a Wellbeing Plan. It is something to refer to and check that you are not relapsing back into a state of being mentally unwell again.

Headings might be:

⚘ Emergency Contacts/Support Persons
  -e.g. jo@samaritans.org / phone: 116 123

⚘ Warning Signs (What happens when I start to feel unwell or relapsing?)

⚘ What negative thoughts am I having?

⚘ What are the Physical/Emotional signs?

⚘ What are the Behavioral signs?

⚘ Taking Action (action required when warning signs are present)

⚘ Keeping Well (what are the things that help me stay well?)

⚘ Completing a plan like this and referring to it now and again will help you know if you are maintaining you mental wellbeing.

_____

Write some answers about you and your life.

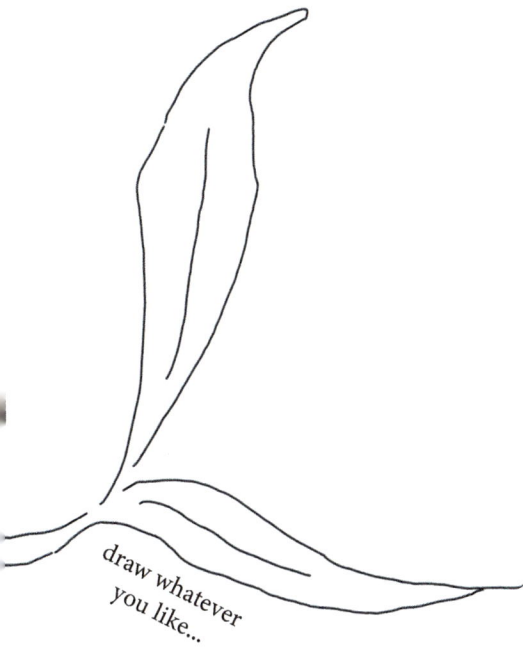

draw whatever
you like...

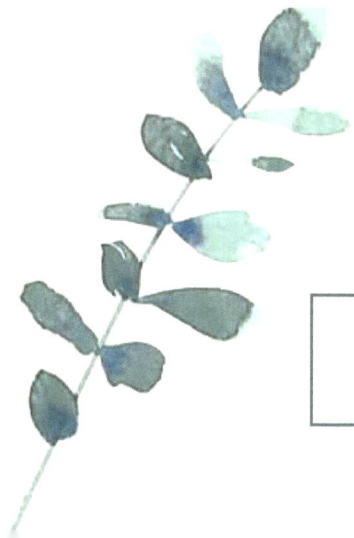

"Art is an outlet of emotion"
Jo Painter

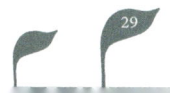

MUSIC & MIND

"Music is a necessity. After food, air, water and warmth, music is the next necessity of life."

Keith Richards, Rolling Stones

One of the easiest ways to ease my headspace is listening to music. Music **meditation** is known for its positive mental effects, and is something that I find can pull me away from stressful thoughts.

I use it when I'm walking along the coast, easing my way into a daily routine and I personally find it a useful outlet for my feelings.

Through treatment, I lost my ability to focus for any length of time. I all but lost the capacity to memorise things, due to the loss of my left anterior temporal lobe, which for example, made it difficult trying to follow a narrative in a book or a film. However with music, I didn't need to as I felt that I could start and finish whenever I wanted, and I hadn't missed anything. A great step back into normality.

Without music, I had no outlet for my emotion.

Music is not just meditation, but has other qualities... science has shown that there may be implicit associations between taste and pitch.

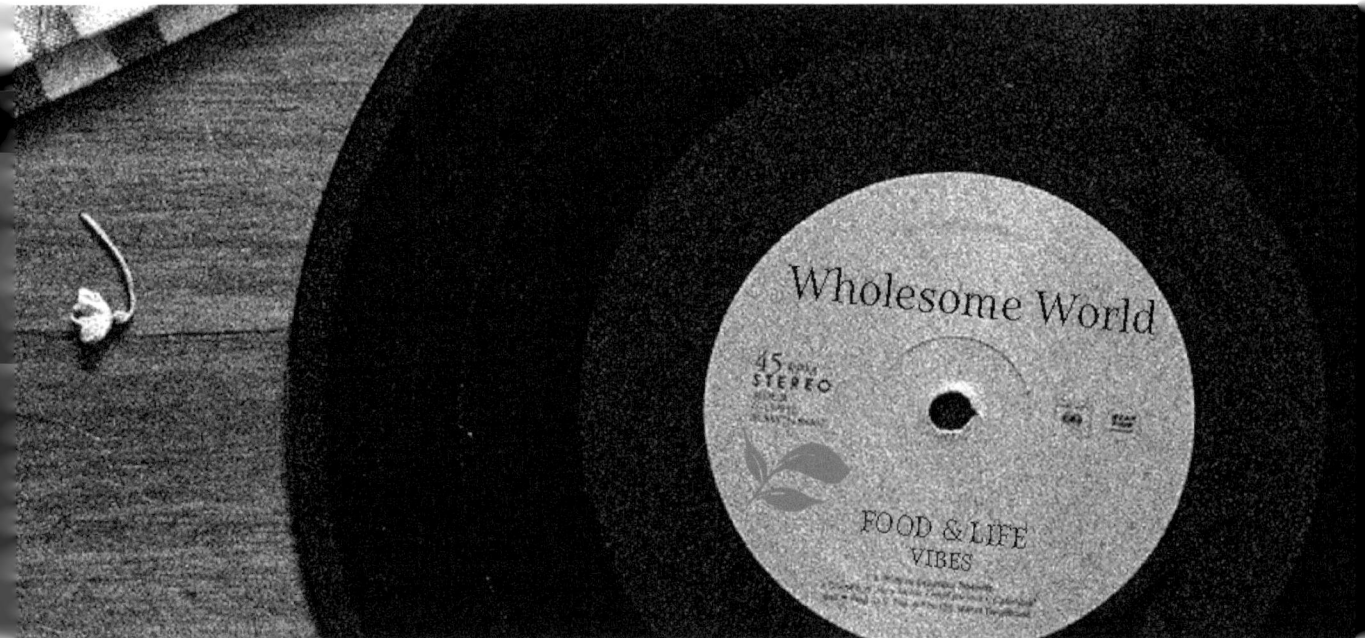

"The use of baroque music has been shown to increase creativity by helping
Meaning that listening to this type of classical music whilst in deep concentration can

According to Experimental psychologist Charles Spence and researchers at the Crossmodal Research Laboratory at the University of Oxford, "there may be implicit associations between taste and pitch. High pitched sounds are mainly associated with sweet and sour tasting foods while low pitched notes are more commonly paired with more bitter and umami tastes.[31]"

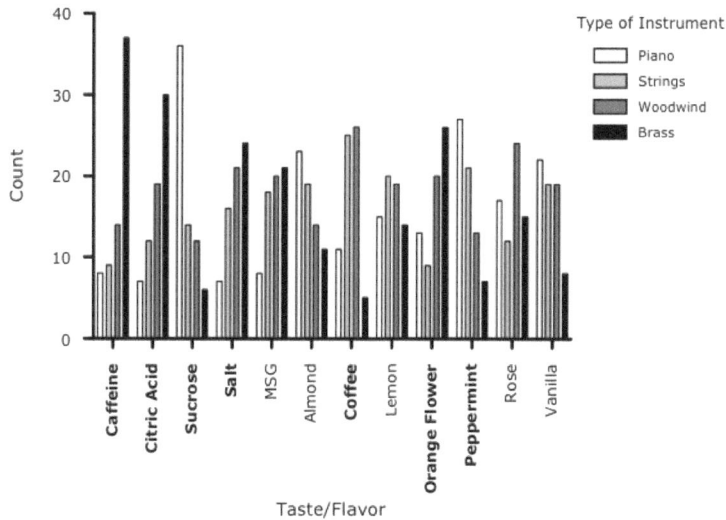

Above: Instruments matched to the tastes/flavours. Maximum count is 68 (34 participants, two trials for each stimulus). Simuli for which there were significant preferences in the choice of instrument are in boldface.

For example, one particular experiment found Spence inviting participants to taste two seemingly different samples of toffee, one while listening to high-pitched sounds, and the other, while listening to lower frequencies. Although the samples were of the same object, subjects "found the toffee sweeter when paired with higher pitches and more bitter when accompanied by lower pitches."

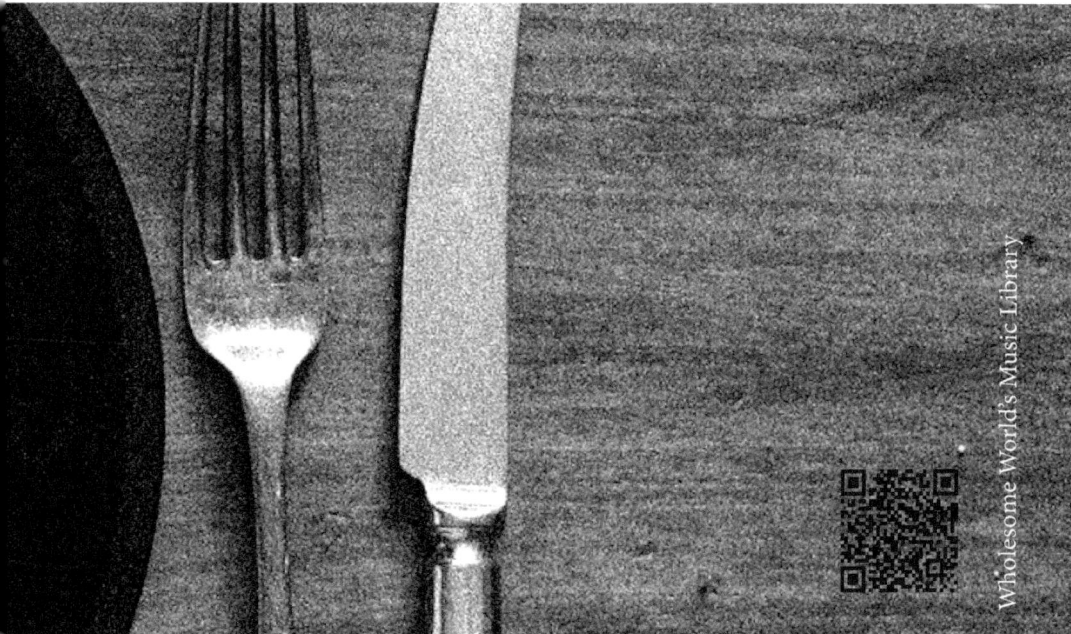

people enter a deep meditative state — sometimes known as the Mozart effect.
help you access higher creative thoughts — some real "aha" or genius moments of clarity.[1]

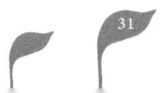

Dr Mayoni Gooneratne

PHYSICALITY

Everyone is different.

This is a beautifully open approach to life so let's just highlight some happy moments in my life and regrowing favourite memories of it.

To start with — as stated earlier, I love being outdoors with fresh air and there are a million ways to do what you want and get where you want. Opening the door to excercise is hard but you can do it.

I feel that the easiest step into this world that is becoming such a solid goal these days is 10,000 steps a day.
I mean, sounds simple, for the general public, but living in a place where you have country roads and sludgy paths and British rain, and even chemotherapy waves here and there, it is quite a hurdle, but a good target to work for. I find, that once you've ploughed through the first week or two, it becomes routine and your body adjusts. My dogs encourage me to open that door, and get walking.

I remember the days that these were impossible whilst going through cancer treatment. Life changes...

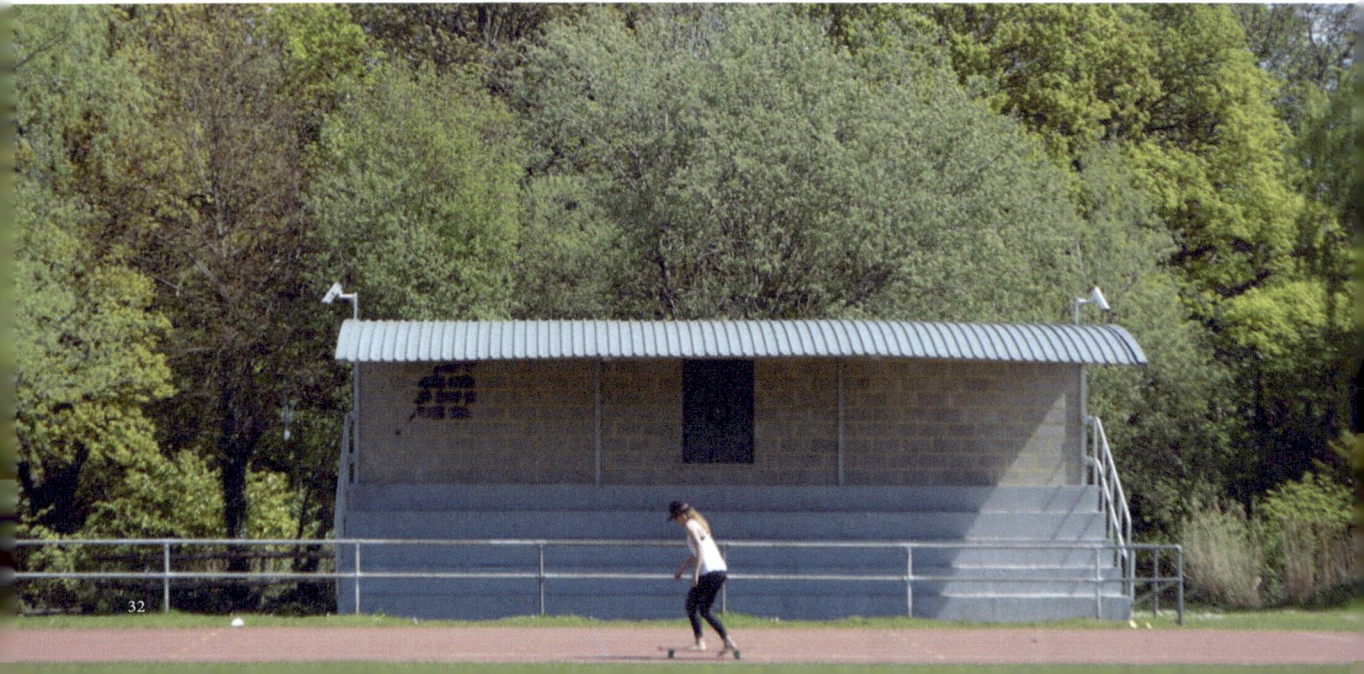

I discussed this with Dr Jonathan Fenn (UK based Sports, Exercise and Wellness Doctor), who agrees with me, here is what he has to say:

Research shows that doing exercise releases feel-good chemicals called endorphins in the brain.

Exercise such as brisk walking, running, cycling, and swimming for 30 minutes causing you to become slightly breathless and increase your heart rate has been shown by extensive research to be beneficial to both your physical and your mental health[1]. We do not all need to become Olympic swimmers or marathon runners to reap the benefits of these types of exercises.

'Couch to 5k' is a brilliant example of how to make a start with exercising and getting past the first few hurdles that stop many of us. I highly recommend downloading the app which that breaks down jogging or running into manageable bite-size chunks. You could even join your local ParkRun.

You may not like the first few runs but I promise you it gets better, and you will reap the benefits of jogging, physically and mentally[1]. The same can be said for swimming, cycling, and brisk walking.

For those with you with pets such as dogs, it can really help to motivate you to go outside to walk the dog, even when the weather is not very good. I know Freyja found this very helpful during her treatment.

When you exercise several neurotransmitters are released, including endorphins, endocannabinoids, and dopamine.

Exercise also promotes neuroplasticity and increases the oxygen supply to your brain. This can help to alleviate some of the aging process of the brain making you healthy in mind, body, and soul. Endorphins act as analgesics which means they diminish one's perception of pain. Dopamine is a feel-good chemical that is important in regulating mood, energy, attitude, and motivation.

Serotonin helps to regulate your mood, but also helps the sleep-wake cycle which is so important. It's also a benefit to your appetite, which can be affected by low mood or illness.

< Skateboarding in London mid treatment, with my dreamboat fitness addict Max Willcocks >

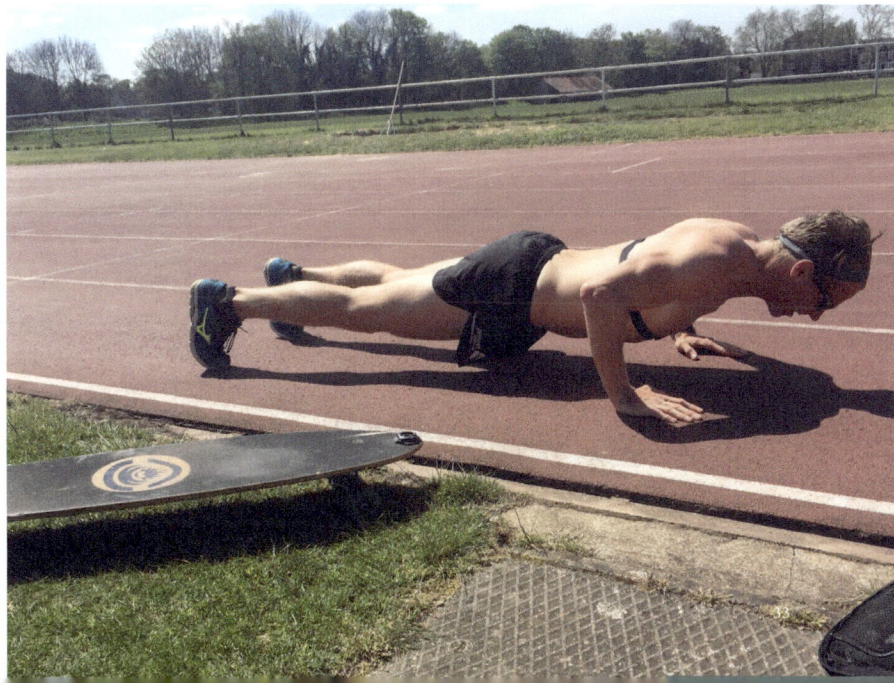

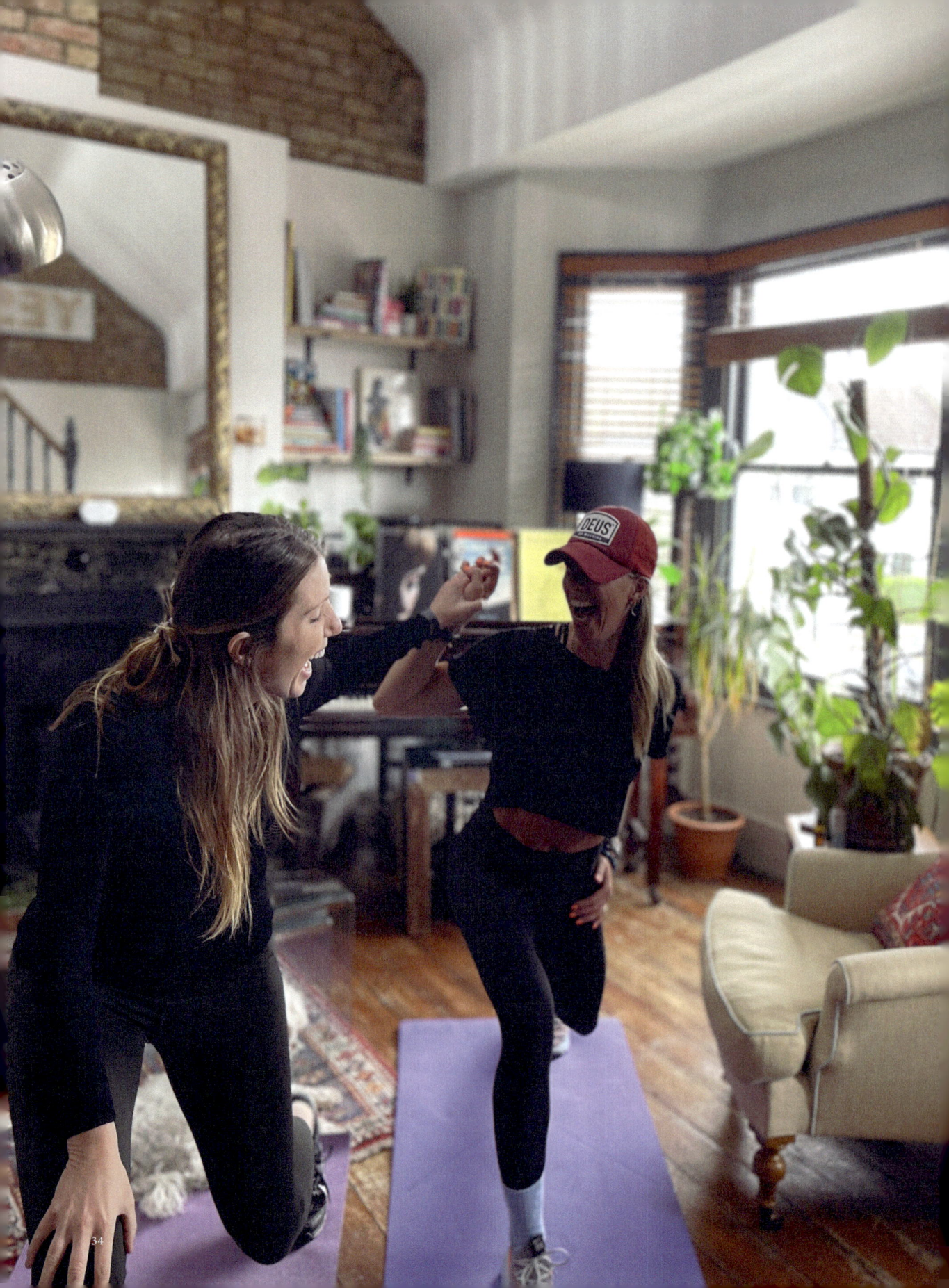

34

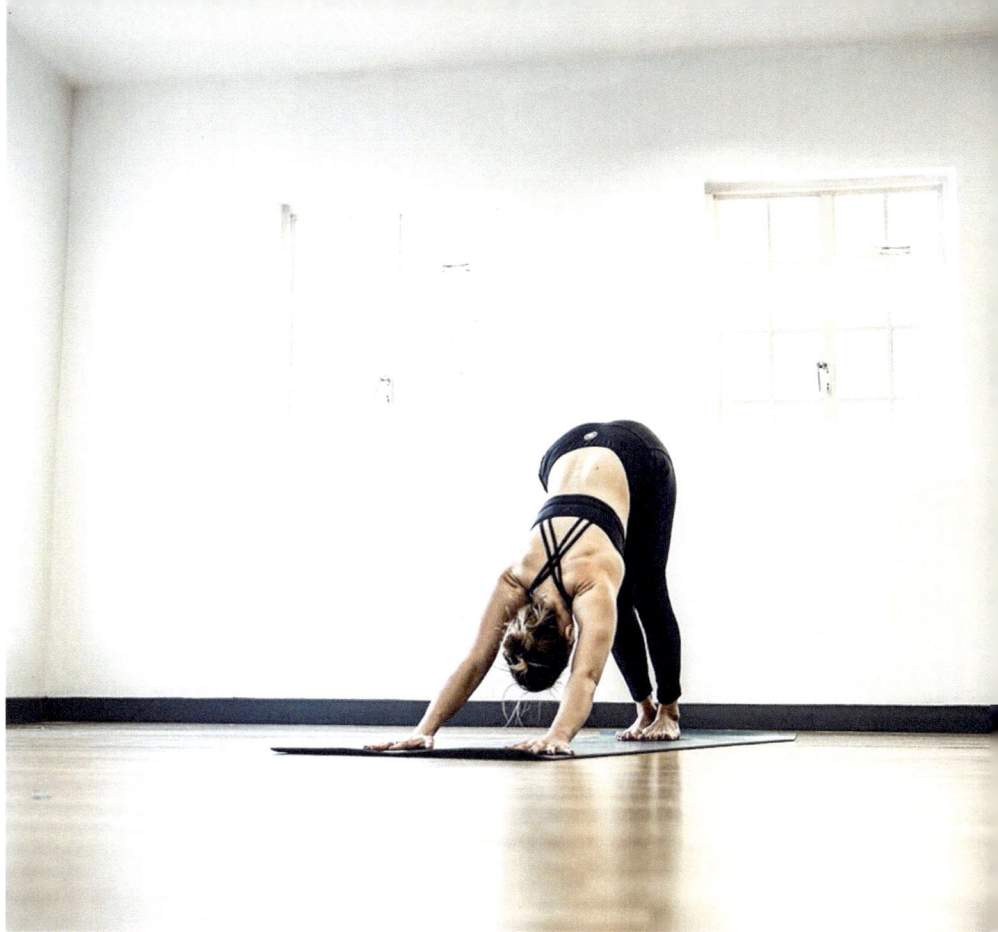

Freyja Hanstein & Bella Campbell, Pilates Instructor

There is a growing movement to get people engaged in community activities and feel connected as human beings. GPs now have a dedicated social prescriber that can now refer you to activities such as gardening, walking groups, and dancing.

All these activities help your mental and physical health and are often a source of support for those who feel disconnected from the community around them.

I find exercise so enjoyable when with good friends.

"Yin yoga is the perfect introduction to meditation which is such an integral part of a yoga practice for holistic well being". I heard this from Katie Johnson, during one of her beautifull yoga classes, which strongly shows the connection between physical and mental heath, and the way they can interlace. "Yin yoga is a gateway drug to meditation."

"Joyful movement can be looked forward to everyday, that brings a smile to your face and unites you with both the present moment and your body. People should be encouraged to use movement that is more healing compared to intense, stressful movement.

This means that we do not increase cellular inflammation which in turn causes chronic diseases like diabetes and heart disease. So, I would encourage things such as Tai Chi, outdoor swimming or yoga as a starting step. I appreciate for some, that running is also a form of mental release too but try to mix it up a bit with more gentler paced activity.

Exercise should not be used as a form of compensation or replacement for other health behaviours.
So - just because you had a take away and a bottle of wine last night,
you can't just exercise the next day to 'make up for it'!"

Dr Gooneratne, Human Health

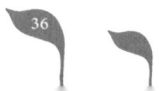

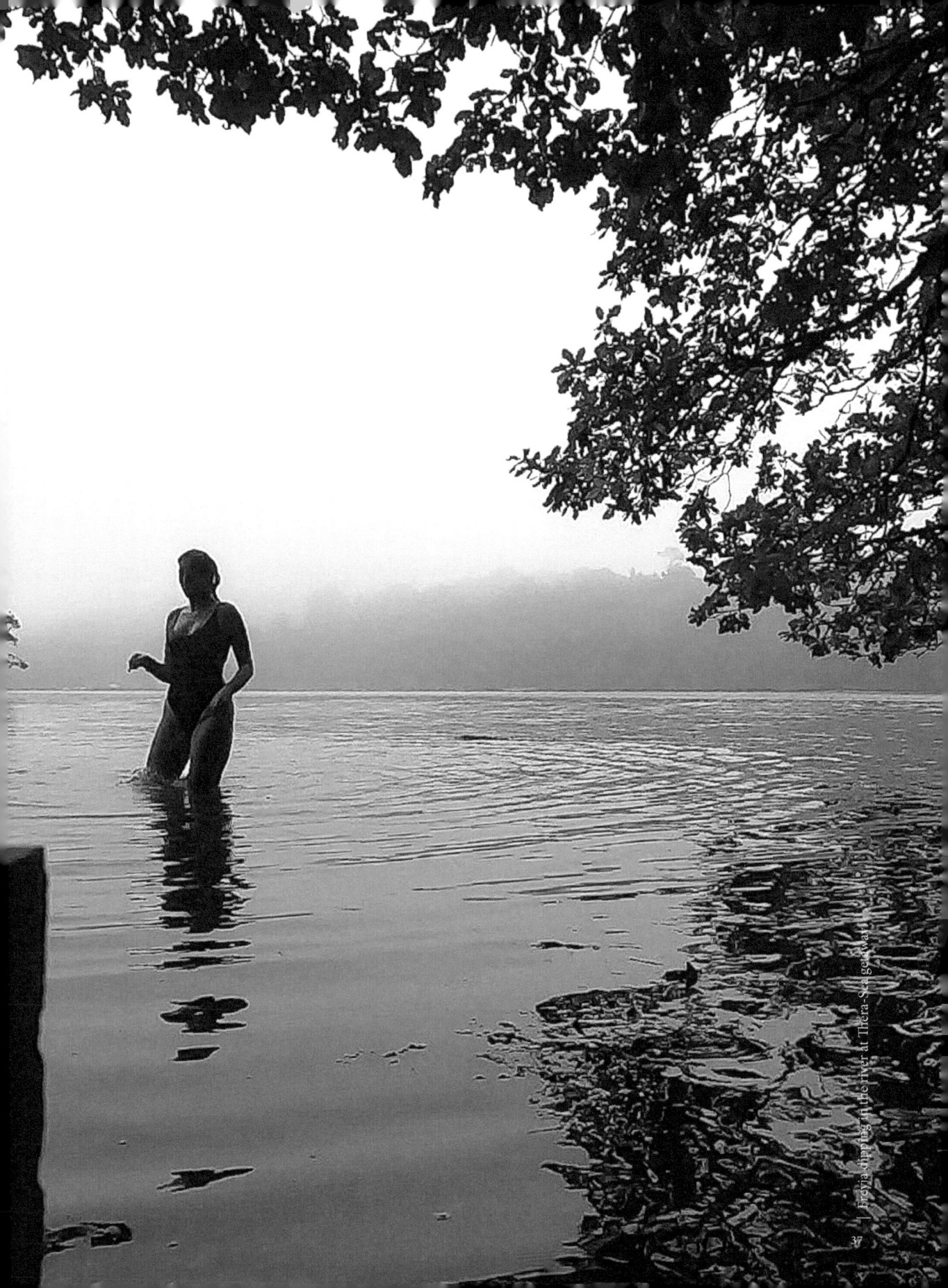

Freyja dipping in the river at Thera. Sea-grey eyes [...]

GROWING HEALTH

Now more than ever, we need to be aware of the importance of living our lives in harmony with nature.

Growing up, I lived in the woods by Heligan [Gardens], in Cornwall. I walked through the fields and woodlands each day to get to the nearest road on the way to school. I revelled in muddy walks, swinging on trees, daily dog walks and building woodland huts. During this time Tim Smit and his partners re-discovered and rescued the Lost Gardens of Heligan, and as children we were able to enjoy and learn from that regeneration. Our families have been good friends since before I was born and we followed with excitement each stage of the restoration.

This natural way of life was the seed for my realisation to prioritising local, seasonal and organic produce from sustainable growers to enrich the salubrity (healthfulness) for both ourselves and the planet.

Following the success of The Lost Gardens, Tim went on to create the awe inspiring Eden Project in a worked-out clay quarry near the South coast of Cornwall, just a few miles from where I now live.

The Eden Project brings the wonders of the world within arms length, and is an amazing place to see and get understanding for seasonal growth across the planet. I share Tim's rationale, to change people's appreciation of natural science.

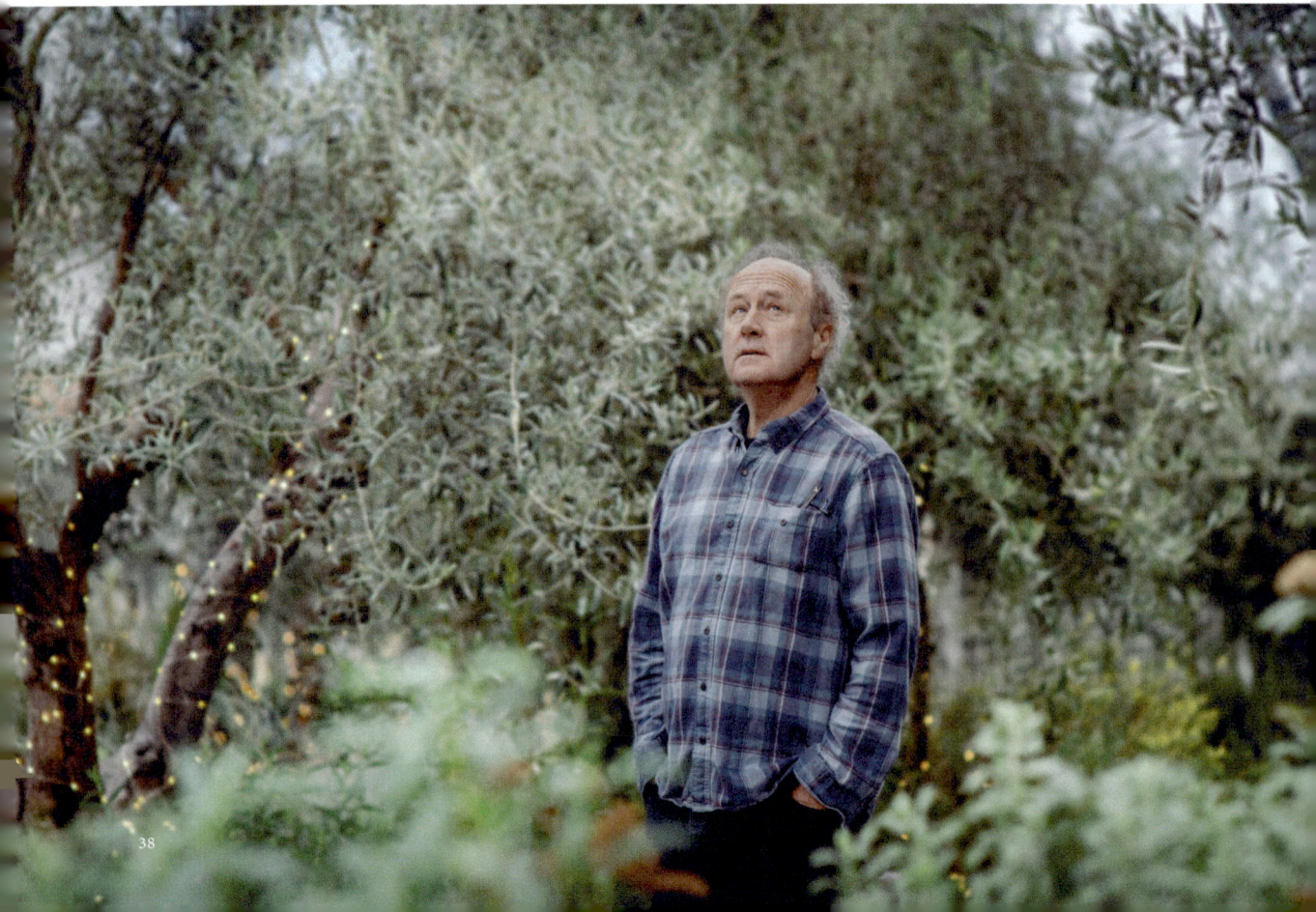

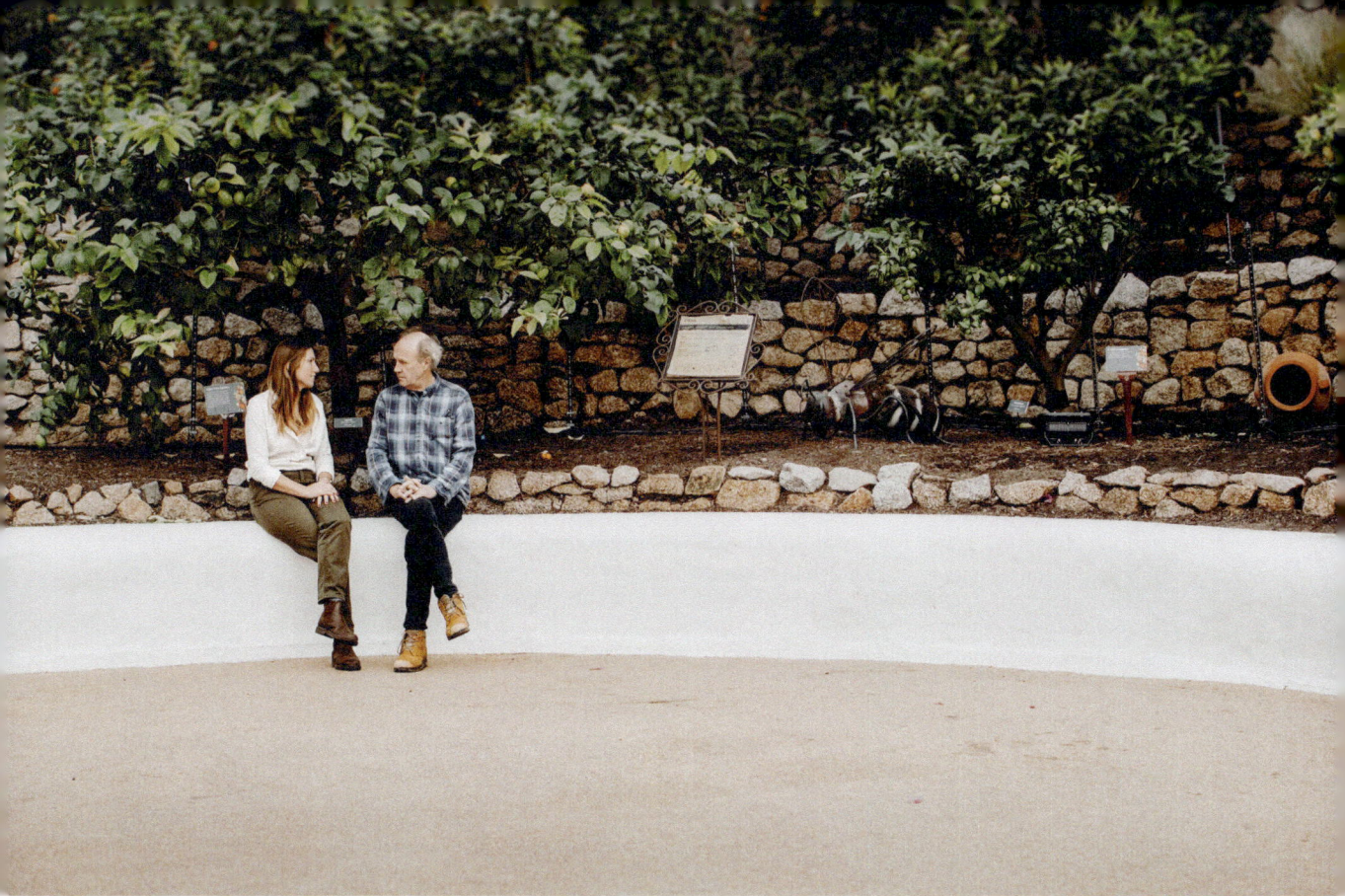

Freyja Hanstein & Tim Smit (above)

Eden Project, Behind the scenes 2021 (below)

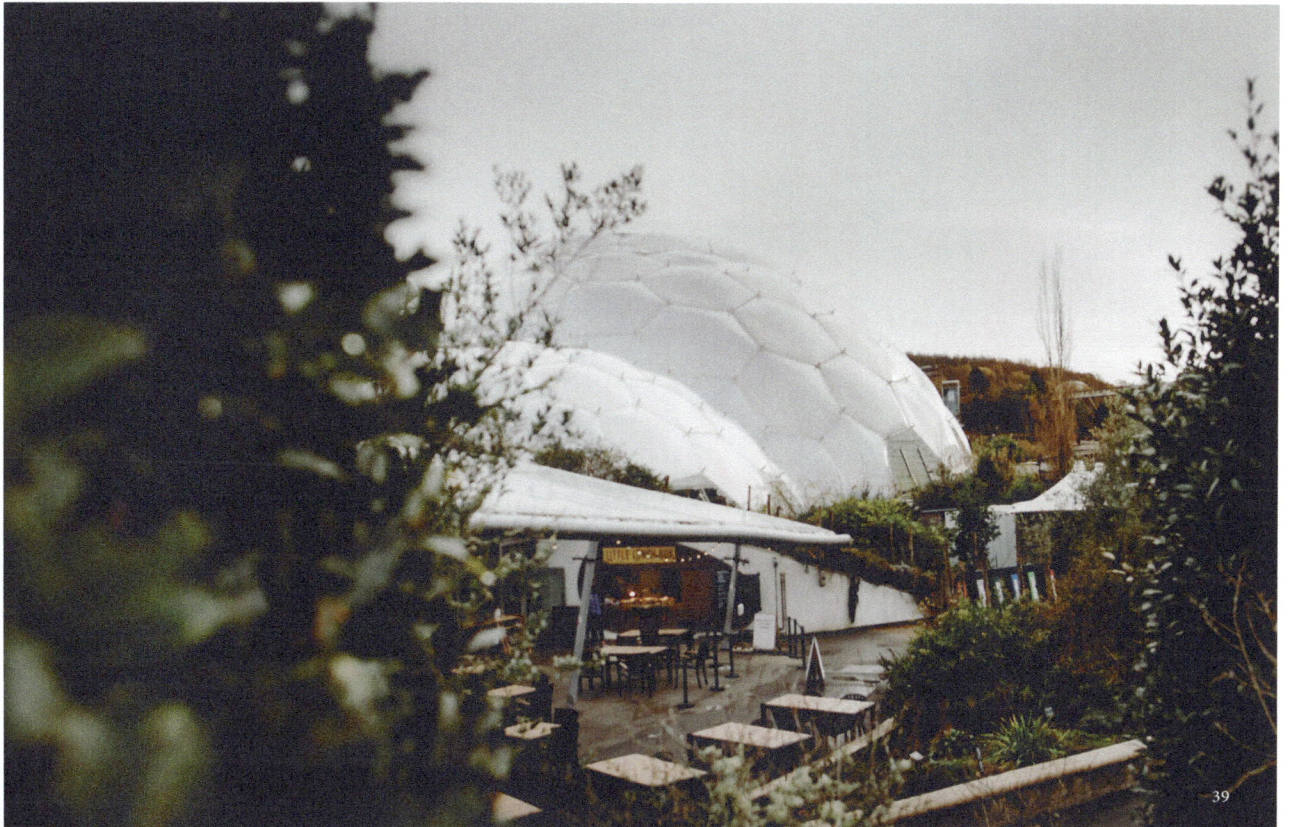

Tim Smit says "Dr William Byrd one of the Founders of Social Prescribing has famously said that he is not so concerned that his patients smoke, drink or take drugs as he is that they don't suffer from the greatest killers of all, loneliness, lack of belonging and sense of safety and purpose."

Food, its preparation, cooking and sharing lies at the heart of so much that takes the mixing of ingredients from being a simple question of nutrition to one of sustenance in its widest sense, that of the body and, of the soul, the widest well-being, in family, friendship and community.

"We are talking here of the actual quality of the nutritional fuel for the body as well as the symbolism and meaning inextricably linked to its consumption. Both ingredients and social meaning are crucial in perfecting this balance".

Click here >
to find out more about
The Eden Project

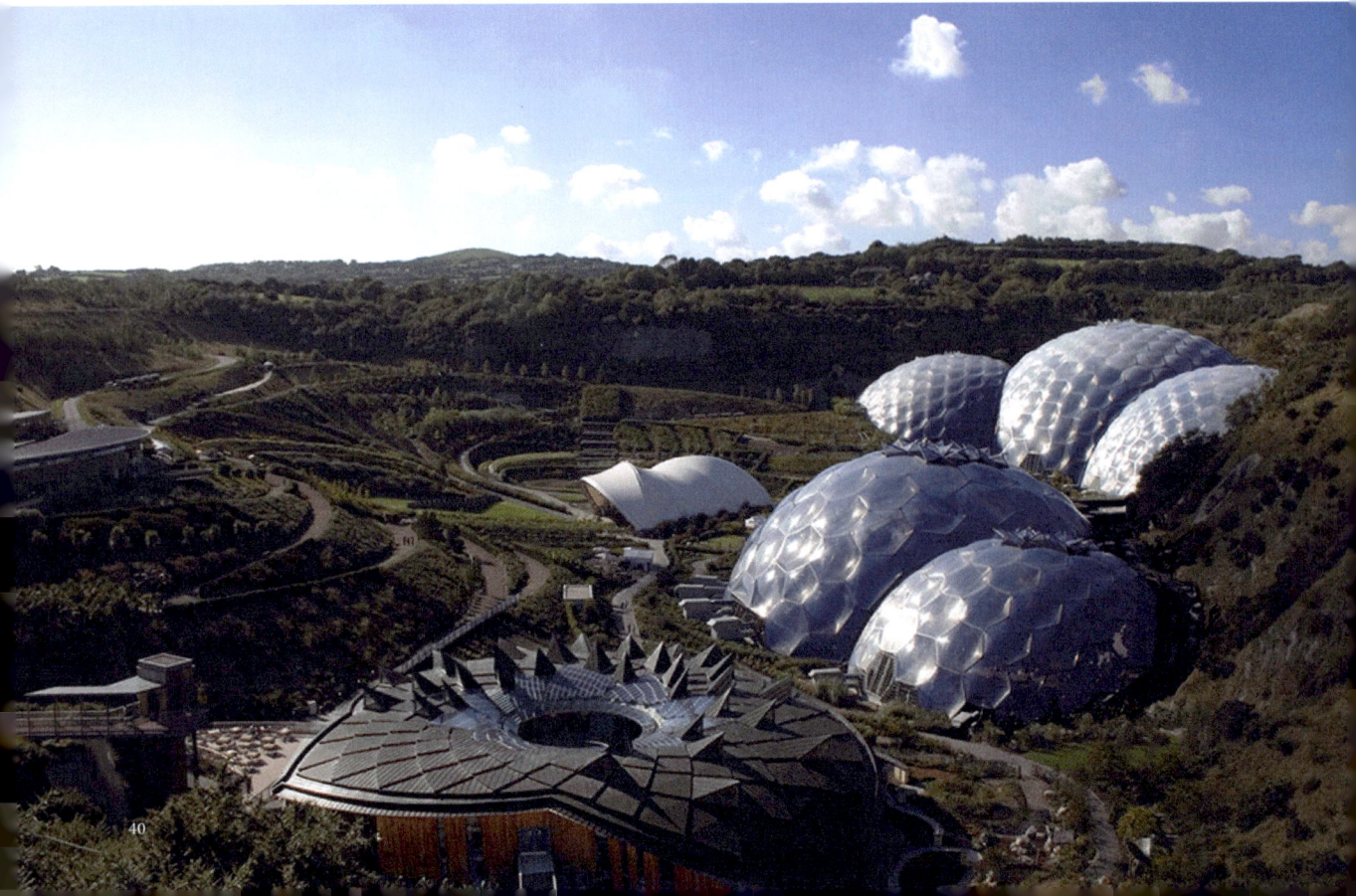

eden project

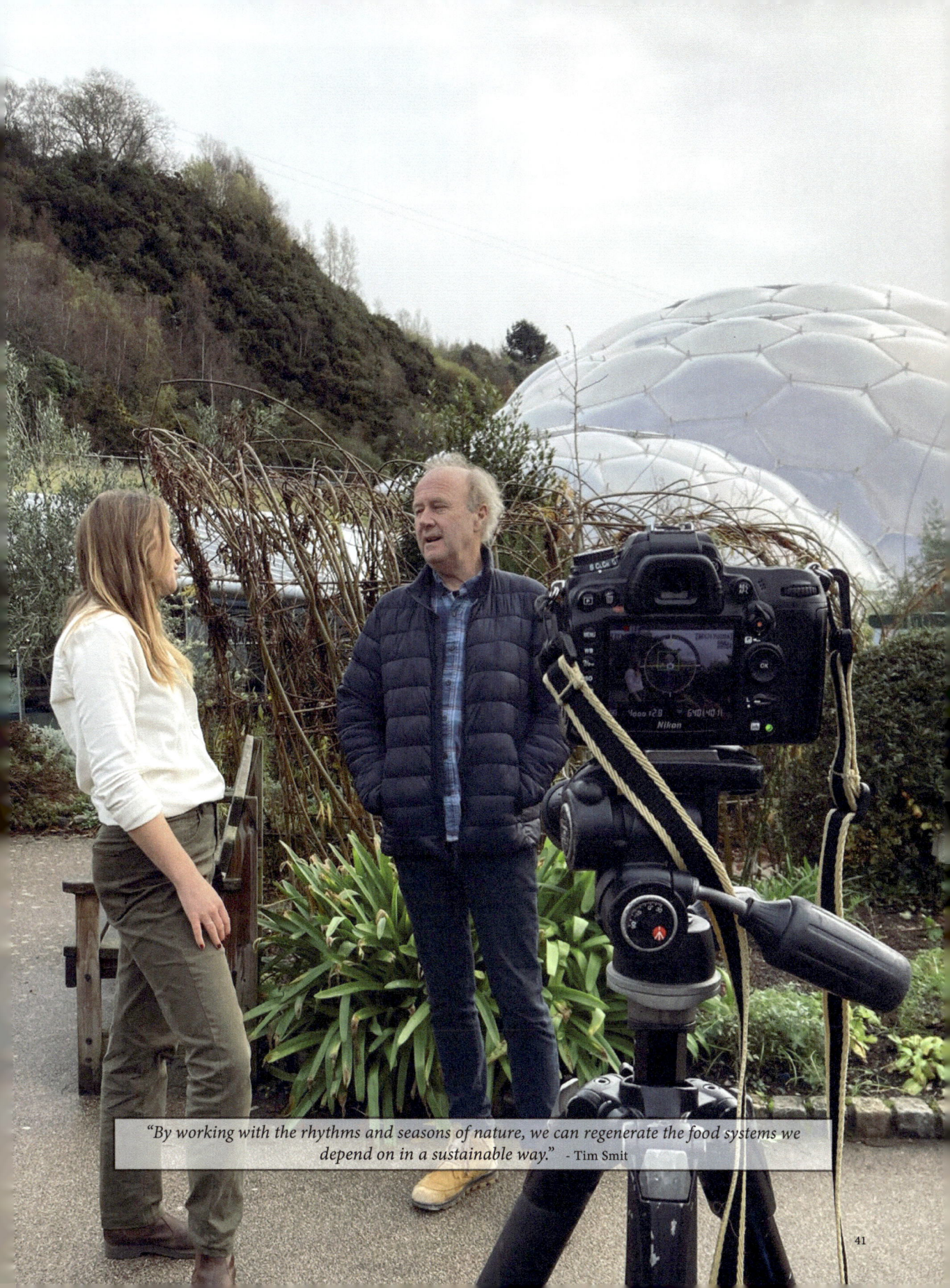

"By working with the rhythms and seasons of nature, we can regenerate the food systems we depend on in a sustainable way."   - Tim Smit

ETHICAL FARMING & EATING

HOW CAN YOU EQUATE THIS TO YOUR HOME LIFE?

I think that knowing the source of your ingredients, your daily intake, the elements that are your body and life, need to be realised. Riverford Organics is a beautiful farm that provides seasonal food, simply grown in an eco and ethical way.

For years I have used them as my foundation for the kitchen, and my health satisfaction base to cook from. Their fresh fruit and vegetables, locally grown, were delivered throughout the cancer treatment and that extra niggly bit of recent life known as COVID.

Through using Riverford Organics, I have found that it is a spark to change the dish monotony, thinking of ways to at least give yourself the freshly delivered ingredients that vary through the seasons. I'd say it was a good pull, to step away from the repetition that was my sole kitchen and ingredient knowledge. It removes the need to check supermarket labels and be swamped by non-eco packaging.

-

Looking into their farming methods, it's interesting to see the differences that spread not only to nutritional health but to invest in ways to reduce their impact on the planet.

Working with nature, not against it.

Riverford have worked hard towards maintaining their organic credentials. They spread from their original farm, to include the local farms and create the 'South Devon Organic Co-operative'. Organic soil aid, zero chemicals and techniques such as crop rotation are used. This allows the earth to evolve a microbiome for sustaining a variety of organisms which keeps the soil nutrient dense; further encouraged by simple techniques such as hedges and strips of grass for 'insect highways'. In the polytunnels, the farm introduced local pest larvae, which once hatched, eat the aphids and control disease.

"Through winter we grow leafy greens with the help of our polytunnels. They're not electrically heated though as this goes against our environmental value, unless solar energy is used."
Emily M. from Riverford

On top of that, to date, more than 50% of their vehicles are electric, which is a phenomenal improvement, whilst working towards switching the HGVs (not a simple feat). But a side-step to the target, is utilising waste-veg bio-fuel. This reduces emissions and balances out the allowance of waste to keep within their environmental status.

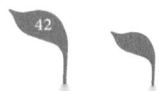

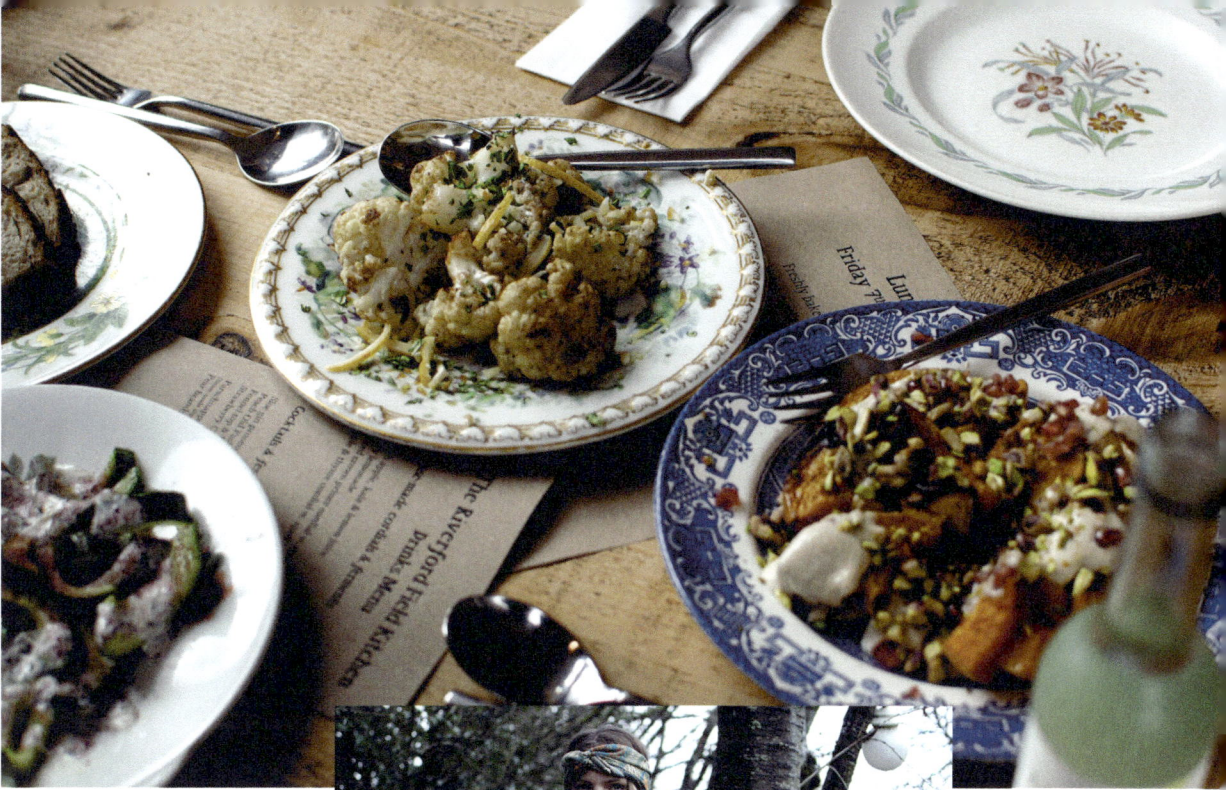

Riverford Farm & Kitchen

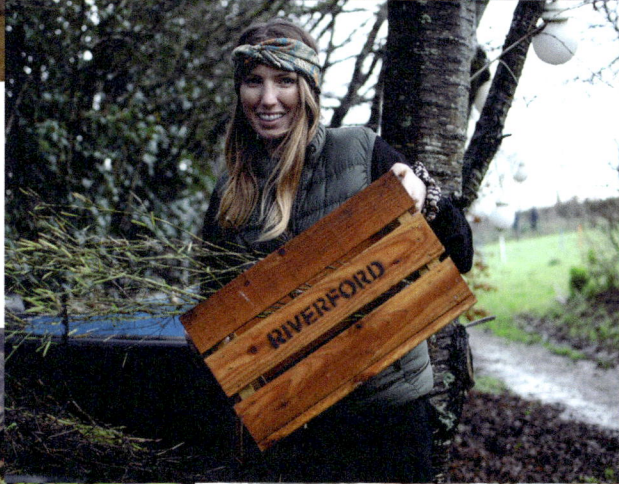

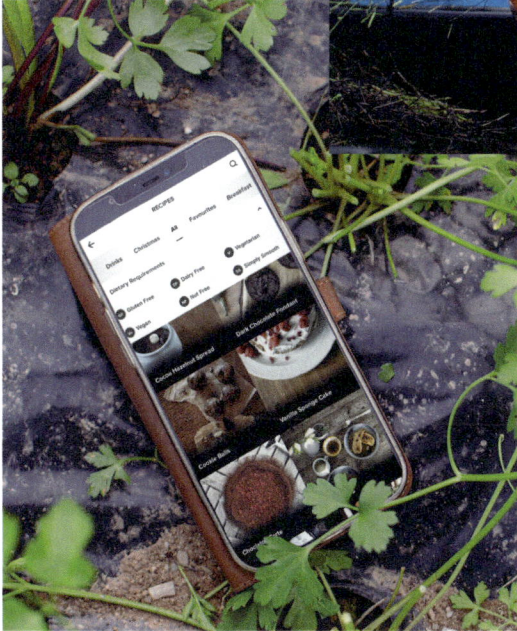

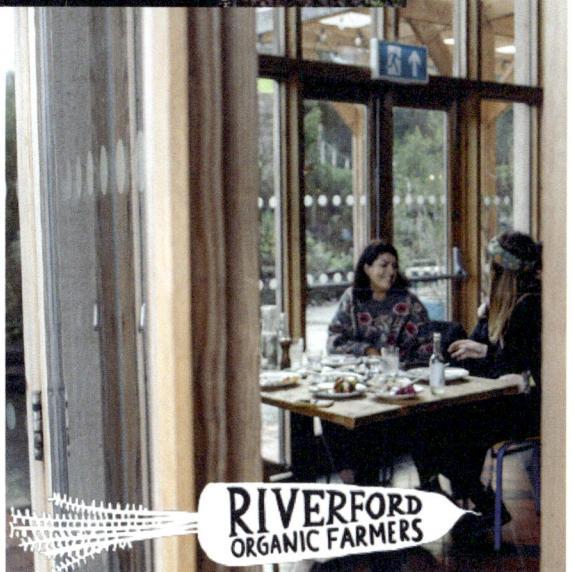

The more diverse you are with the plants that you eat, the healthier your gut, ultimately enhancing your wellbeing. In terms of growth aid and contamination, produce likely to carry the most pesticides, known as the 'Dirty Dozen', which you can be found on p54 — try to eat the organic version.

How your food is grown or raised can have a major impact on your mental and emotional health as well as the environment.

Organic foods often have more beneficial nutrients, such as antioxidants, than their conventionally-grown counterparts. People with allergies to foods, chemicals, or preservatives may find their symptoms lessen or go away when they eat only organic foods.

LIVESTOCK

Their principles of ethical farming are directly transferred to their animal and livestock welfare too. The livestock live in small groups, which lowers the quantity per farm, and of course raises the price. But this is reflected in the flavour, texture and life of the animal, especially chickens. Battery hens are filled with antibiotics to prevent diseases often created by the harsh and inhumane conditions they are forced to endure. I'd choose organic every time.

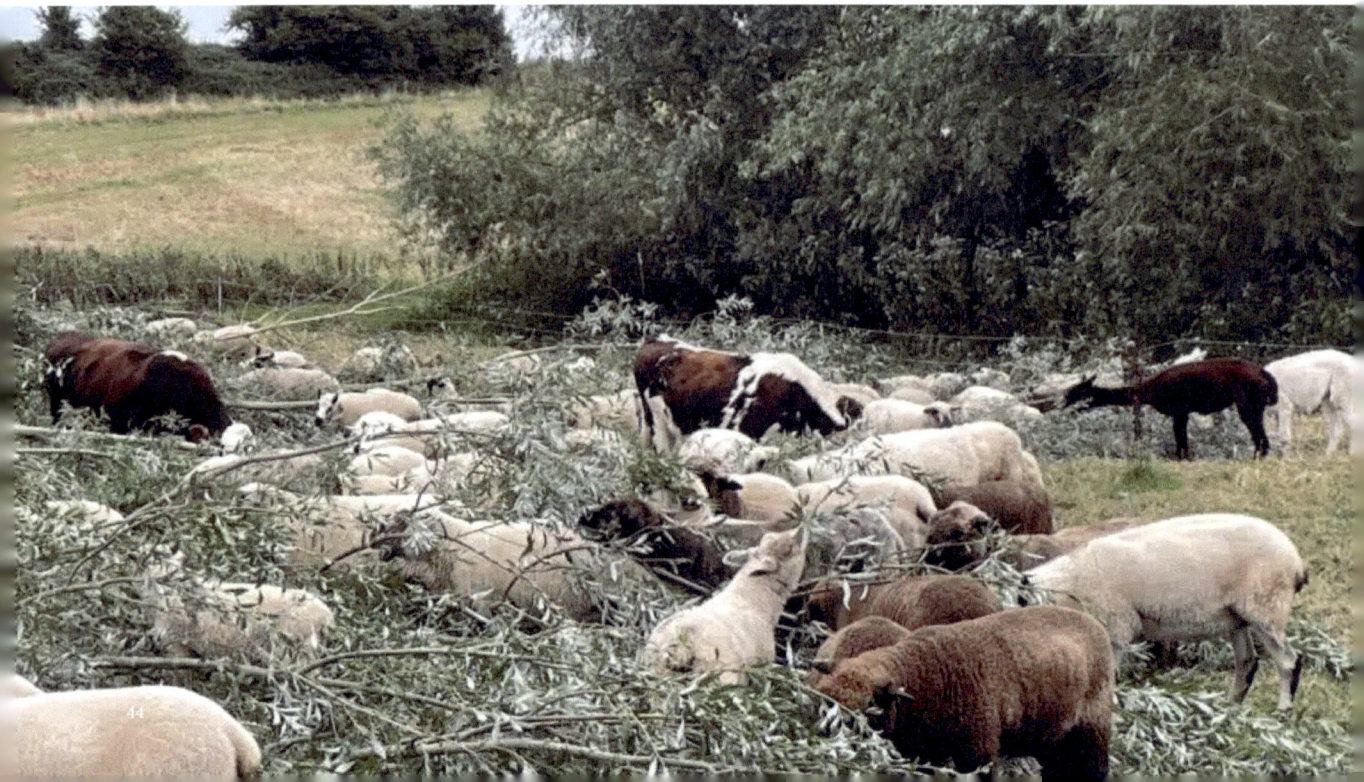

THE PROBLEM WITH PESTICIDES

There are so many reasons to choose seasonal and organic produce, but primarily for our health and the environment. The health of our soil is of fundamental importance to future sustainability. The use of soluble nitrogen and intensive farming methods is eroding the nutrient levels and the all important microorganisms within it.

If we think of our gut microbes as the soil in our body we can imagine how pesticides, herbicides and fungicides can upset the balance just as they can upset the balance of the earth's soil. They kill off some of our beneficial bacteria and are inflammatory, this can lead to less attachment sites for our gut microbes on the gut lining. We must look after our bodies and the earth with care, they are a finely balanced ecosystem.

SO WHAT ARE THE BENEFITS OF EATING SEASONALLY AND, EVEN BETTER, ORGANICALLY?

To start with seasonality, those vegetables and fruit grown close to home do not clock up the food miles that produce grown abroad will do. Food miles are not just bad for the environment but mean that the food may be less fresh when it reaches us. It will no doubt have been picked when it was underripe and refrigerated on its journey. Often this produce will need to be ripened in a hot house once it reaches its destination. This often reduces the flavour and texture and certainly reduces the nutritional content. In particular, green leafy vegetables should always be eaten as close to picking as possible to ensure optimal nutritional value. They begin to leach their nutrients very quickly once picked.

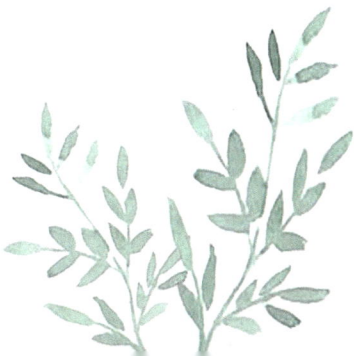

RIVERFORD
ORGANIC FARMERS

IF YOU HAVE A GARDEN
AND A LIBRARY YOU
HAVE EVERYTHING YOU
NEED

MARCUS TULLIUS CICERO

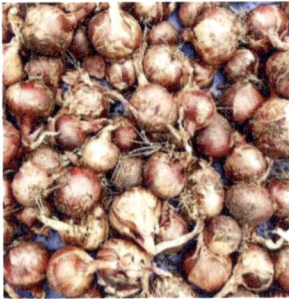

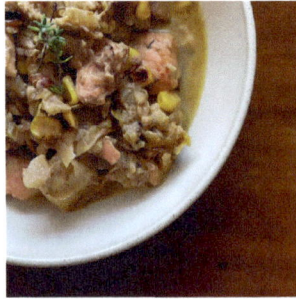

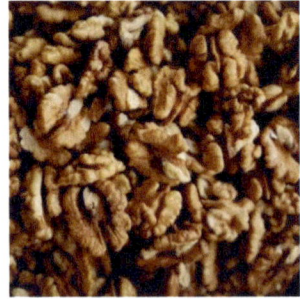

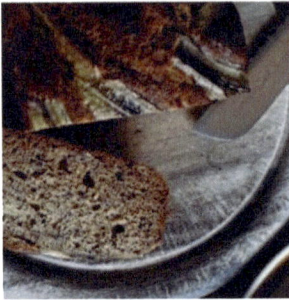

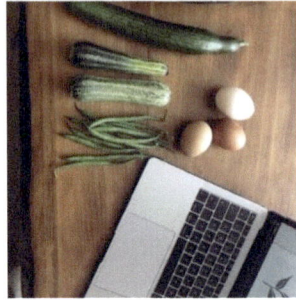

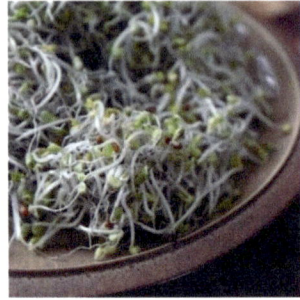

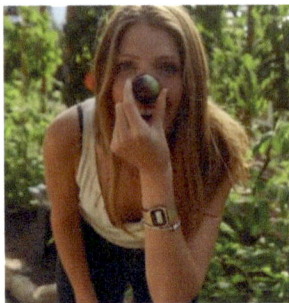

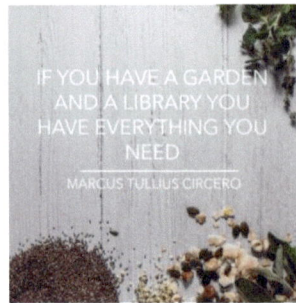

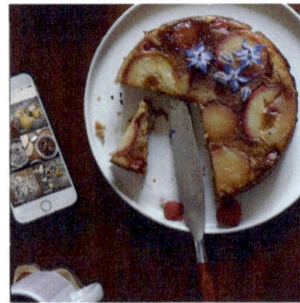

Optimal Anticancer Diet: Research has shown that those who eat a diet high in veg and fruit, but particularly green leafy veg, lower their risk of cancer.[1]

FOOD NOURISHMENT FOR OUR CELLS

Food has changed significantly over the last 50 years or so and often doesn't resemble anything that our ancestors would have eaten.

Highly refined, manufactured foods are not what our bodies were designed to use for nourishment. Much food now is just fodder to supply us with energy and not quality nutrients. There is also concern that putting the wrong type of food into your body i.e. unnatural processed food may be more detrimental than not eating enough healthy food.

If we want our body to work optimally, we must nourish it well and that begins with the choices we make when we source our food. Think of food as information for our cells. Given nutritious food in its natural state our digestive processes break down the food effectively and the nutrients are sent to our cells to keep them healthy.

If we are giving our cells the information they need, they work efficiently, communicate to each other, behave well and are less likely to mutate into cancer cells.

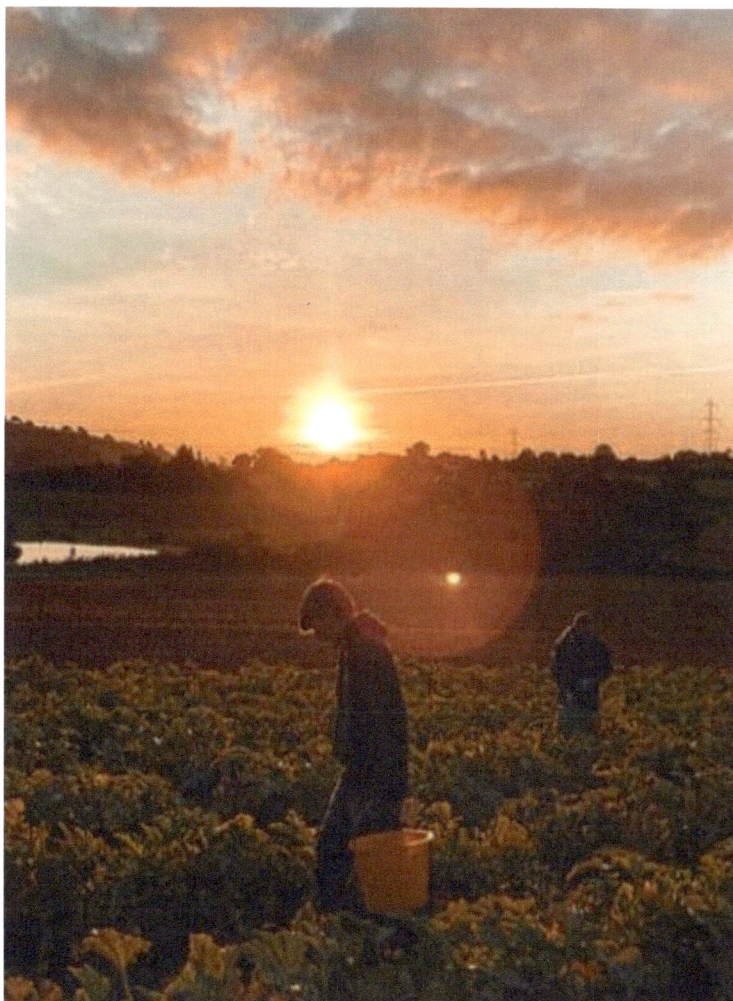

UNDERSTANDING THE RELATIONSHIP BETWEEN HUMAN NEEDS AND WELLBEING

The relationship between human needs and wellbeing particularly around food and nutrition can be nicely illustrated by using the principles of Maslow's Hierarchy of Needs

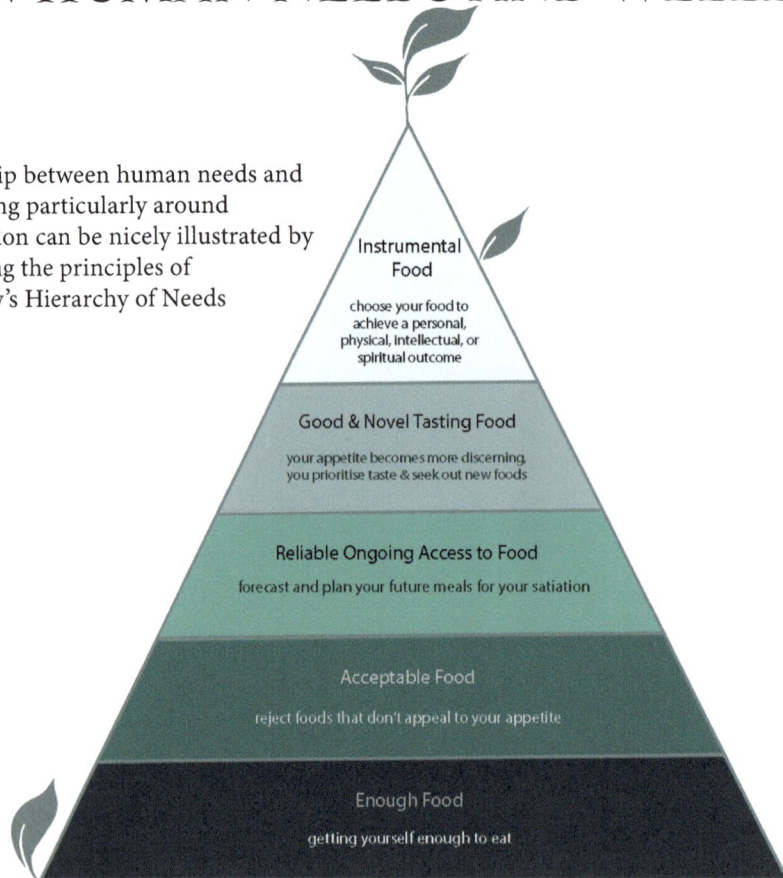

Instrumental Food
choose your food to achieve a personal, physical, intellectual, or spiritual outcome

Good & Novel Tasting Food
your appetite becomes more discerning, you prioritise taste & seek out new foods

Reliable Ongoing Access to Food
forecast and plan your future meals for your satiation

Acceptable Food
reject foods that don't appeal to your appetite

Enough Food
getting yourself enough to eat

(Maslow A.; 'A theory of human motivations.' Psychol Rev. 1943;50:370-396.) nutritionally updated by Dr Satter (Ellyn Satter, MS, RD, LCSW, BCD* Ellyn Satter Associates, Madison,Wisconsin (J Nutr Educ Behav. 2007;39:S187-S188))

This is a beautiful platform that shows the hierarchy of nutritional needs as an understanding of which needs are being met in our life and which are not. It helps us work out what changes in our life might improve our well-being.

As you can see from the image above, at the most basic level we needs enough air, warmth, food and water to survive.

Needs at each level must be satisfied before those at the next higher level can be experienced and addressed. I related my life to this ladder after my emotional and physical hits from losing Lars and my cancer treatment.

In terms of food and the quality thereof, once these basic needs to sustain life are met we can start exploring the opportunities for moving from mere survival i.e. from enough food to more body- and mind- beneficial foods.

Once our most basic needs are continually met in this way — once we have satisfied the primary levels — we open the door to the apex of the pyramid where we are choosing food for instrumental reasons, for example, to prevent disease, prolong life and reinforce mental and emotional functioning. Mental, physical and nutritional benefits are all intertwined.

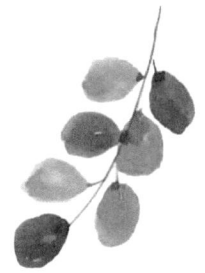

"To transform the biological necessity of feeding into a flow experience, one must begin by paying attention to what one eats. It is astonishing — as well as discouraging — when guests swallow lovingly prepared food without any sign of having noticed its virtues."

Mihaly Csikszentmihalyi, Hungarian-American psychologist

HOME NUTRITION

LARDER BASICS

The big swap – give your cupboard and fridge a spring clean and fill it with only healthy options to reduce the temptation to eat rubbish. If it's not in your home you cannot eat it!
(see p.80)

INGREDIENT SWAPS FOR HEALTHIER EATING
LOW TO HIGH NUTRIENTS

Refined Sugar	Raw Honey / Maple syrup / Blackstrap molasses / Dates / Stevia
Refined Oils e.g Sunflower Oil	Coconut / Rapeseed / Olive oil
White Rice, Pasta & Bread	Quinoa / Cauliflower / Brown, Wild, Black Rice Wholewheat / Veg Pastas Wholewheat sourdough / Rye / Seed / Nut Bread
White Flour	Spelt, Rye, Buckwheat, Wholewheat Flour / Ground Nuts, Seeds & More
Margarine Spread	Organic Butter / Coconut Oil / Nut Butters
Non-Organic Milk	Organic Milk OR Oat / Almond / Coconut Mylks...
Refined Breakfast Cereals	Porridge Oats / Homemade Granola / Muesli
Low Fat Yoghurt	Full Fat Yoghurt
Crisps / Bread Sticks	Homemade Seedy Crackers
Black Tea / Coffee	Green / Herbal Teas
Table Salt	Unrefined Sea Salt / Himalayan Salt

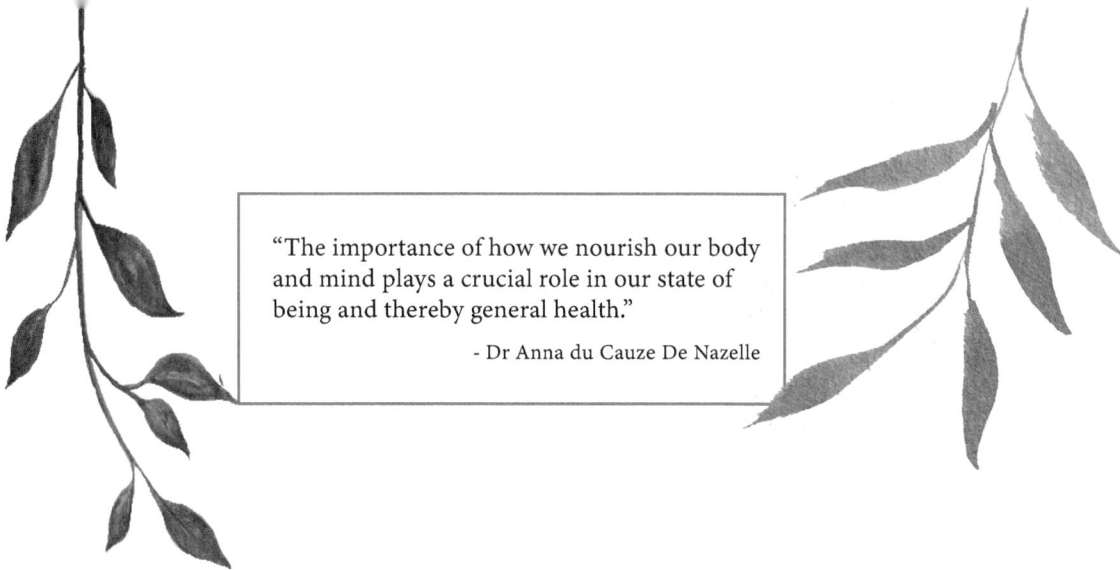

> "The importance of how we nourish our body and mind plays a crucial role in our state of being and thereby general health."
>
> - Dr Anna du Cauze De Nazelle

Still sugars but more nutrient dense as opposed to empty calories

Avoid refined oils, as some are damaged fats, high in pro-inflammatory omega 6 *(read more p256)*

Higher in fibre, nutrient dense, lower glycaemic effect

Lower pesticide residues, higher in fibre & nutrients

Free from damaged fats

Free from antibiotics & pesticides, healthier fat content

Whole grains, rich in fibre, lower glycaemic effect

Healthier fat profile, less processed

Lower glycaemic effect, nutrient dense

Low or no caffeine, calming on the gut

Table Salt is bleached, has added anti-caking agents
& is depleted from the natural minerals

Seasonal Food Chart

Although we find much of this produce in our shops all year round, if we adhere to seasonality we will be supporting the environment along with our budget. Obviously some foods will need to be grown abroad and naturally we enjoy eating them, but again, eating within the season means that they have hopefully not been grown in a hot house or under plastic. The most obvious step away from this is the use of eco earth heating, solar panels, the creation of hotbeds, undersoil hot water heating.

We are so lucky in the UK that so many different crops can be locally grown.

Spring
March - May

Leek, parsnip, Jerusalem artichoke, spring greens, cauliflower, wild garlic, rhubarb, spinach, carrot, broad beans, peas, cabbage, celeriac, watercress, nettles, spring onion, bananas

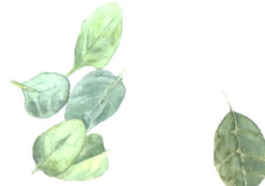

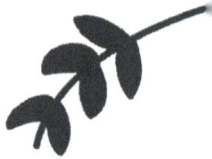

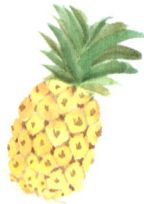

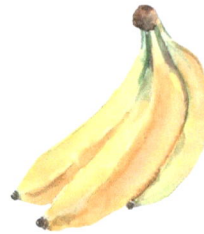

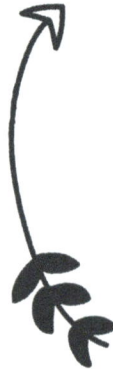

Winter
December - February

Cabbage, leek, celeriac, parsnip, Jerusalem artichoke, kale, purple sprouting broccoli, beetroot, swede, greens, cauliflower, Brussel sprouts, onions, apple, celery, sweet potato, turnip, pineapple, orange, pomegranate, pumpkin

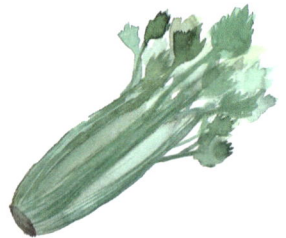

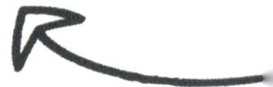

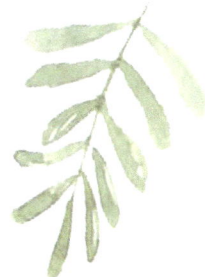

Summer
June - August

Sugar snap peas, lettuce, asparagus, aubergine, blackcurrants, apricot, courgette, fennel bulb, globe artichoke, gooseberries, mangetout, nectarine, new potatoes, pak choi, radish, rhubarb, runner beans, spinach, spring greens, watercress, blackberry, garlic, kohlrabi, peach, pepper, raspberries, redcurrants, samphire, Swiss chard, tomato, melon, blueberries, bananas, cherries, strawberries, wild nettles, cucumber

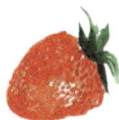

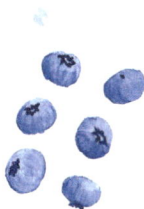

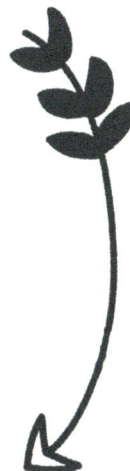

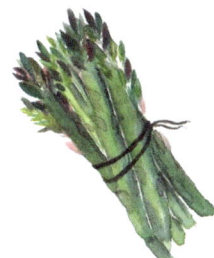

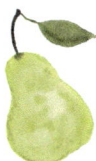

Autumn
September - November

Apple, apricot, aubergine, beetroot, blackberries, broad bean, broccoli, Brussel sprouts, cabbage, cucumber, carrot, cavolo nero, celeriac, celery, chestnut, chicory, clementine, courgette, elderberries, fennel bulb, fig, globe artichoke, kale, kohlrabi, leeks, lettuce, pear, peppers, plum, pomegranate, pumpkin, quince, radish, rocket, raspberries, runner beans, salsify, sweetcorn, Swiss chard, shallots, tomato, wild mushrooms, bananas

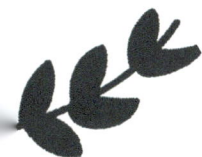

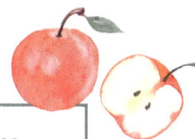

Frozen fruit or veg is the perfect plan so you can extend your seasons.

- Buy (unpackaged) frozen ingredients, or just do it yourself.

Top of the list is LOCAL...

...Just check where it comes from.

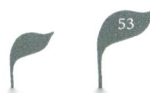

Organic produce is farmed without the use of man-made fertilisers, pesticides, fungicides, hormones, antibiotics and livestock feed additives. The food is also not allowed to be irradiated or GMO and the food that livestock are fed, must be 100% organic.

Organic food cannot claim to be more nutritious as this is really down to the soil it is grown in but it is probably fair to say that if the soil is healthy then the nutrient uptake of the plants will be greater. Many soils around the world are severely depleted in minerals such as iodine and selenium, along with many other trace minerals. Sadly, this is directly impacting the nutrient density of our food.

If organic is unavailable or budget does not allow it, here are foods that are not generally heavily sprayed with pesticides, but it really does depend on where it is grown. Remember eating plenty of veg and fruit is the most important thing.

> Eating organic means you can preserve
> vitamins by eating the peel.

WW - DIRTY 12
-----

1. Grapefruit
2. Celery
3. Strawberries
4. Lemons
5. Pears
6. Spinach
7. Grapes (& raisins / sultanas)
8. Tomatoes
9. Herbs
10. Oranges (& soft citrus)
11. Peaches & Nectarines
12. Salad Leaves in Plastic Packaging

WW - CLEAN 15
-----

1. Broccoli
2. Cauliflower & Cabbage
3. Aubergine
4. Kiwi
5. Pineapple
6. Asparagus
7. Honeydew Melons
8. Sweetcorn
9. Onion
10. Mushrooms
11. Avocados
12. Papayas
13. Bananas
14. Mango
15. Peas

The Dirty Dozen
Best eaten organically

(adapted from ref: pan-uk.org & ewg.org)

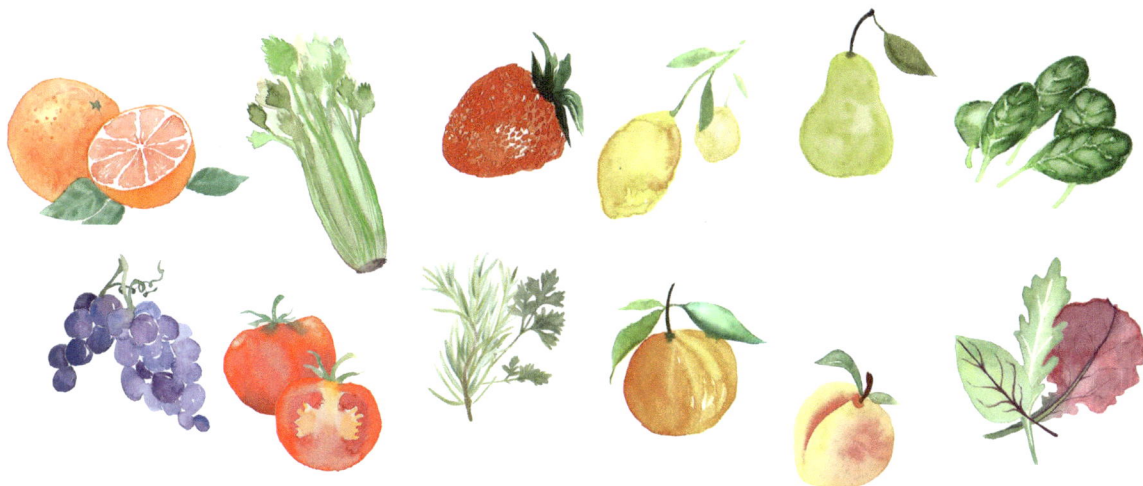

The Clean Fifteen
Top ingredients that have less non-organic health issues

(adapted from ref: pan-uk.org & ewg.org)

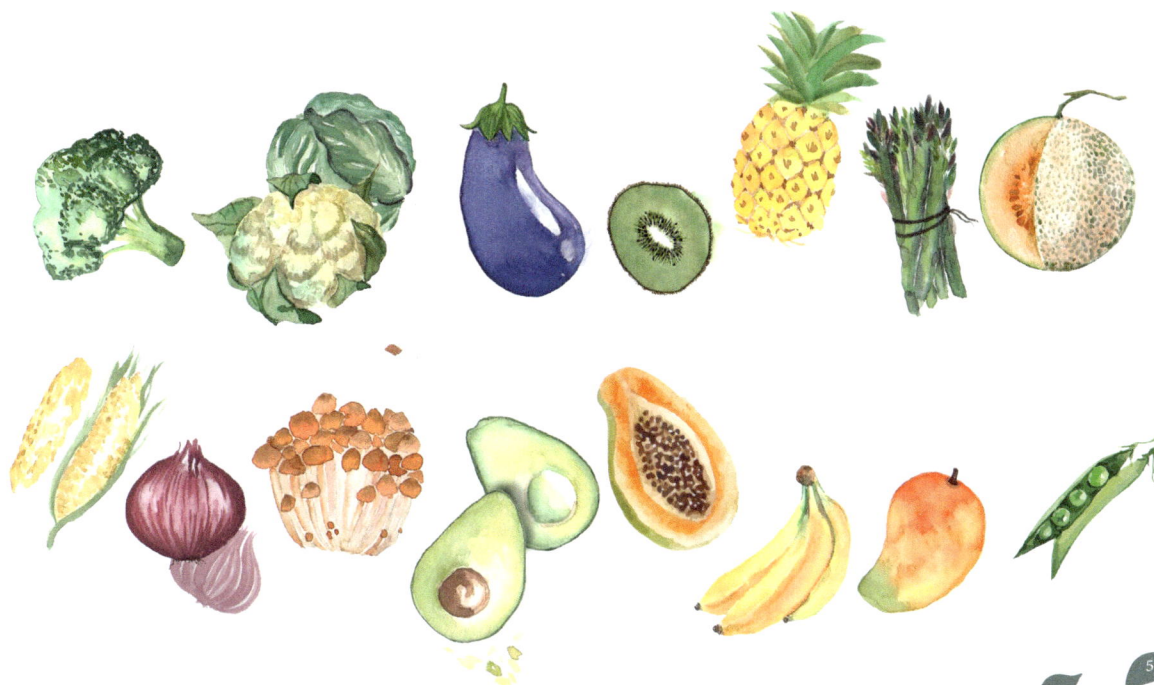

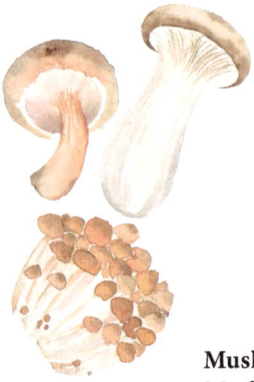

MY TOP TEN

Mushrooms

Mushrooms are a good source of protein as they contain all the essential amino acids. The different mushroom types offer slightly different health benefits from the variety of soluble fibre called beta glucans. Mushrooms are one of the few food sources where the precursor to vitamin D occurs naturally, a big benefit..

Cruciferous Veg

These have been found to be particularly high in the anticancer compound sulphoraphane. Studies have shown that those who eat at least one portion of cruciferous vegetables a week compared with those with no or occasional consumption had a significantly reduced risk of certain cancers.

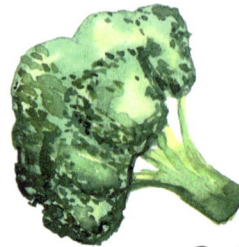

Berries

Dark coloured berries provide many antioxidant benefits and can be extremely anti-inflammatory. They have been shown to stimulate the immune system, block angiogenesis, aid detoxification and reduce cancer cell proliferation.

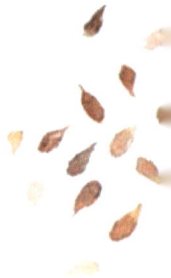

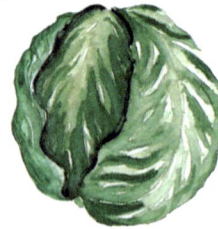

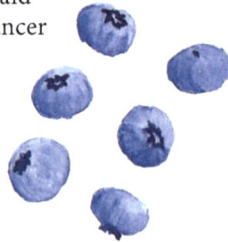

Green Leafy Vegetables

Leafy green vegetables are an important part of a healthy diet. They're packed with vitamins, minerals and fiber but low in calories. Eating a diet rich in leafy greens can offer numerous health benefits including reduced risk of obesity, heart disease, high blood pressure and mental decline.

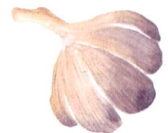

Garlic & Onions

The sulphur compounds in garlic and onions mean that these foods are strong detoxifiers and so help to reduce toxicity. Once chopped, crushed or chewed they release enzymes which have strong therapeutic properties. They are highly anti-microbial too so can help guard against bacterial infections, but best eaten raw.

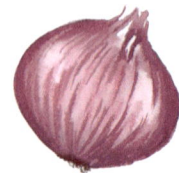

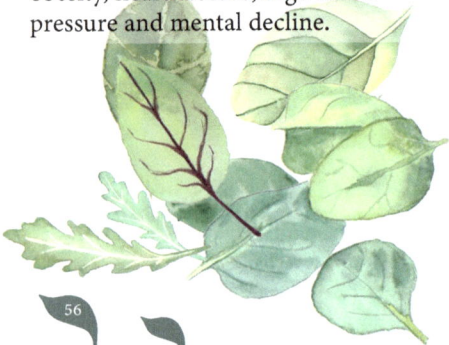

INGREDIENTS

Seeds

Seeds are valuable sources of fibre and provide us with a wealth of healthy fats, vitamins and minerals. Because seeds are so nutrient-dense, you don't need to eat that many to reap the benefits.

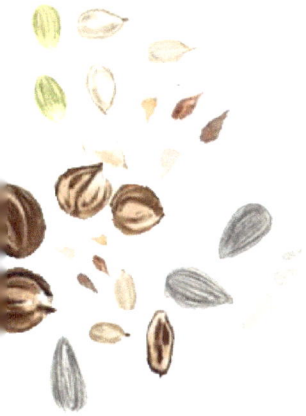

Spices

So many spices have been found to have very important anticancer and anti-inflammatory benefits. They are known to contain high levels of antioxidants, vitamins, minerals and polyphenols, which help support digestive function, healthy circulation, relaxation and sleep and counter inflammatory responses.

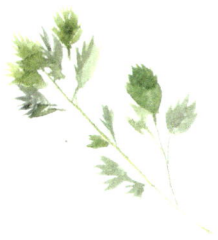

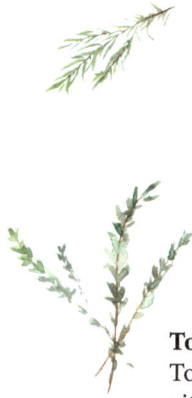

Herbs

Most have a carminative *(anti-flatulent)* effect on our digestive tract due to the volatile oils, impressive anti-inflammatory and anti-bacterial properties. They are also excellent sources of nutrients.

Tomatoes

Tomatoes are a great source of vitamin C, biotin and vitamin K and a very good source of manganese, potassium and vitamins A, B6 & 3 and E. Tomatoes are a carotenoid rich food, the benefits of which have been shown to be more bio-available to the body when they are cooked with olive oil.

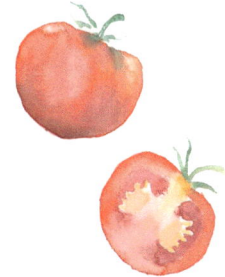

Nuts

Nuts are laden with antioxidents, including the polyphenols in nuts, can combat oxidative stress by neutralizing free radicals — unstable molecules that may cause cell damage and increase disease risk. They're healthiest raw or toasted. Store them at room temperature or put them in the fridge or freezer to keep them fresher for longer.

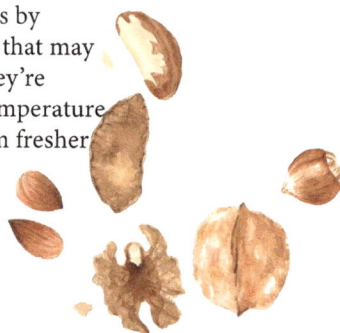

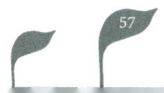

Nourish Yourself

For me, having a healthy mind, body and soul is crucial.

I believe that nutrition is an important place to start and an accessible way to start taking control.

Simply adding one beneficial bite or meal to your day is a bonus, or in my mind, equals a good food moment. It will raise both your satisfaction as to what you have achieved and ease your body into physical enrichment. Detoxing your wellbeing through your diet is important and every little effort counts.

The sooner you embark on a life-long journey of a wholesome foods diet, the greater the effects will be on your mental and physical health.

Wholesome World is my way of sharing some options that have helped me. So many of us don't pay enough attention to life; I've seen it first hand, and I want people to nurture and celebrate their health.

TIPS

The simplest step is to improve your bodys hydration. Drink enough H_2O to increase satiety and boost your metabolic rate. Your brain is made mostly of water, so it helps you think, focus and concentrate better and be more alert. I drink about 4-5 pints per day.

To support your health through food; remove refined sugar and bleached carbohydrates from your diet. A light swing toward a Paleo (caveman) diet, focusing on the health benefits given by fresh vegetables is how I improve my wellbeing.

A simple starting step is to follow the Wholesome recipes; I have broken down the nutrition for each one, so you can build yourself up and improve your immune system. Even if it's a tiny part of your diet, it benefits your health.

Try Wholesome World Granola, Simply Stuffed Dates or Hemp, Cacao nutri-balls.

These are great starting steps.

By eating whole foods and avoiding processed foods you can support your brain function.

I recommend that you buy your fresh produce locally, and keep it organic and seasonal when possible. There are steps towards this though, different fruit and vegetables absorb and retain pesticides and chemicals at different levels (read more p42)

All of the above can help your physical and mental health. Enhanced by the fact you made it yourself, it contains health nutrients and you know there are no additives. Every Step counts.

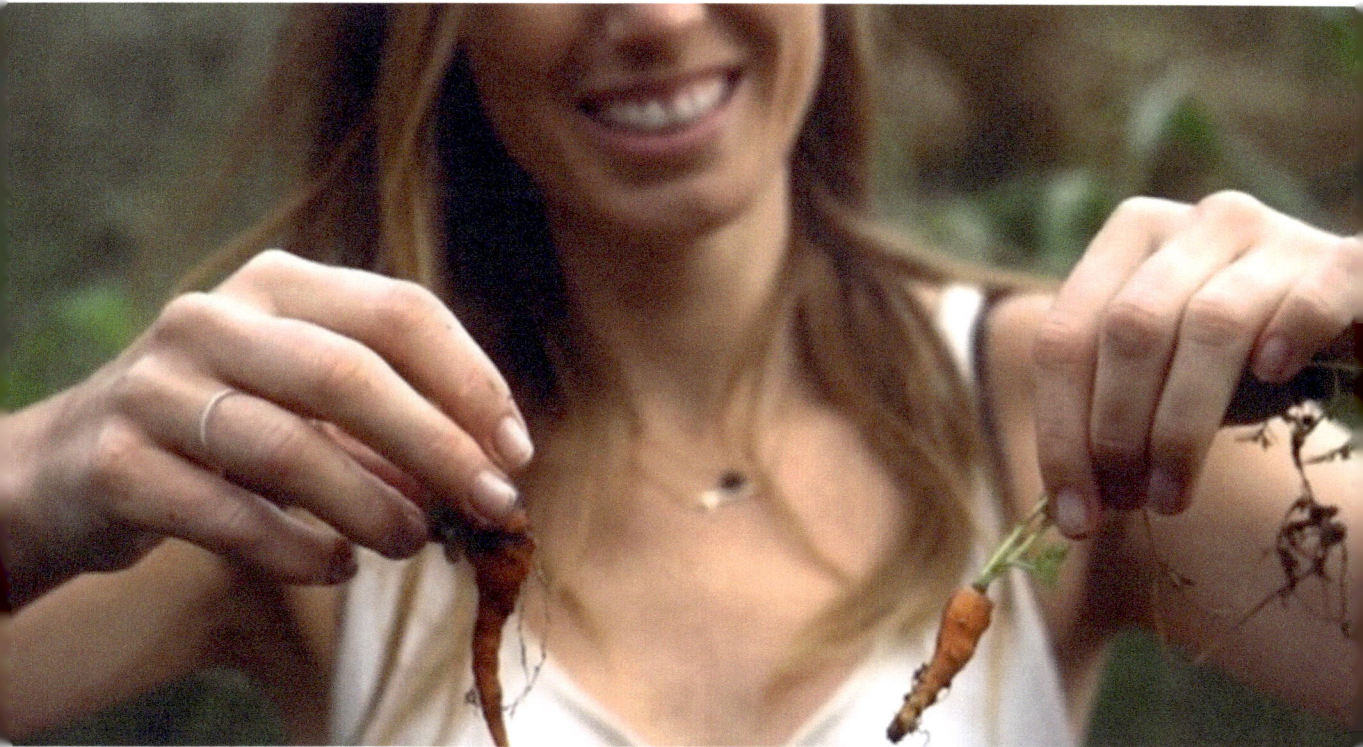

Tea Benefits

Aligning this aspect of life helps you realise the benefits of pharmacopoeial-grade herbs, which can be readily absorbed by the body in the form of tea.

'Ayurveda' is a good path to understand the benefits of tea, and effectively translates as ayu (life) and veda (knowledge)[1].

According to Ayurveda, there are three fundamental states of a being such as the physical (including physiological), mental, and the spiritual. Health is a balance of all these three states and their relationship with the outside world[2].

You need to take time out and consider what you're doing and how you're doing it, and take time to develop yourself.

Black teas have high anti-oxident properties which benefit your overall health and boost the immune system[3]. They fit well with heavy, hearty dishes such as our Aubergine Lasagne (p158).

Green teas act as a beautiful benefit to brain health, due to its low, but beneficial caffiene and amino acids. They are the least processed tea type, made from unoxidised leaves[4]. They're perfect for light, spring and summer salads and seafood, due to its beautifully strong tastes, and go well with our Coastal Chowder (p132).

White teas are rich in anti-oxidents, particularly polyphenols, which protect cells from damage caused by free-radicals.[5] The subtle aroma and taste of white tea is best enjoyed with lightly flavoured desserts. Try with our Maple Pears dessert for the perfect end to dinner (52).

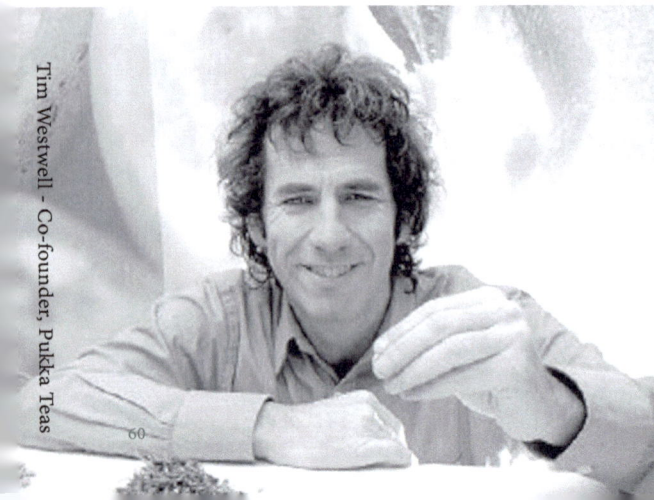

Tim Westwell - Co-founder, Pukka Teas

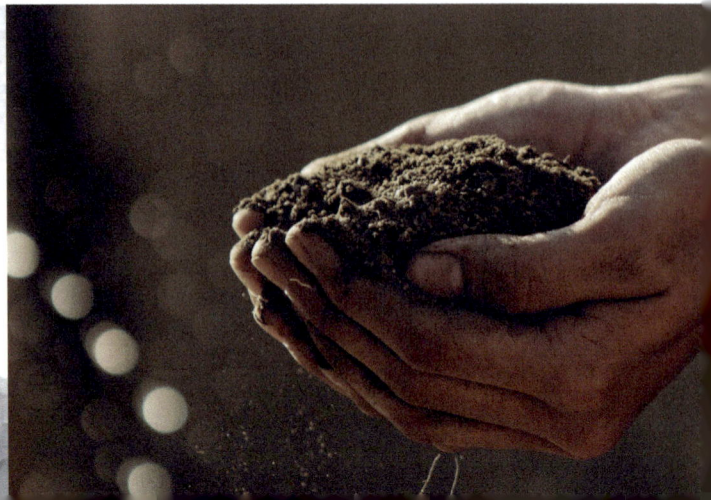

- FORAGE -
LOCAL NETTLE TEA

Foraging for fresh nettles and boiling them into a tea has many health benefits, not least getting out in nature and secondly providing a free source of a nutritious vegetable.

Nettles are high in vitamins A, C, and K, and the minerals iron, selenium, zinc, calcium and magnesium, along with an abundance of antioxidants.

- To make a nettle tea -
Steep 2-3 teaspoons of dried nettle leaves in 1 pint of boiling water for 10 minutes.

*If you can, simply use fresh nettle leaves, picked from the top few leaves.

*Herbal & fruit teas provide such a wealth of nutrient benefits.

To feel the full benefits of tea nutrition, it should be sourced from ecosystems built upon organic farming. This gives a simple foundation to amplify your health, regenerate people and their communities as well as the plants and our environment.

'Organic farms deliver more wildlife, healthier soils, climate mitigation, protection against flooding, clean water, lower pesticide use, lower antibiotic use, more jobs and better food security'[6].

Realise what is your taste preference, what flavour enahnces your mood, and with teas, you can add this to both improves the benefits from your intake of nutritious food and increase your biodiversity.

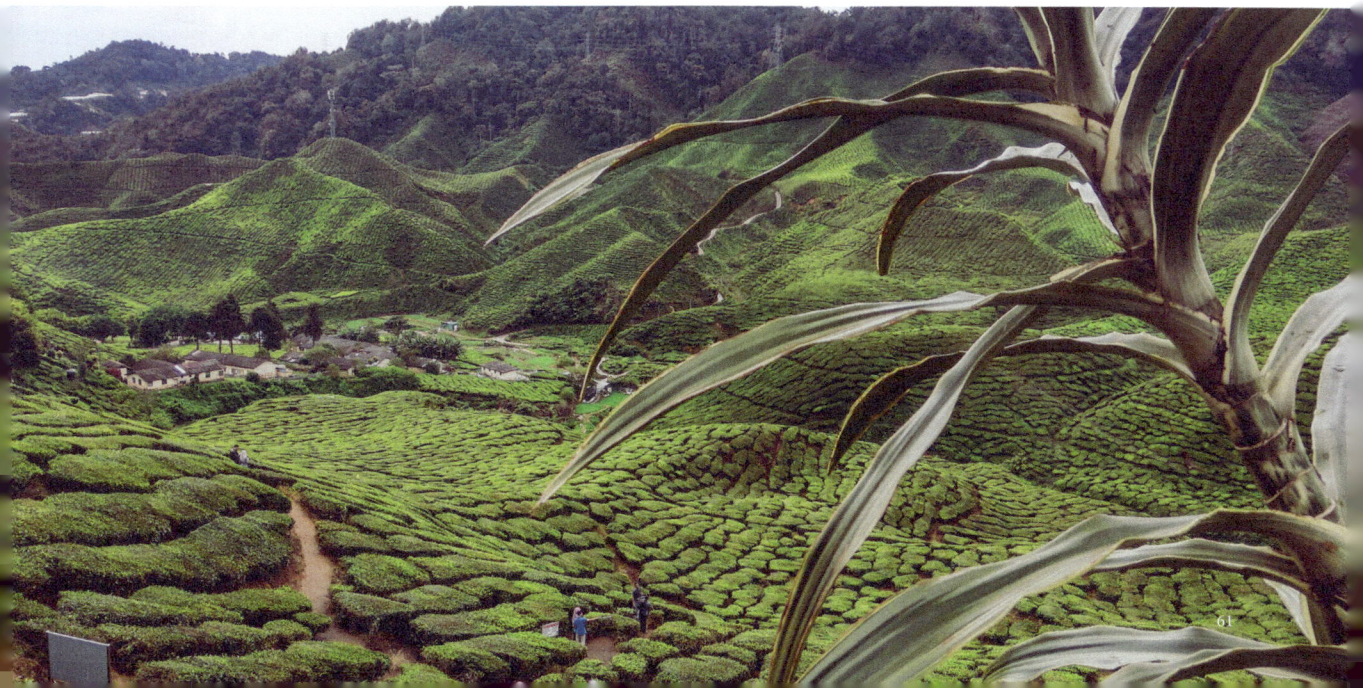

When time is short... let life flow...

Frozen food can be healthy convenience food. Frozen vegetables which have been snap frozen (quickly frozen after being picked) have generally retained their nutrition so peas, spinach, carrots, broccoli can be useful items for when fresh is unavailable.

A few vegetables and some homemade stock can make a quick and healthy soup. Have red lentils, or tinned pulses to hand which cook quickly and can be added to make it even more nourishing and giving a boost to the protein and fibre level.

If you have a glut (surplus) of vegetables or fruit, chop them up and freeze them yourself ready for a rainy day. Freezing retains most nutrients. Home freezing reduces the environmental impact of plastic packaging,

NB: You can reduce enivromental impact from plastic by sourcing dry and frozen goods through what I call 'naked shopping', package free.

To avoid relying on ready meals when time is short, choose your frozen ingredients or a pre-chopped stir fry vegetable pack to which you can add fish, chicken, tofu etc. or chop excess veg you may have and store in the fridge or freezer for quick additions to stir-fries.

So so worth it.

If you do buy a ready meal, best to buy one that is **not in a plastic container,** but if it is, decant it into a oven proof dish and put a lid on top to cook, using the oven if you have time.

You only need a windowsill to grow a ready supply of herbs. Fresh herbs are extremely nutritious and anti-inflammatory. Get into the habit of adding some herbs to your recipes whenever you can. Herbs also freeze well, so chop fresh herbs when you have them and freeze in small, labelled containers or bags; see p106.

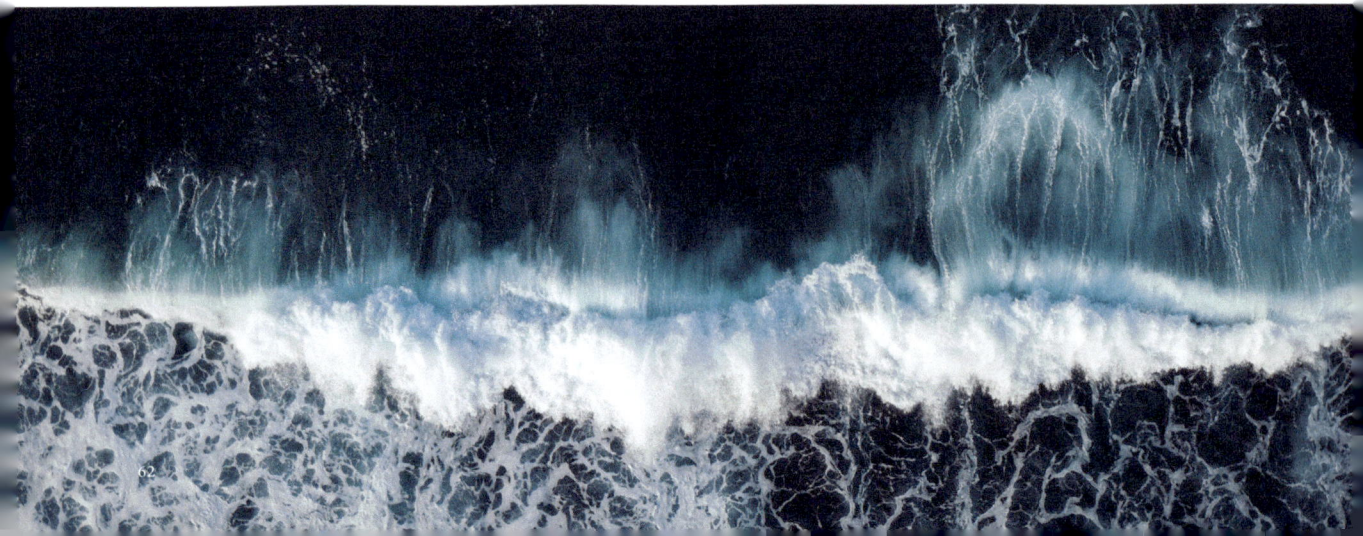

KITCHEN CONVERSION CHARTS

WEIGHTS

G	OZ	LB
58	2	
114	4	
170	6	
226	8	½
340	12	
454	16	1

LIQUIDS

ML	PINTS	FLUID OZ
28		1
140	¼	5
285	½	10
425	¾	15
570	1	20
850	1½	30
1100	2	40

1 fluid cup U.S. - 230ml

OVEN HEAT

GAS	°C Norm / Fan	° F
1	140 / 120	175
2	150 / 130	300
3	170 / 150	325
4	180 / 160	350
5	190 / 170	375
6	200 / 180	400
7	220 / 200	425

SPOONS & SIZES

1 tsp	teaspoon (tsp)	5ml
2 tsp	dessertspoon (dsp)	10ml
3 tsp	tablesoon (tbsp)	15ml

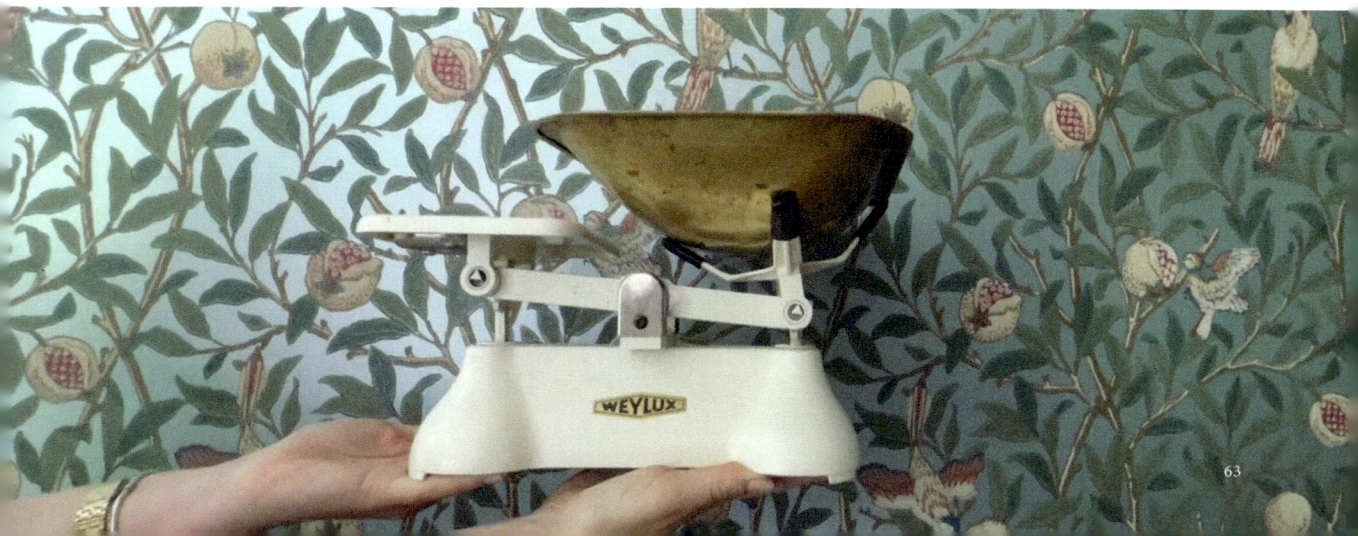

WELCOME

TO MY WHOLESOME RECIPES

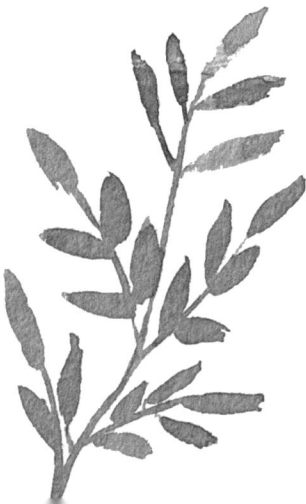

Basic Kitchen Goods

Here are some good foods used in the recipes, so stock up.

--

Give your cupboard and fridge a spring clean to refresh it, and fill it with healthier options to reduce the temptation to eat less healthy food.

Vegetables

Horseradish	Asparagus
Kale	Beetroot
Mushrooms	Avocados
Onions	Broccoli
Peppers	Carrots
Pumpkin	Cauliflower / Romanesco
Spinach	Chillies
Sprouted seeds	Cabbage
Salad leaves e.g. Rocket	Fennel
Sweet potatoes	Garlic
Turmeric	Ginger

Fruit

Apples
Berries galore (*fresh or frozen*)
Grapefruit
Lemons
Oranges
Pears
Pomegranates
Tomatoes
Watermelon

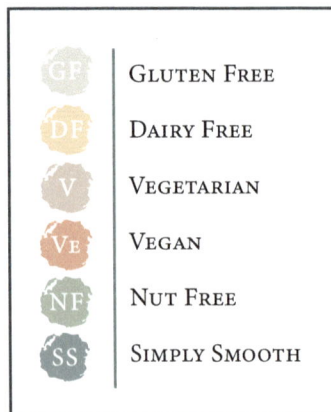

GF	Gluten Free
DF	Dairy Free
V	Vegetarian
Ve	Vegan
NF	Nut Free
SS	Simply Smooth

* All oven temperatures are for non-fan ovens.
See p63 to find alternate temps.

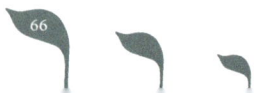

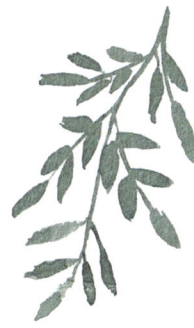

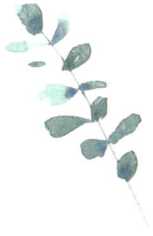

Little things, like thinking about the
packaging makes a difference.
Save your jars and boxes and discover
non-packaged dry goods in eco-stores.

Oils

Avocado oil
Olive oil
Virgin coconut oil
Ghee

Nuts and Seeds

Almonds
Walnuts
Brazil nuts
Cashews
Pistachios
Pecans
Pumpkin seeds
Sunflower seeds
Chia seeds
Quinoa
Sesame seeds
Linseeds

Dried and Tinned Goods

Brown / Basmati / Wild rice
Blackstrap molasses
Bouillon powder / Organic stock cubes
Cartons of chopped / Whole tomatoes
Coconut milk & cream
Carob nibs / Raw cacao / Cocoa
Tomato paste
Alternative mylks
Spices
Herbs (best fresh)
Himalayan / Sea salt
Dried lentils

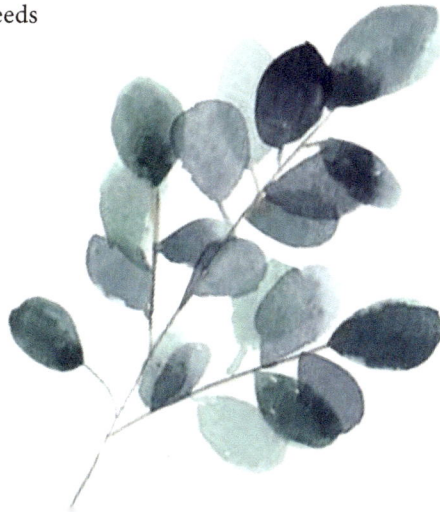

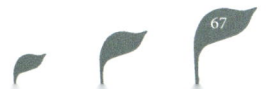

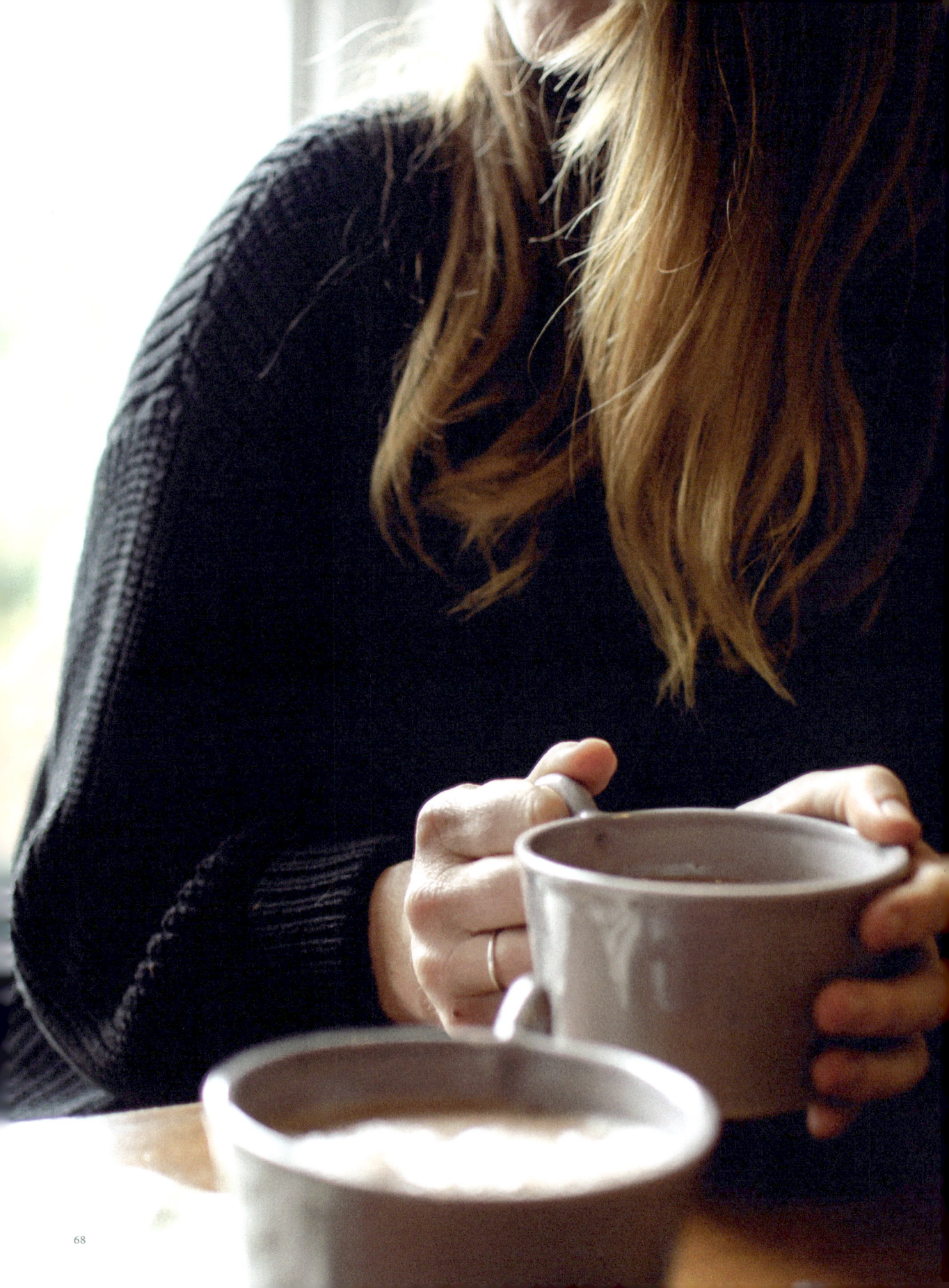

DRINKS

GREEN HULK SMOOTHIE

SERVES 2 | ⏲ 10 MINS | GF DF V VE SS

"I sometimes like a small squeeze of lemon to freshen it up! But the standard Green Hulk is strong. Did you know that an avocado a day may match the cholesterol lowering effects of statins, as it contains high levels of sterols and stanols. It also contains a good level of healthy fats."

Use bananas that are less ripe for less sugar and more health benefits.

Spinach adds to the array of anticancer nutrients that green leafy veg provide, vitamins A, B6, B9, C , E, K and the minerals folic acid, iron, magnesium and calcium. Add a squeeze of lime to help preserve the abundance of antioxidants and complement the alkalising effects. It is a surprising fact that green leafy veg contain healthy omega fats but the addition of avocado and peanut butter increases this significantly. It is good for fighting off infections.

Choose a wholesome peanut butter with no added sugar or oils. Other nut butters could also be used. Nuts provide some all important protein.

By putting kale into smoothies, the chopping, crushing action can help to release the sulphoraphane, a potent antioxidant which has been shown to have impressive anticancer properties.

INGREDIENTS

1	Banana
½	Avocado
1 handful	Spinach
2 handful	Kale
2 tbsp	Peanut butter

EQUIPMENT

Blender

METHOD

1. Peel the banana and skin the avocado.

2. Pull the greens apart so they fit in the blender.

3. Then add about 125ml of water and add the peanut butter.

4. Blend until smooth and serve.

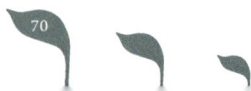

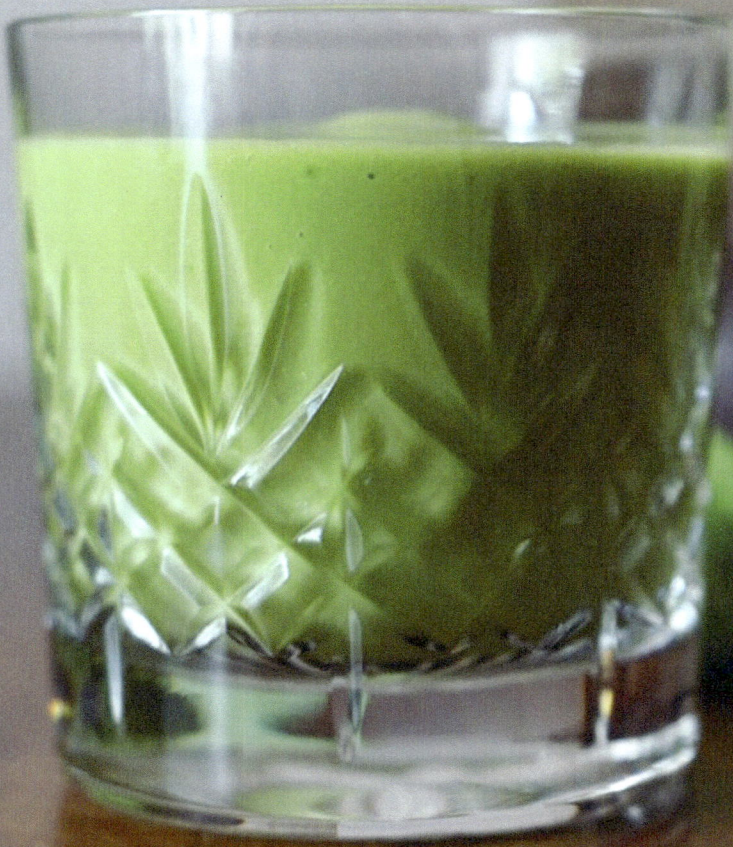

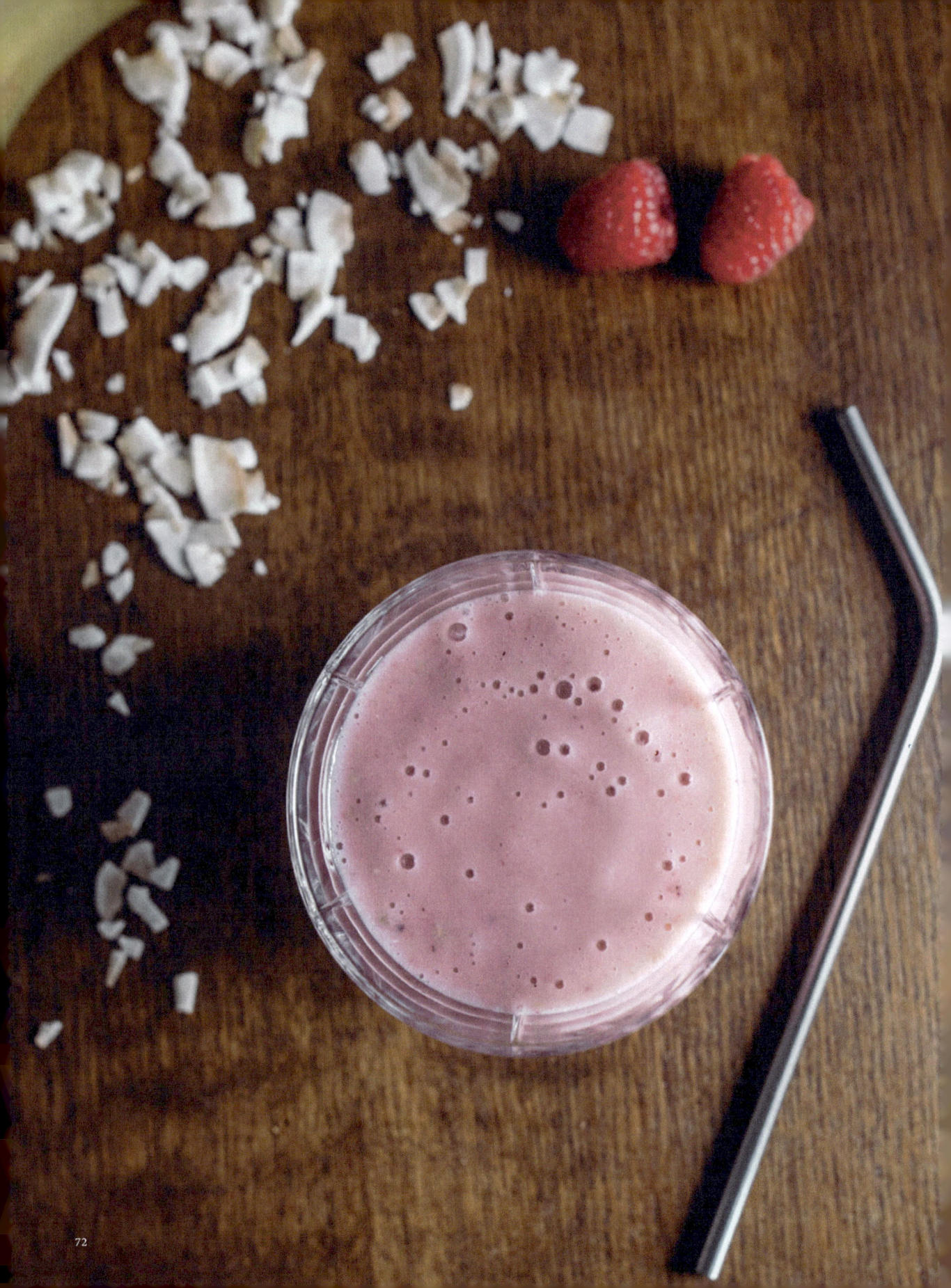

Pink Island Smoothie

SERVES 2 | 🕐 10 MINS | GF DF V VE NF SS

"This is one of the sweeter smoothies in this book, but it is perfect for when you need a sweeter day."

A treat when you want to spoil yourself with an indulgent smoothie.

Raspberries are packed with antioxidants to make that indulgence worthwhile. Bananas provide fibre and several antioxidants and nutrients.

Less ripe bananas are healthier as they contain more resistant starch and so less sugar and higher levels of pectin, which benefits our gut microbiota and can improve gut transit time and nutrient absorption.

Choose a coconut milk with no added sugar and raw honey for its added value.

INGREDIENTS

200g	Raspberries
1	Banana
400ml	Coconut milk
2 tsp	Honey / Agave syrup

EQUIPMENT

Blender

METHOD

1. In a blender place the raspberries, banana, tinned coconut milk and honey.

2. Whizz until smooth and creamy, if too stiff, add a little water.

3. Serve with ice on a hot day.

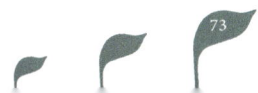

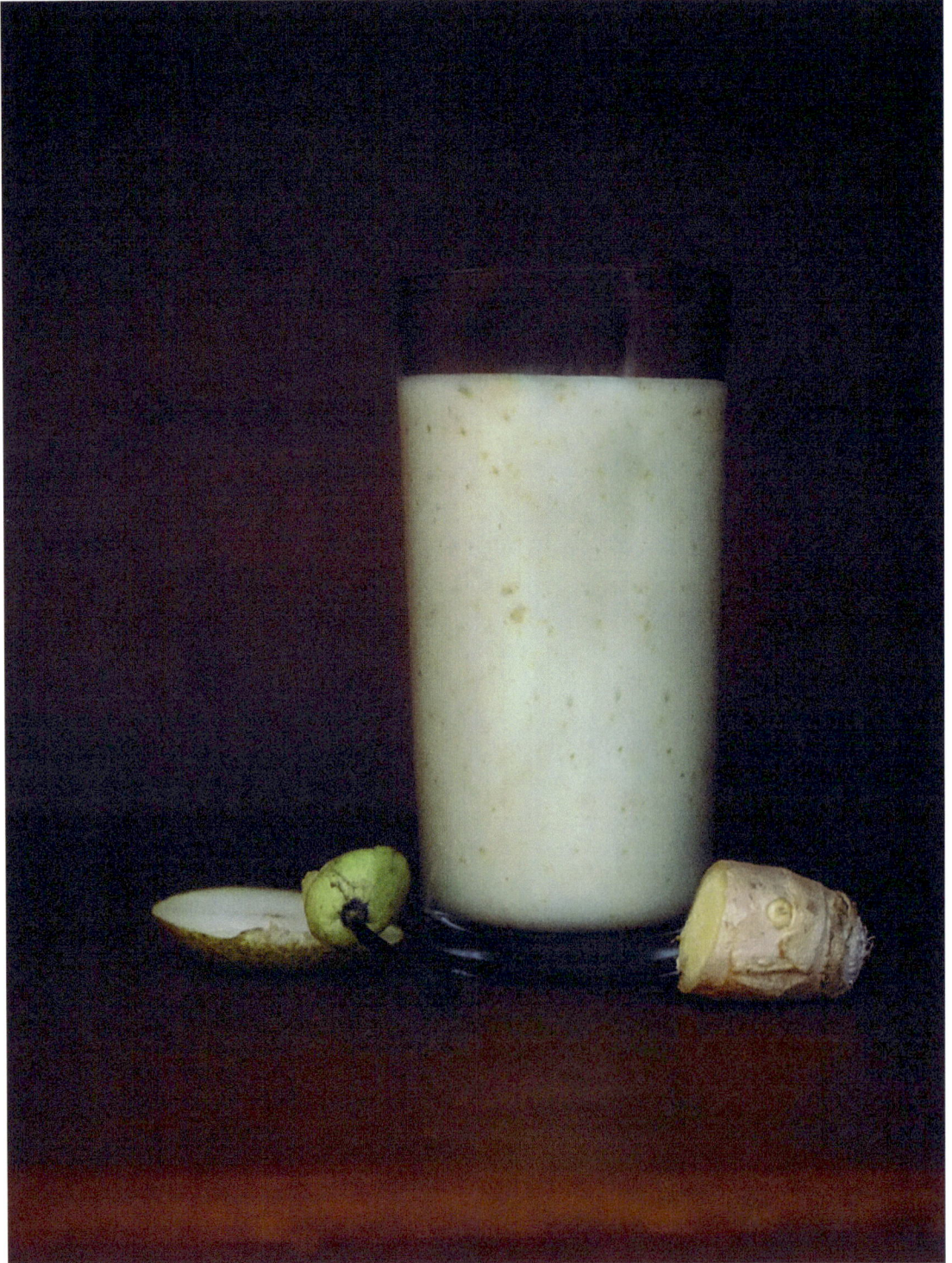

GINGER, PEAR & APPLE SMOOTHIE

SERVES 2 | ⏱ 5 MINS | GF V NF SS

*"So I have hugely productive apple trees and miniscule baby pear trees out in the garden.
They act as an inspiration and a reminder that there is so much local fruit and growth that I should be throwing my arms out for."*

Pears contain a valuable source of soluble and insoluble fibres but much of this is in the skin. If the skin isn't too leathery then I would whizz them up skin and all, for it is these fibres which give pears the reputation of being good for constipation. It is the pectin that also acts as a prebiotic, helping to feed and maintain our gut flora.

Added to this, pears have been shown to contain vitamins, minerals, and plant chemicals such as anthocyanins and quercetin, that add up to the all important anti-inflammatory and anticancer properties.

Ginger is one of our top anticancer foods (see ingredients) containing even more anti-inflammatory compounds. With some live yoghurt too, this is yet another fabulous smoothie that will do wonders for your gut health.

"Make sure that the apple juice is simply juice, with no added sugar."

INGREDIENTS

2	Pears
½ tsp	Ginger
200ml	Apple juice
50ml	Natural yoghurt

EQUIPMENT

Blender

METHOD

1. Peel and roughly chop the pears.

2. Cut ½ a tsp of ginger, and grate it.

3. Add the pears, ginger, apple juice and natural yoghurt into the blender.

4. Whizz until smooth.

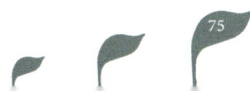

Banana, Honey, Oat Smoothie

SERVES 2 | 🕐 10 MINS | DF V NF SS

"This is a great morning smoothie. Thick and filling, but with different breakdown time ingredients, keeping you energised as long as possible. I personally was a banana bread and morning porridge girl; beautifully filling start to the day, which holds back the hunger properly, but this is now the replacement. Simple and delicioso."

Bananas provide fibre and several antioxidants and nutrients. Less ripe bananas are healthier as they contain more resistant starch and so less sugar and higher levels of pectin which benefits our gut microbiota and can improve gut transit time and nutrient absorption.

Organic local honey is best. Check other sources of honey for added sugar before you buy.

INGREDIENTS

2	Bananas
2 tsp	Runny honey
600ml	Oat mylk
35g	Oats

EQUIPMENT

Blender

METHOD

1. Peel the bananas and add to the blender with the honey, mylk and oats.

2. Blitz until smooth.

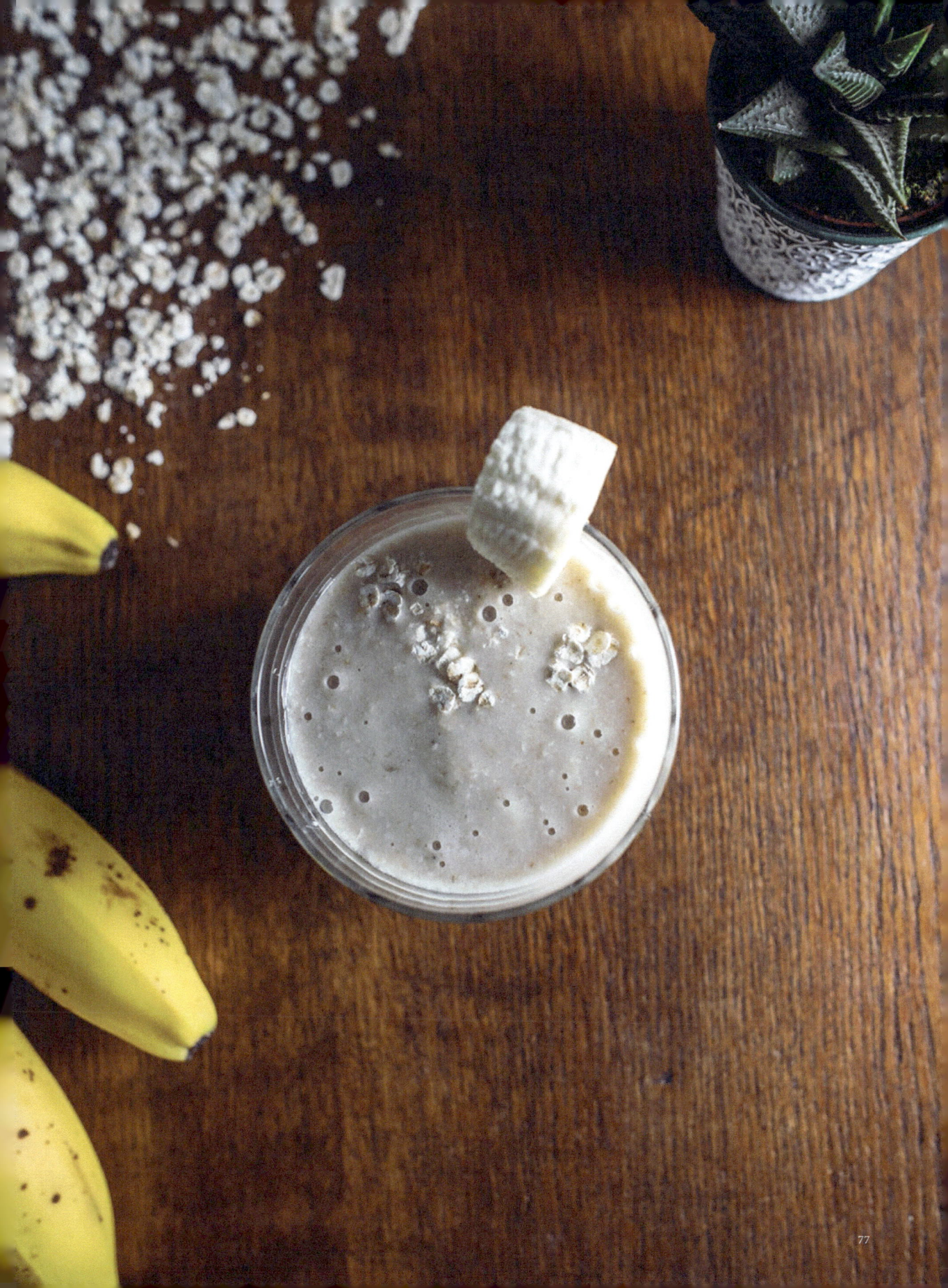

FRESH GREEN ZING JUICE

SERVES 2 | ⏲ 10 MINS | GF DF V Ve NF SS

"Years ago I grabbed some green tart cooking apples from the garden trees, and fell in love. To keep it fresh and less sharp, the cucumber was a perfect addition, as it always has been, I ate cucmber as a child in every way possible."

Apples and cucumbers contain a therapeutic array of antioxidants that counteract the damaging effects of free radicals.

A squeeze of lemon juice into anything increases vitamin C intake and aids digestion.

The capsaicin in cayenne pepper adds to the antioxidant and anti-inflammatory benefits of this juice.

INGREDIENTS

2	Green apples
1	Cucumber
½	Unwaxed lemon
Pinch of	Cayenne pepper

EQUIPMENT

Blender

METHOD

1. Remove the core and seeds, and chunkily chop the apple.

2. Chop the cucumber to fit the juicer.

3. Halve the lemon, de-pip and de-skin.

4. Add all of the above to the juicer, then stir in the cayenne pepper spice when serving.

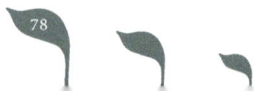

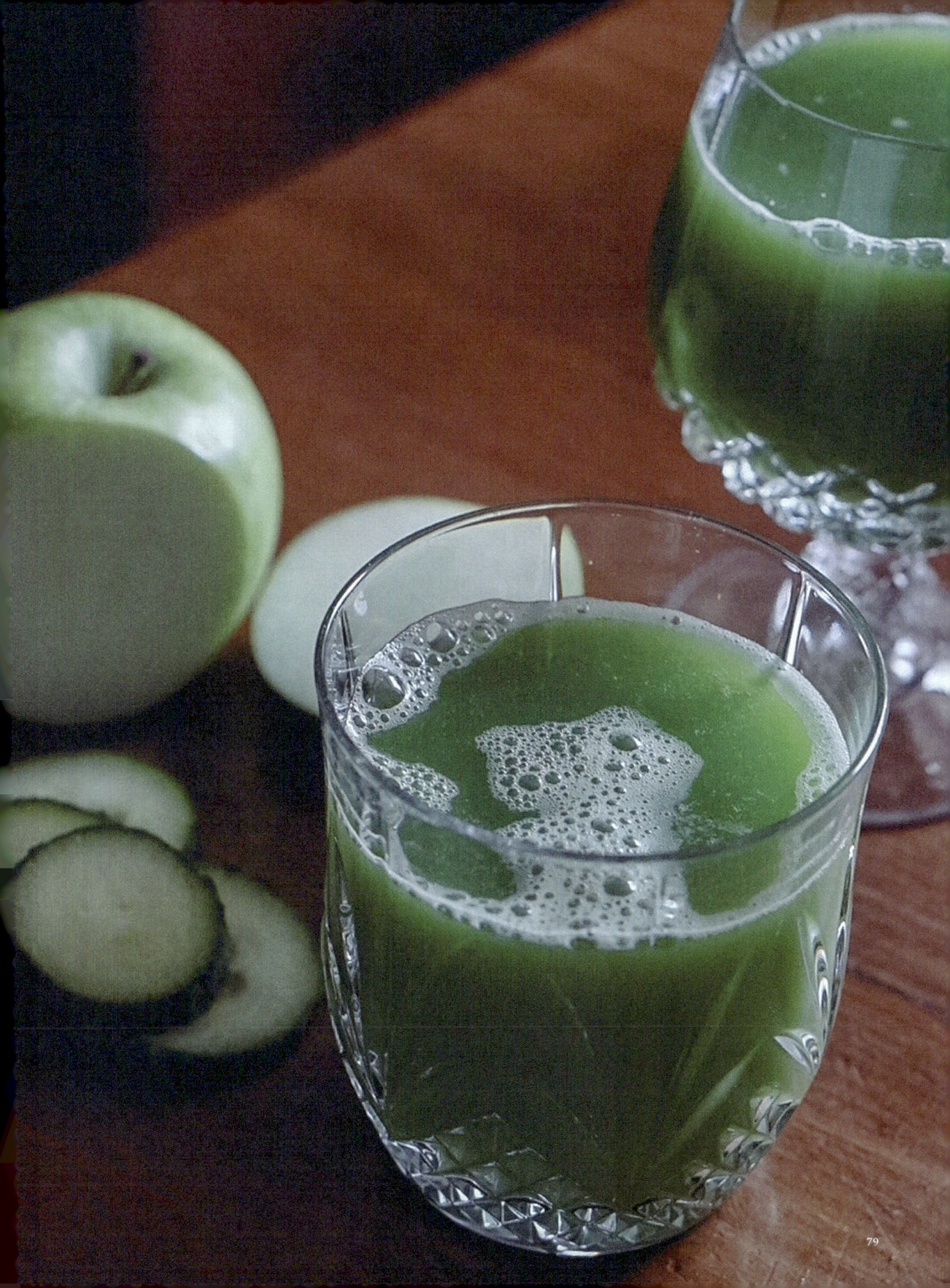

Cacao Carob Smoothie

SERVES 2 | 🕐 10 MINS |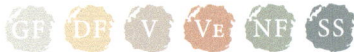

"Sneaking cacao into your daily diet is a good step towards absorbing healthy nutrients as it contains more antioxidants per gram than blueberries, goji berries, red wine, raisins, prunes and even pomegranates. I find it a solid way to start the day. This Cacao Carob Smoothie is definitely super, super healthy. Top with cacao nibs for decoration and extra taste satisfaction."

The cauliflower and courgettes ramp up the vitamins and minerals and anticancer plant chemicals. Aka, they add nutrition, bulk but no flavour!

The avocado creates a wonderful creaminess and adds in some essential healthy fats too. Cacao and carob powder add more potent antioxidants, including gallic acid which has been shown in studies to have anti-inflammatory and anticancer effects.

Ginger and cinnamon are super spices to aid digestion and blood sugar balance. Great if you're struggling with digesting fructose.

INGREDIENTS

75g	Cauliflower
50g	Courgettes
250ml	Soya mylk
¼ tsp	Avocado
½ tsp	Cinnamon
½ tsp	Ginger powder
½ tsp	Vanilla extract
1 tsp	Carob powder
1 tsp	Cacao powder
25ml	Agave syrup

METHOD

1. Chunkily chop and steam the cauliflower and courgettes for 5-7 mins.

2. Once cooked, add to a blender with the soya mylk, and all of the other ingredients and blitz until it's super creamy.

- *Add more soy or water to perfect your consistency.*

EQUIPMENT

Blender

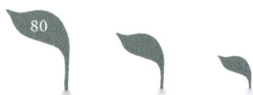

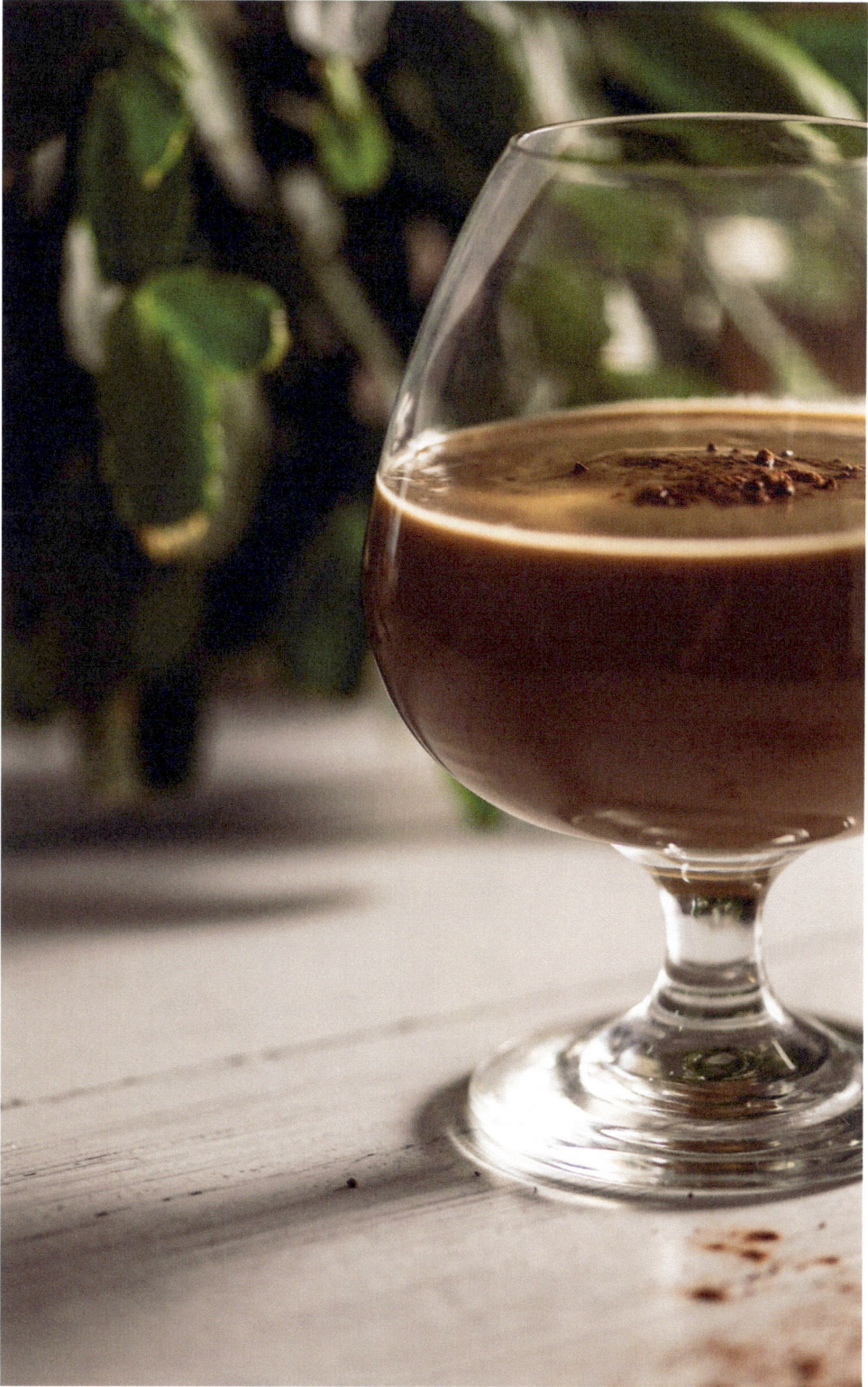

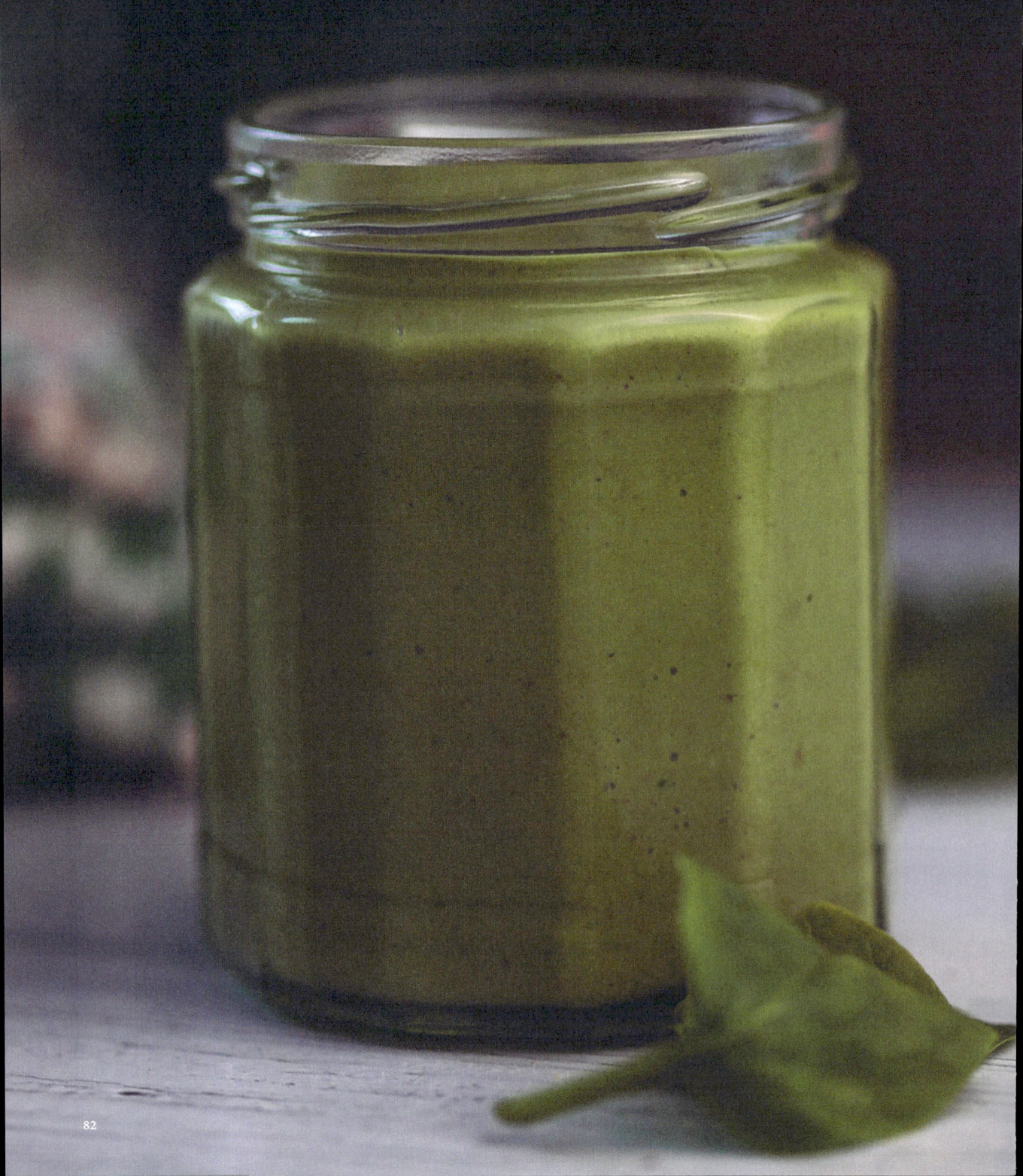

GREEN ISLE SMOOTHIE

SERVES 2 | 🕐 10 MINS | GF DF V NF SS

"It's no secret that avocados are a good source of healthy fats and an excellent addition to your daily diet. But it's worth noting that they have a high carbon footprint as they are mainly grown in tropical regions and then flown far and wide due to their global popularity. Help out the planet and go easy on your avocado consumption. I restrain my consumption and go for the organically, sustainably sourced avo, to keep the world a teeny bit better."

Spinach provides you with your all important green leafy veg for vitamins A, B6, B9, C, E, K and the minerals folic acid, iron, magnesium and calcium.

Avocado contains a good level of healthy fats so this can be a good smoothie to have as part of a 'build-up' diet when weight gain is needed.

Add a squeeze of lime to help preserve the abundance of antioxidants and enhance the alkalising effects.

INGREDIENTS

1	Avocado
200ml	Almond mylk
1 dsp	Honey
Handful of	Spinach
½	Lime

EQUIPMENT

Blender

METHOD

1. De-skin and destone the avocado.

2. Simply throw all ingredients into a blender, except the lime, just add the juice.

3. Check the consistency and if too thick for your liking, add some water and whizz again.

4. Decant into a glass and garnish with a slice of lime when serving.

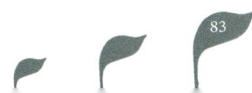

83

COCONUT CHAI LATTE

SERVES 2 | 🕐 10 MINS | GF DF V NF SS

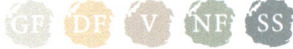

"A combination of complementary spices derived from the traditional masala chai blend. I classically enjoy this beautifully warming flavour and aroma next to an outdoor fire in the summer evenings or to cosy up with after a cold winter's surf. This is how I placate myself; warm, deep and worth it in every aspect. I love to top with cacao nibs or ground cacao."

For the healthiest choice choose the best almond and coconut mylks with the least amount of additives, particularly sweetners. Mixed with all these wonderful spices makes it a warming but calming drink for the gut.

INGREDIENTS

200ml	Full-fat coconut milk *(½ a can)*
200ml	Almond mylk
2 tsp	Cinnamon *(ground)*
½ tsp	Cloves
¼ tsp	Cardamom *(ground)*
½ tsp	Ginger *(ground)*
½ tsp	Mixed spice
½ tsp	Vanilla extract
2 dsp	Agave syrup

METHOD

1. Start by mixing the coconut milk and almond mylk, lightly heating them in a pan. Quickly sneak approx 3 tbsp to the side, before it heats, to a mug.

2. Stir the spices into your cupped mylk and mix, followed by the vanilla extract and agave syrup.

3. Stir the paste into the warmed mylk and simmer for 5 minutes.

4. Using a hand-held frother, froth the mylk for an extra creamy latte.

5. Serve sprinkled with a dash of cinnamon!

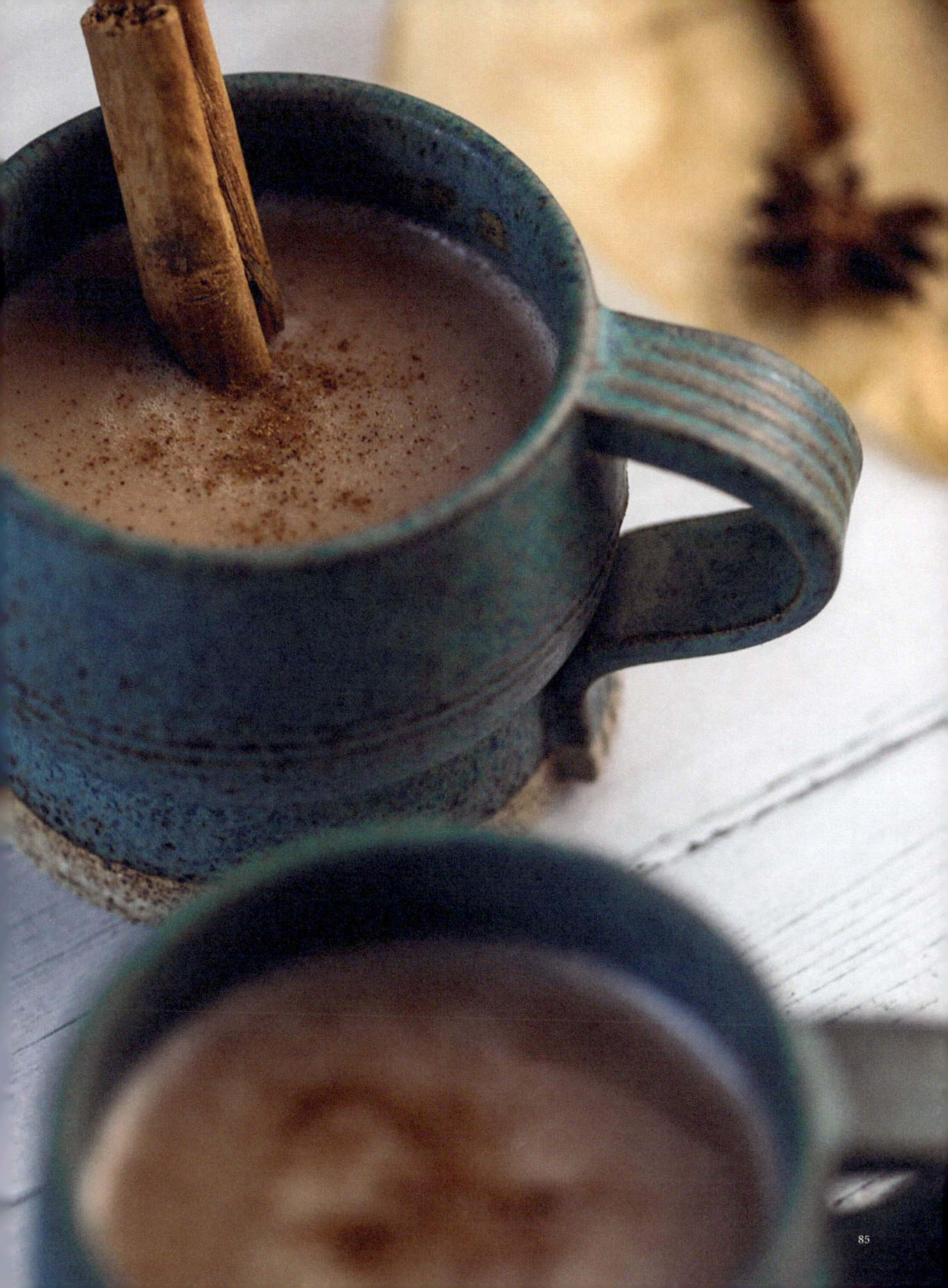

Wholesome Kombucha

SERVES 10 | 🕐 20 MINS (14+ DAYS) | GF DF V Ve NF SS

"A fermented tea derived from a living culture, similar to the sourdough theory, that you can flavour to suit your palette. Use a good quality green tea that will be high in antioxidants, organic is even more beneficial. SCOBY (symbiotic culture of bacteria and yeast), is just 'alive' with active yeast and bacteria, it is the 'extra' ingredient that you can buy online."

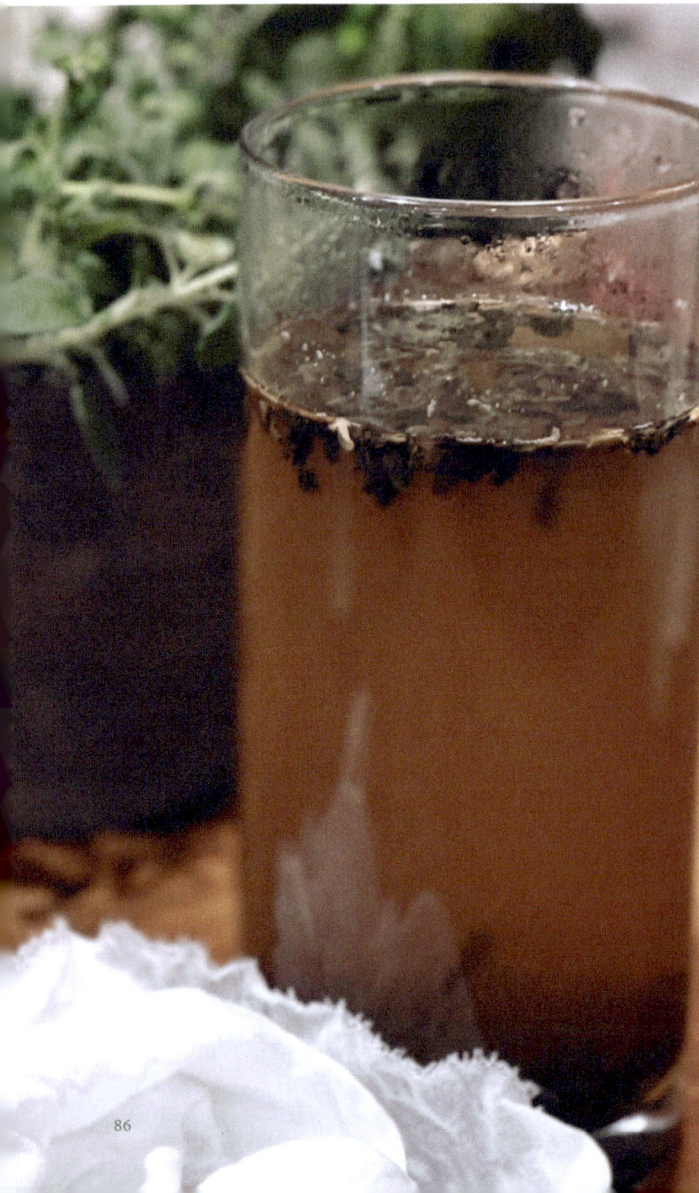

"Here are my top types of this sumptuous juice;

Spring/Summer	*Redberries; 100g of your choice, strawberries, raspberries, blueberries, cherries.*
Autumn/ Winter	*Ginger and Turmeric; 75g finely sliced ginger, 75g peeled and finely sliced turmeric."*

-

Kombucha simply is a fermented tea, a blend of tea, water, sugar, SCOBY. It's low in sugar and contains acetic acid and antioxidant polyphenols which are natural and good for the gut.

The acidity of the kombucha will develop over these days and this is a very personal thing, if you want to take total scientific control of your fermentation use litmus paper / ph strips and test. Ideally it should sit around 3.0ph.

Use a good quality green tea that will be high in antioxidants. Add some nutrient rich berries, equally full of antioxidants to the kombucha.

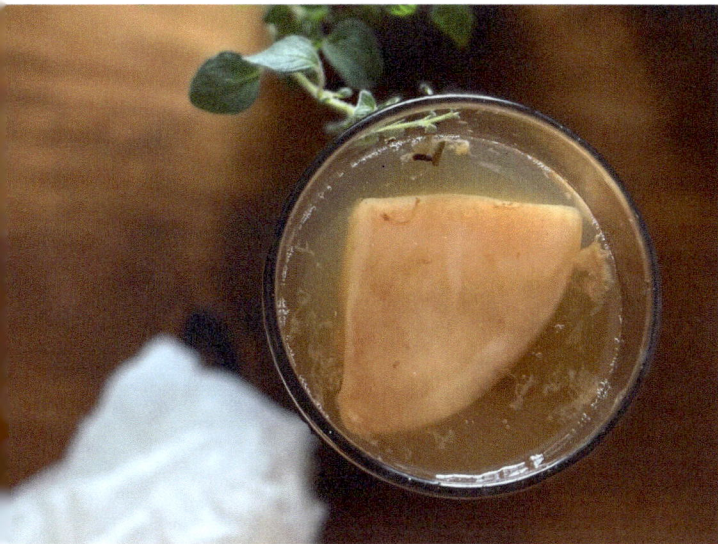

INGREDIENTS

1	SCOBY *(or 200ml quality Kombucha)*
-	
5 teabags	Green tea
175g	Granulated cane sugar
2 tsp	Redberries; *strawberries raspberries, blueberries cherries*

METHOD

1. Boil 500ml of water. In the jar place the tea bags and sugar, add the boiled water, mix well, and leave to cool for 10 minutes.

2. Remove the teabags (if loose tea was used strain until all the tea leaves are removed) return the sweetened tea to the sealed jar such as a Kilner jar.

3. Add 1.5 litres of room temperature water and mix in; the liquid should be tepid (below 29°C) before you add your SCOBY or 200ml kombucha.

4. Cover with the cotton / linen cloth, secure with a rubber band and place in a warm airy place that is between 23°C-27°C, possibly an airing cupboard and leave to brew for 10-15 days.

5. Stir the kombucha daily with a slotted spoon to add air to the mix. if you did not use a SCOBY to start and just some good quality kombucha you should start to see a fragile film build up. Don't worry this is the start of you home grown SCOBY!

6. When this is achieved remove the SCOBY and 200ml of the kombucha to start your next brew.

7. Bottle the remaining kombucha, and add your summer berries and leave standing to steep for 4 - 10 days. See more favourite flavour choices in the 'overview'.

8. The longer you steep it the more bubbles will start to arise in your kombucha. If the weather is warm do take care to burp your bottles; ie open them for a moment, to release a build up of gasses.

9. Store in the fridge and this will stop the the fermentation and deliver you a delicious and refreshing drink.

Plum & Banana Kombucha Smoothie

SERVES 2 | 🕐 10 MINS | GF DF V VE NF SS

"I think that plums are perfect in this one, a light summer, autumn feeling which pulls you through the day. It's easy to switch to peach, or if you want to swing through the year, go for anything from rhubarb, red fruits like strawberries and raspberries to delicious Cornish gooseberries.

Kefir can be made with basically ANY sort of milk, but classically dairy. If you're looking for vegan, I recommend rice, coconut or soy."

The combination of kombucha, yoghurt and kefir (fermented foods) makes an ideal gut restoration tonic.

Plum contains the anticancer compound ursolic acid and plenty of vitamins A, C & K, so good for bones and healing. Plums tend to be tart so an added benefit is that they do not have a significant effect on blood glucose levels.

INGREDIENTS

1	Banana
1	Plum
50ml	Kombucha *(berry)*
1 tbsp	Yoghurt *(dairy or not)*
100ml	Kefir *(dairy/vegan)*

EQUIPMENT

Blender

METHOD

1. Place all of the ingredients in a blender.

2. Whizz until smooth.

3. Simply taste and enjoy.

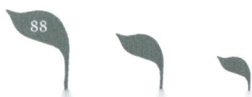

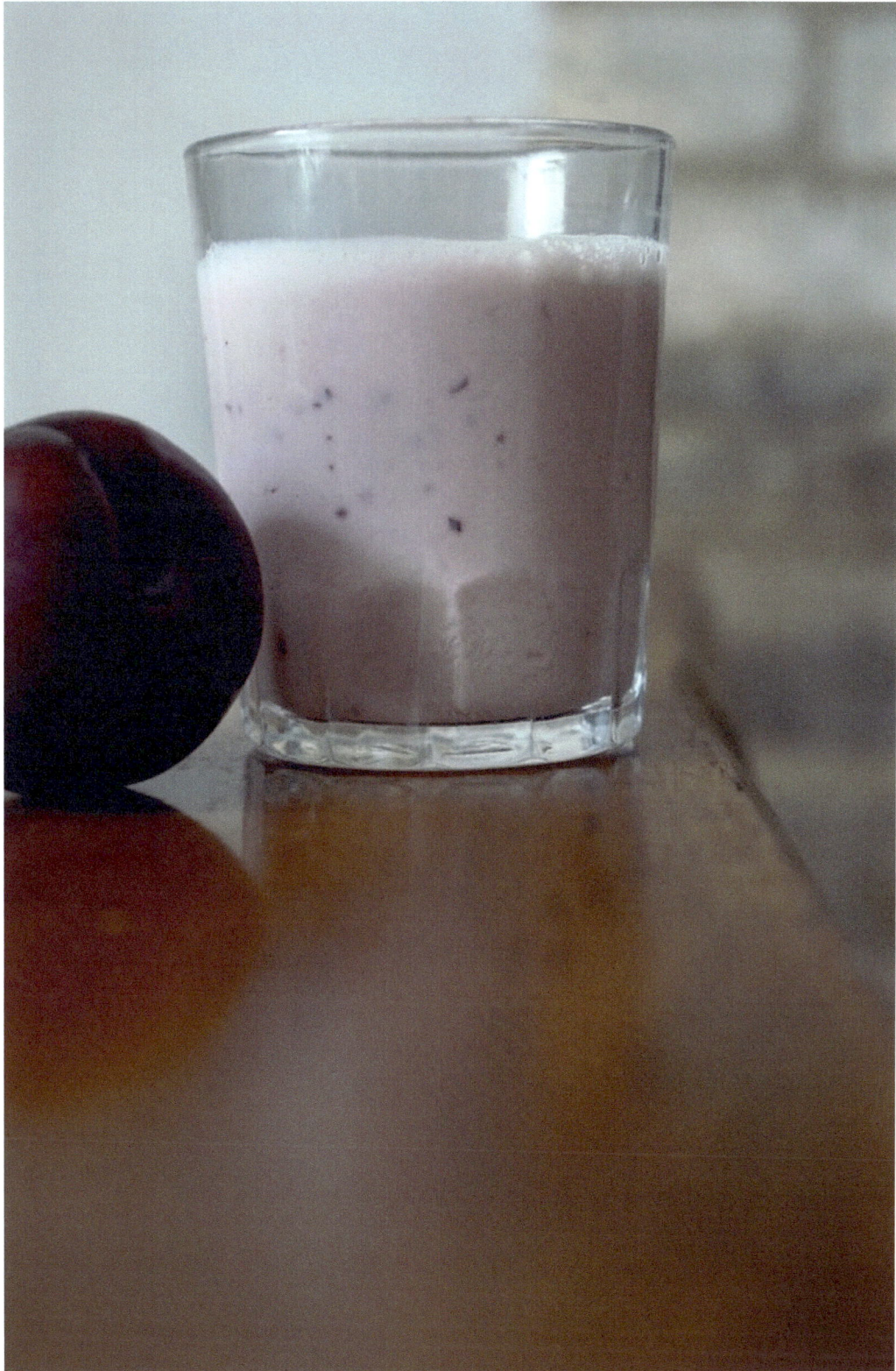

ROSE & CARDAMOM HOT CHOCOLATE

SERVES 2 | 🕐 10 MINS | GF DF V NF SS

"I've gone for soya, as it tastes sweet in the perfect way. A SOFT sweetness and it's that little bit thicker, though all milks and mylks work brilliantly. Soya mylk for this is best as the sweetened version — but only if sweetened with apple juice — which you can do with a splash at home if difficult to find. Well worth it.

Rose water is a heavenly touch to the hot chocolate. The recipe was discovered whilst working an amazing Christmas market in Germany with Carina Hildebrant and her beautiful alpaca clothing back in the day. She inspired the blend of it to mix well with the chocolate drink, when she ran out of normal honey and found a stall selling rosewater-infused honey; a delicious twist to the cardamom hot choc."

Cocoa is one of the richest sources of polyphenols which have amazing anticancer, anti-inflammatory, anti-diabetic and anti-thrombotic properties. Choose high quality cocoa, as some are highly refined. The less refined the cocoa is, the higher its health benefits.

Choose organic soya mylk as otherwise it can be high in pesticide residue.

INGREDIENTS

700ml	Soya mylk
2	Cardamom pods
2 tbsp	Cocoa powder
2 tsp	Creamy honey
1 tsp	Rose water

METHOD

1. Heat the mylk with the crushed cardamom in a pan.

2. Add your cocoa and follow up with a heaped teaspoon of thick creamy solid honey.

3. Finally when ready to pour in your mug, add the rose water.

You can either remove the cardamom pods before slurping, or just avoid them and let them warm the flavour as you go.

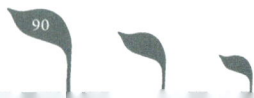

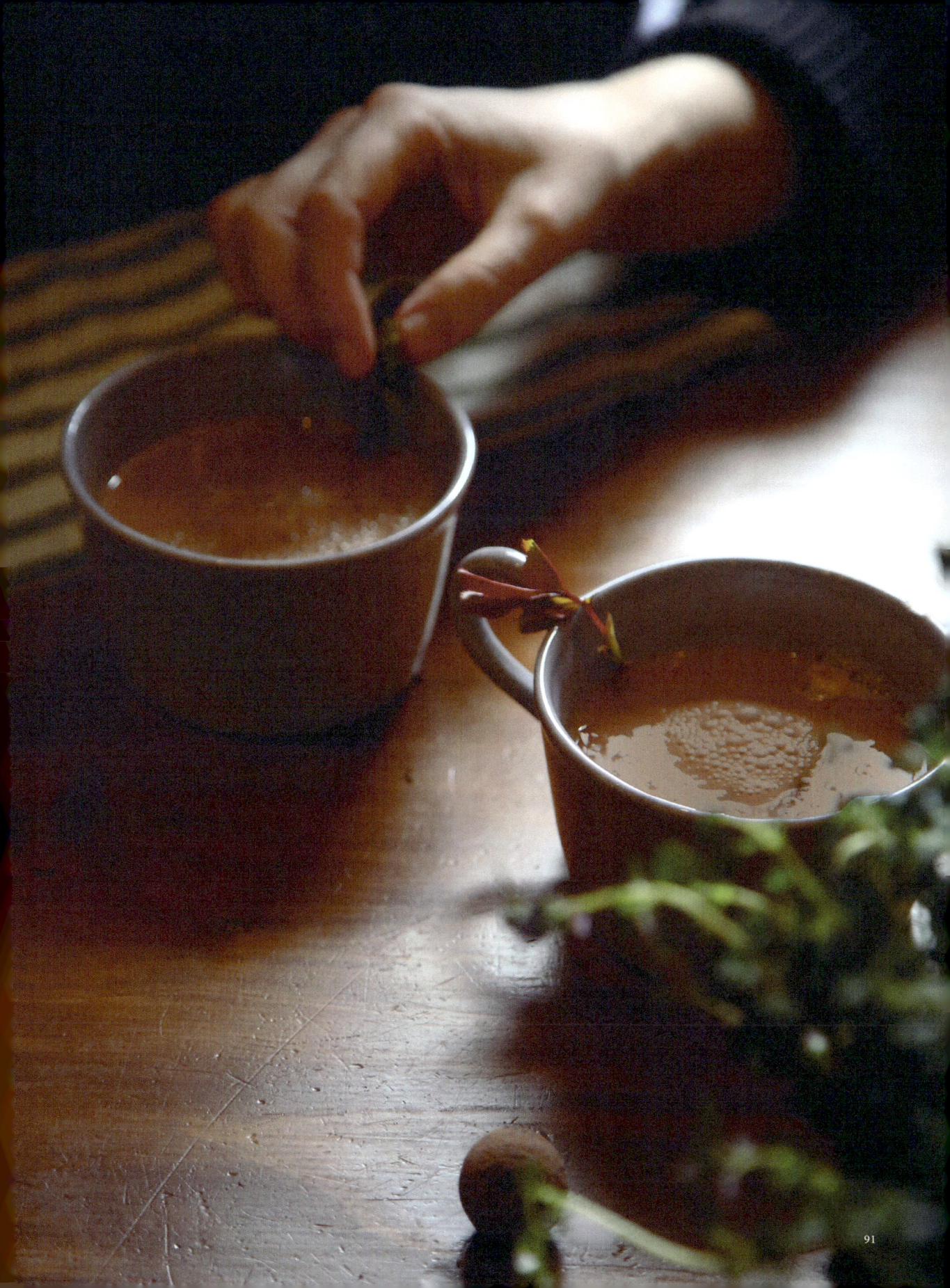

IMMUNITY BOOSTER SHOT

SERVES 14 | ⏱ 10 MINS |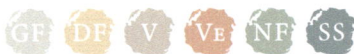

"I think this is one of the strongest drinks that I regularly wake myself up with. Morning Glory to boost the start of the day. Never underestimate what we can do to support our immune system through diet. This shot is a concentrated blast that will surely have your immune cells zinging."

Ginger, Tumeric and Garlic all have important immune strengthening properties. Lemongrass contains several antioxidants to protect the body, one of note being chlorogenic acid. It also has anti-microbial and anti-inflammatory benefits which are known to protect against viruses and the damage they cause.

Chillis contain many vitamins and minerals known to support the immune system such as vitamins A, B6 and C along with potassium and various antioxidants which can have added antiviral benefits which can help scavenge free radicals in your body that may cause disease.

Lemon or lime juice should be added where possible to food and drinks as it has numerous benefits, not least providing a concentrated intake of vitamin C, a key immune boosting vitamin.

INGREDIENTS

100g	Fresh ginger
60g	Turmeric
1	Garlic clove
1 stick	Lemongrass
½ -1	Red chilli
	(medium heat)
½ tsp	Black pepper
2	Lime

EQUIPMENT

Blender

METHOD

1. Wash all the ginger and turmeric well. No need to peel them; chop into chunks and place in a blender.

2. Peel the garlic, roughly chop the lemongrass, remove the green tops from the chillies, cut in half, and add all to the blender and grind the black pepper in.

3. Peel the lime zest and add it to the blender — squeeze the juice in too.

4. Cover the contents with water, and add another 4cm to your blender and blitz until smooth and blended to a liquid (approximately 500ml).

5. Sieve the liquid, and adjust its consistency by adding more water if needed for flavour and and consistency to suit your palette.

6. Store in the fridge, covered and sealed, and aim to take at least one shot a day.

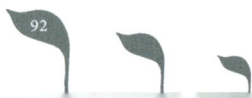

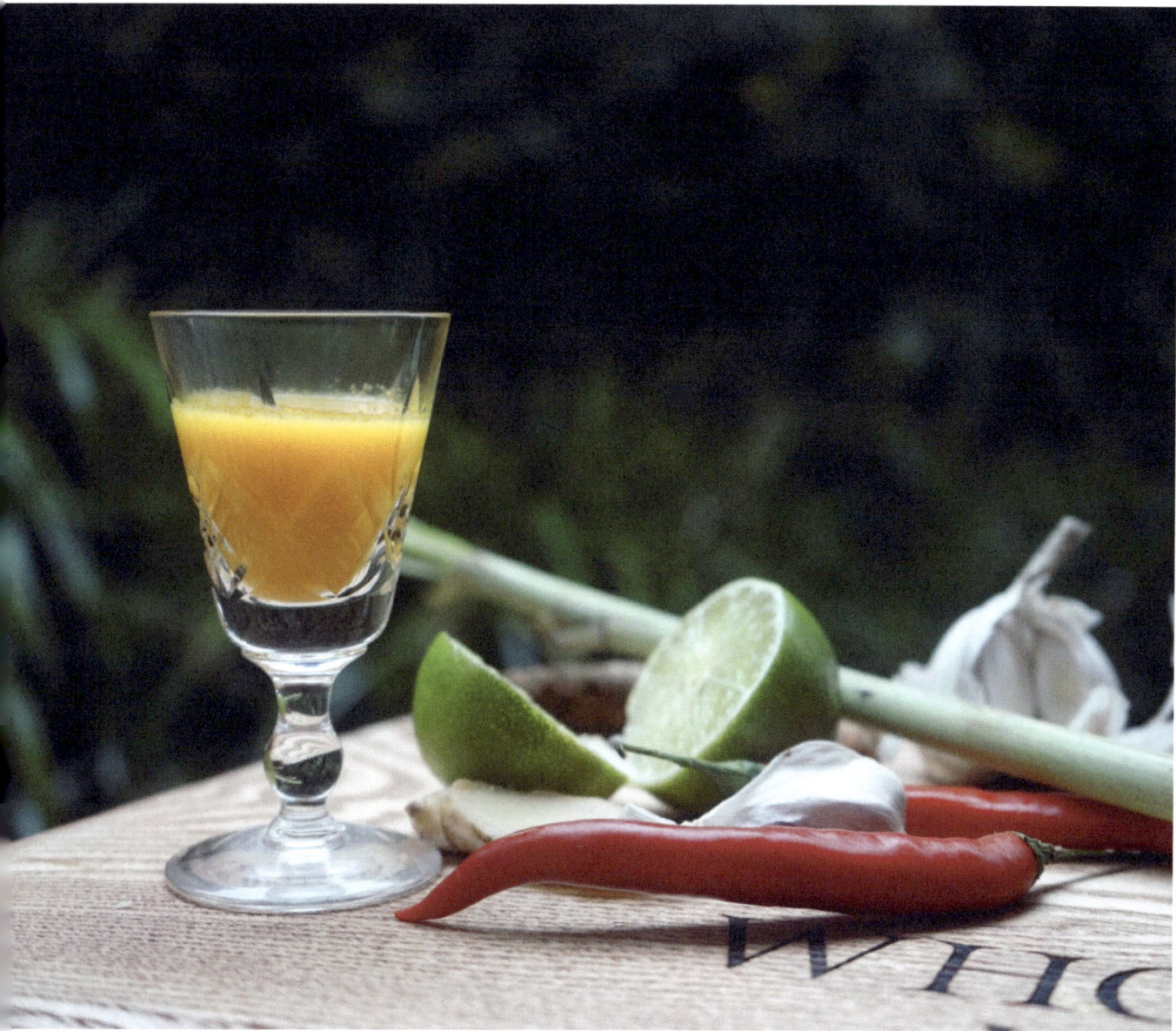

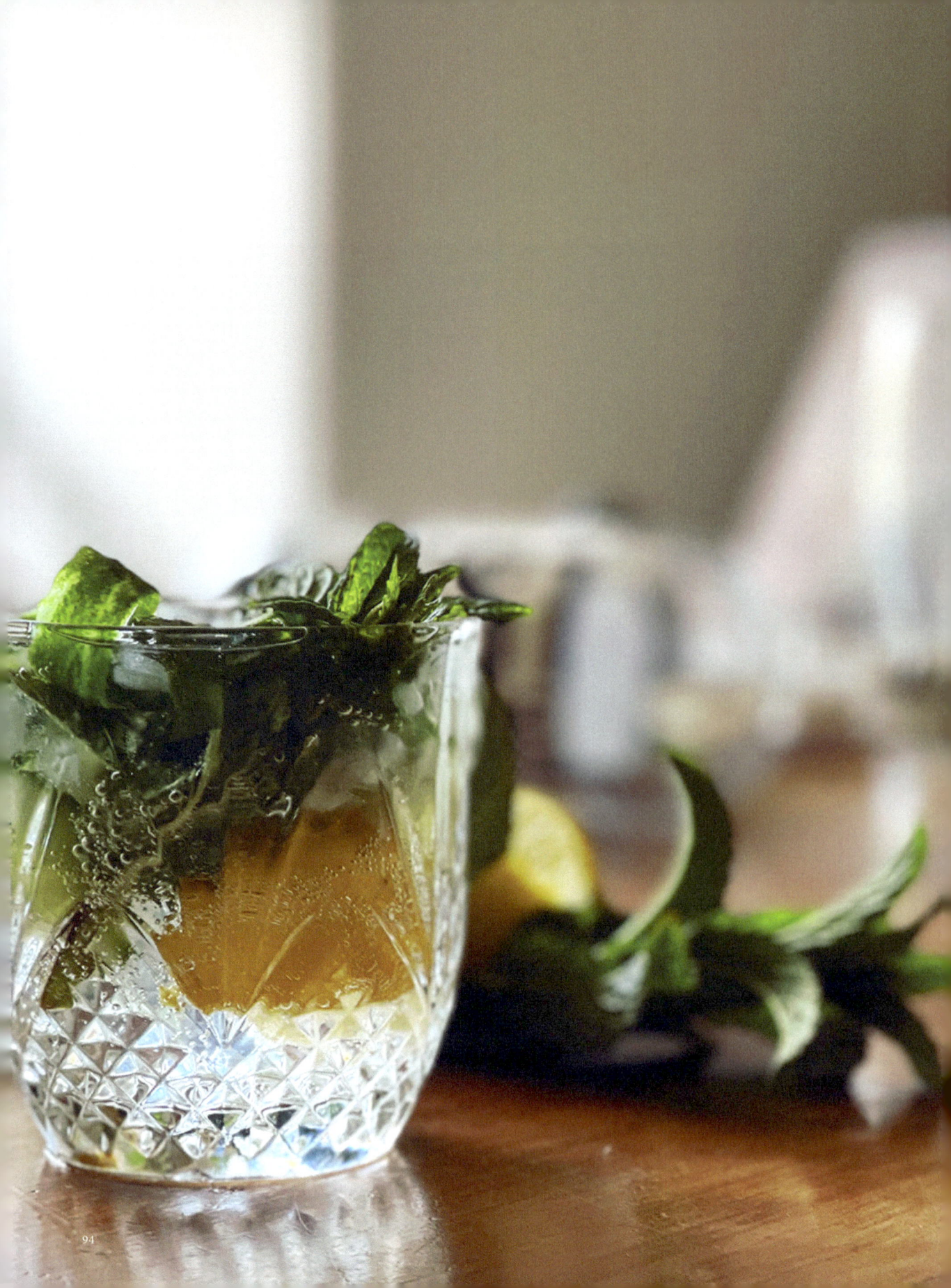

LOVER MOCKTAIL

SERVES 2 | 🕐 2 MINS | GF DF V Ve NF SS

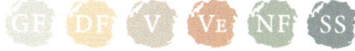

"If I'm wanting to up the game to a cocktail, just simply adding a shot of gin is my route. My father has a distillery, based in beautiful Sweden, and I love the classic light organic herbed, Jüst Gin, infused with wild dill which has a beautiful ethos, 'Not too little. Not too much. Just right.'"

Elderflower is commonly used in medicine to help with the common flu, and swelling in the sinuses. You can find in-depth benefits of elderberry through Healthline.

Mint is high in nutrients, and similar to lemon, it helps indigestion and can improve brain function.

Cucumber contains antioxidants and improves hydration and also improves the skin.

INGREDIENTS

500ml	Soda water
5ml	Elderflower syrup
½	Lemon
5cm	Cucumber
Pinch of	Fresh mint

METHOD

1. Start with a glass of your choosing. Fill half the glass up with crushed ice cubes.

2. Pour 500ml soda water into the glass and follow that by pouring in 5ml of elderflower syrup.

3. Cut half a lemon up and really squeeze it into the glass... Get all those juices!

4. Chop the cucumber into 1cm square-ish chunks and place them in the drink.

5. Finish it off with a pinch of fresh mint and mix all together!

6. If you are feeling creative, you can place a cut up sliced cucumber on the glass for a fancy garnish!

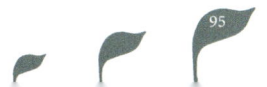

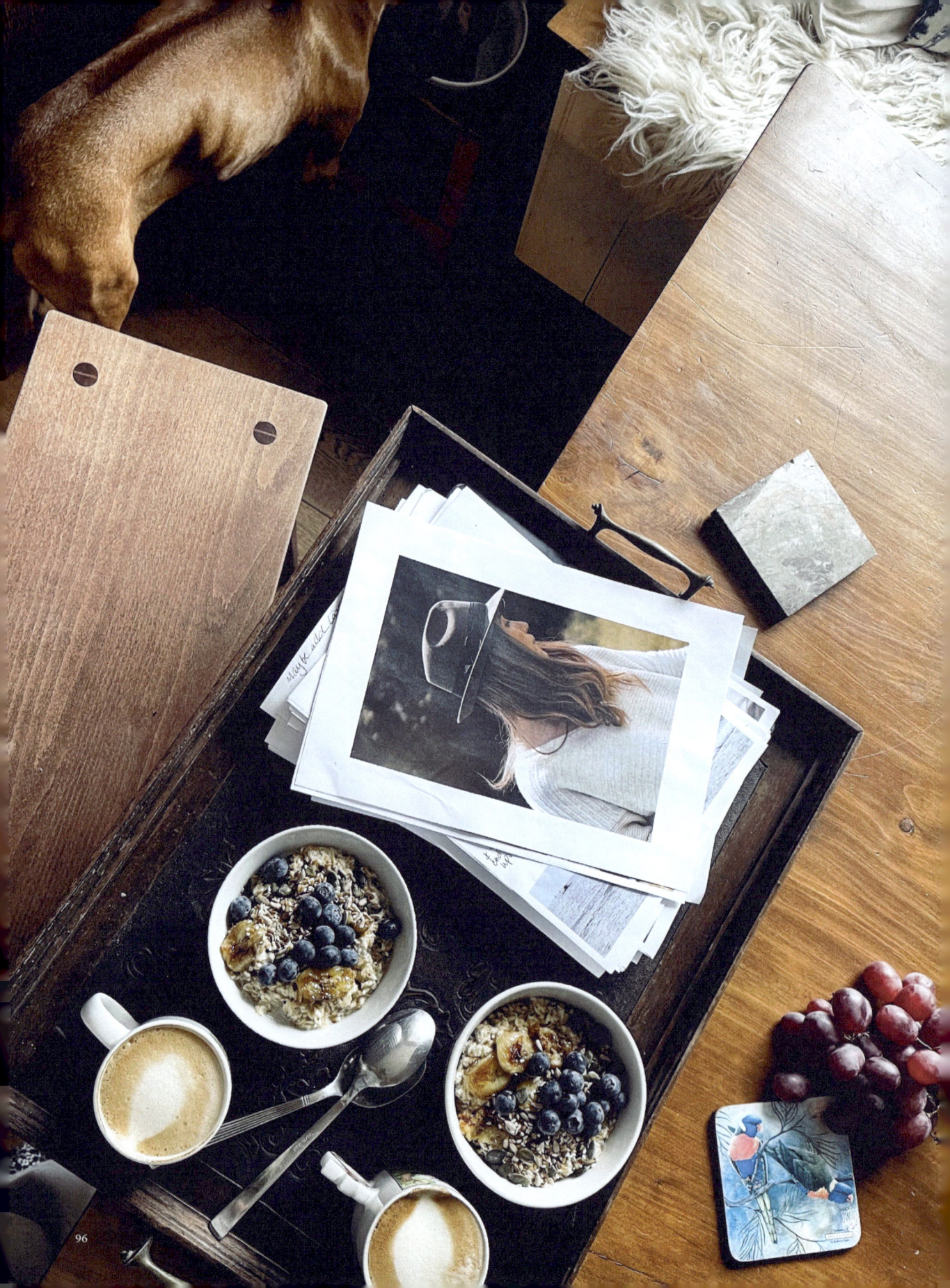

BREAKFAST

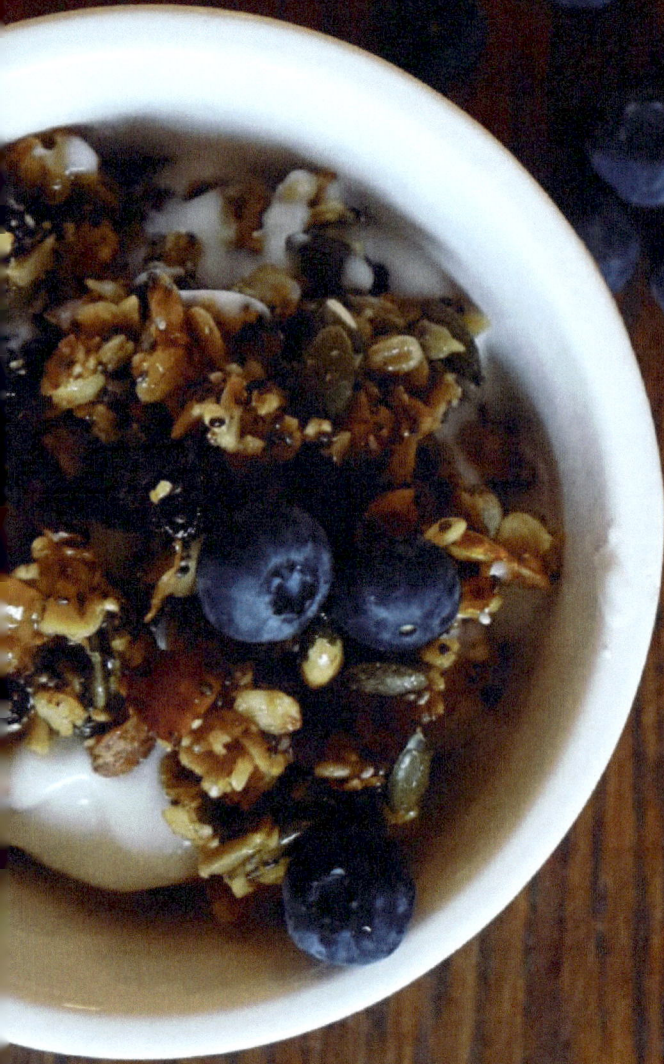
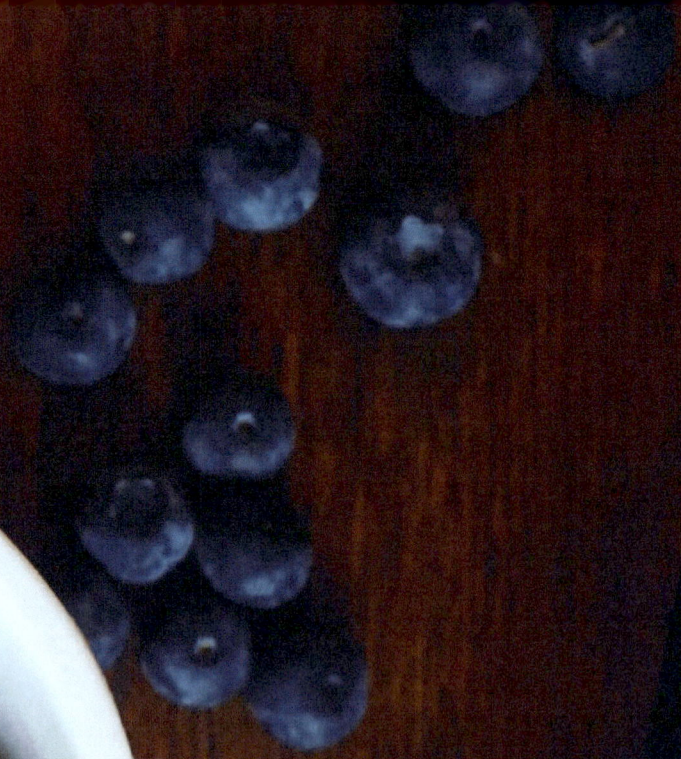
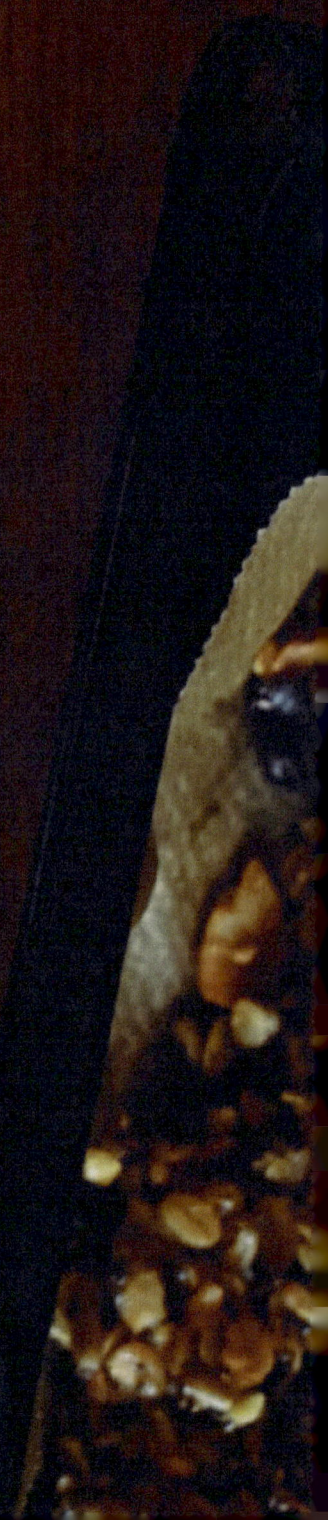

WHOLESOME CRUNCHY GRANOLA

SERVES 20 | 🕐 45 MINS | GF DF V

"This is so much healthier than shop bought granola which is generally overly laden with sugar. You can tailor the ingredients to your own taste but this combination serves up a super balance of omega fats from the nuts, seeds and oils. Even more satisfaction to start the day than the succulent taste! Versatile with its allowance for any seasonal fruit toppings, and I standardly add it to live yoghurt."

Chia seeds and walnuts provide excellent levels of omega 3. The ingredients provide oodles of fibre especially from the cholesterol lowering oats. Oats are also great prebiotic fibre to keep your beneficial microbiota healthy. Use a good quality honey if possible although heating it will negate some of the benefits of raw honey so don't use a very expensive product.

INGREDIENTS

125g	Olive oil
230g	Honey
230g	Oats (GF if needed)
85g	Sesame seeds
100g	Sunflower seeds
60g	Pumpkin seeds
60g	Chia seeds
55g	Coconut flakes
50g	Walnuts
45g	Hazelnuts
100g	Raisins

METHOD

1. Heat the oven to 180°C.

2. Place the oil and honey in large mixing bowl, and stir.

3. Stir in the oats, sesame, sunflower, pumpkin, chia seeds, coconut and lightly chopped walnuts and hazelnuts. Save only the raisins 'til later.

4. Evenly divide the mix onto two baking trays and brown in the oven for 20-30 mins, checking every 5-10 mins, mixing well to get an even golden colour throughout.

5. Remove from the oven and allow to cool.

6. Once cooled add the raisins and mix through.

7. Store in an airtight container to retain the lovely crunch.

Mushrooms on Toast with Hazelnuts

SERVES 2 | 🕐 10 MINS | GF V

Mushrooms are one of our top anticancer foods and are known to be supportive of the immune system. Using an array of different types of mushrooms (wild, chestnut, button, portobello, horse... the list goes on...) will provide you with slightly different health benefits from the variety of soluble fibre called beta glucans. Look out for vitamin D mushrooms in the shops!

Hazelnuts are rich in healthy fats, calcium, magnesium, B vitamins and vitamin E.

Piled onto spelt sourdough bread provides a healthier addition than normal wheat bread and is much tastier.

Add a dollop of full fat creme fraîche, once lightly cooled if you have the tummy for it and want a thicker creamier sauce. It's so delicious and worth it. I add a dessert spoon per person.

INGREDIENTS

300g	Mushrooms
2	Garlic cloves
Small bunch	Fresh parsley
1 tbsp	Coconut oil
Pinch of	Sea salt
2 slices	Soughdough bread
	(*or GF)
20g	Butter
20g	Hazelnuts
Crack of	Black pepper

METHOD

1. Rinse the mushrooms, pat dry and chop into evenly sized slices.

2. Crush one of the garlic gloves and just cut the remainder in half, keep separate.

3. Finely chop the parsley approx. 1 tbsp. In a large pan heat the coconut oil, add the mushrooms, sautée on a high heat frequently moving around, sprinkle with salt to draw out the moisture.

4. Toast the sourdough and when toasted rub with the halved garlic cloves, spread with butter and place onto plates.

5. Add the remaining garlic, parsley and hazelnuts to the mushrooms cook for 1 minute.

6. Spoon onto the toast top with a twist of pepper to taste.

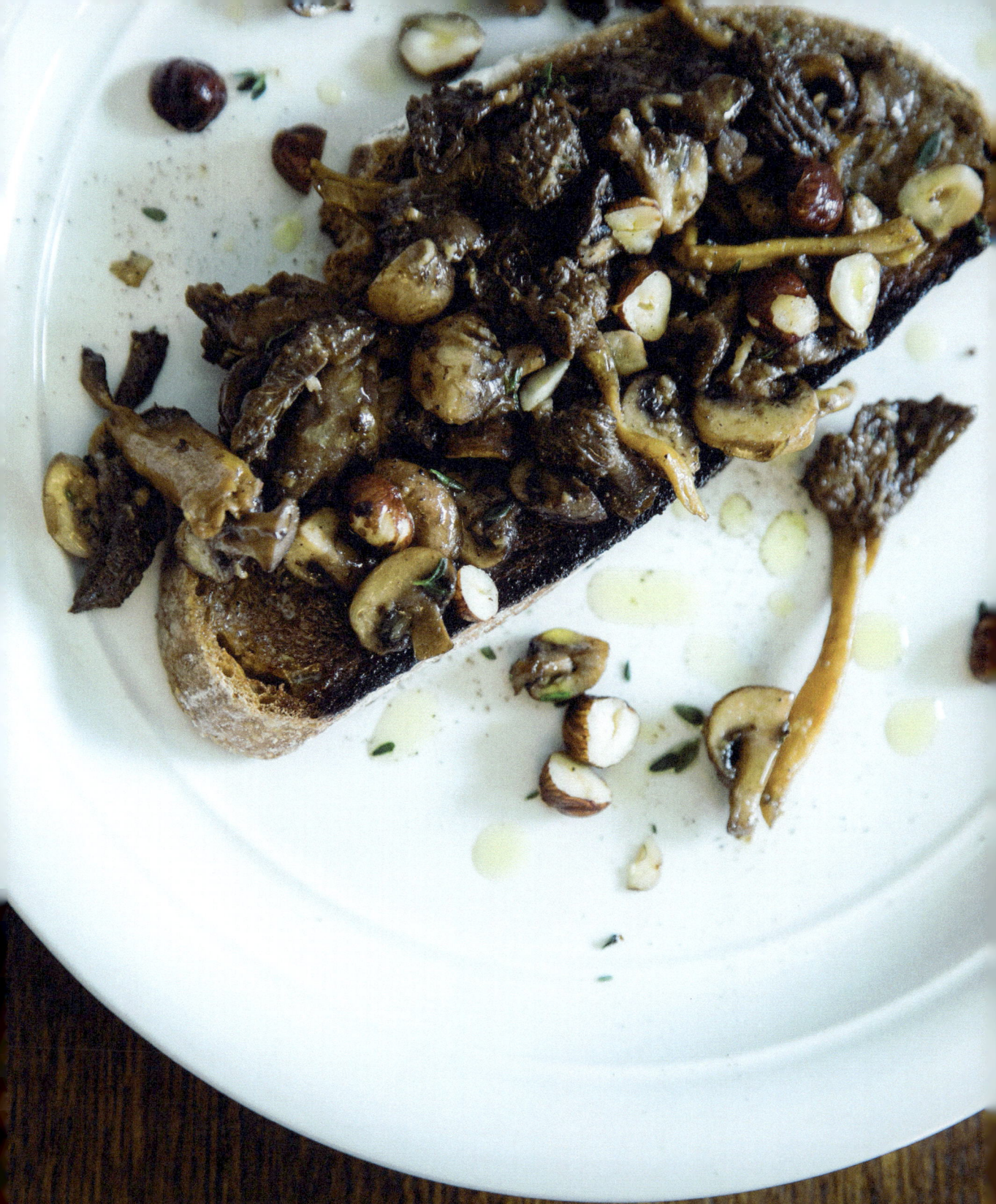

HERBS

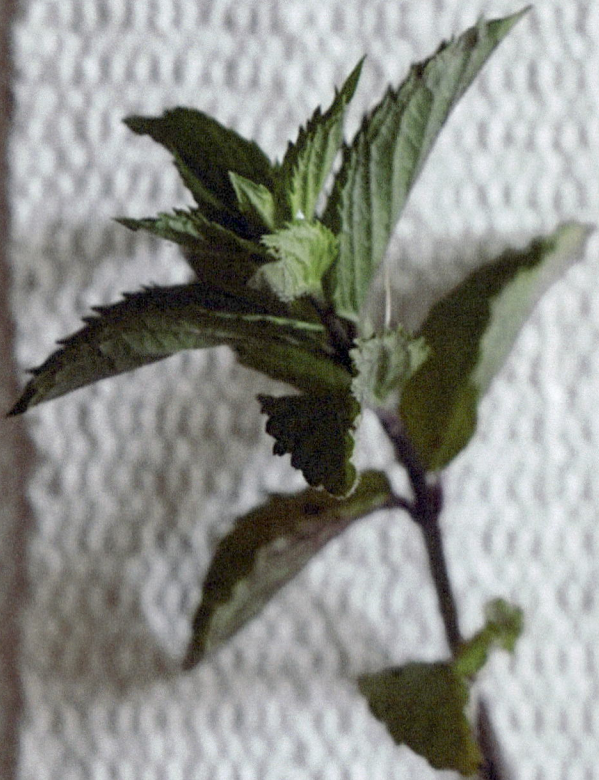

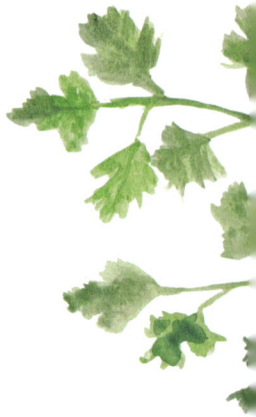

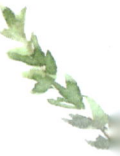

PEPPERMINT

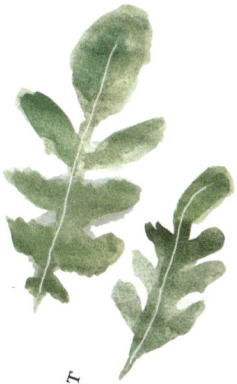

ROCKET

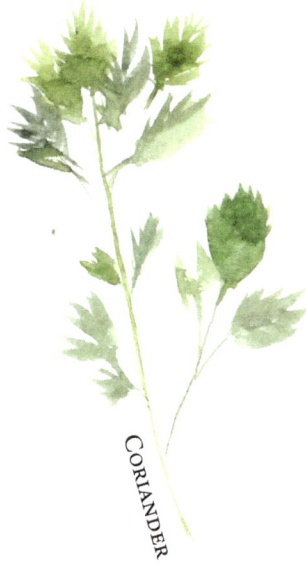

CORIANDER

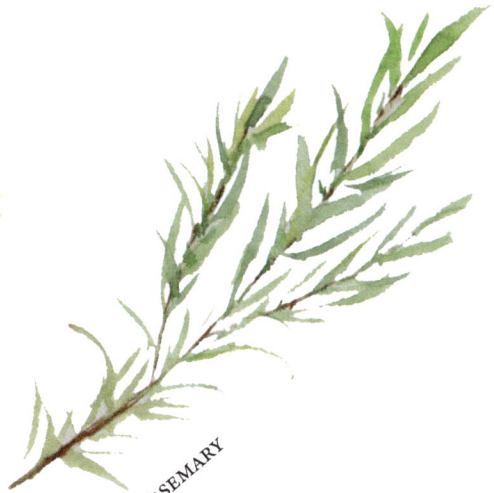

ROSEMARY

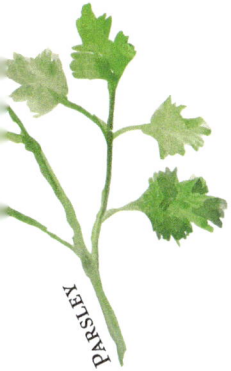

PARSLEY

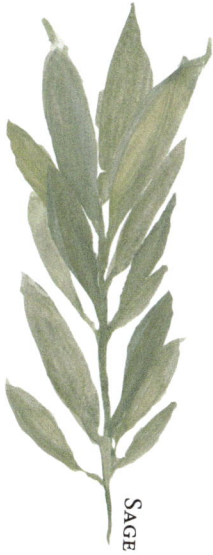

SAGE

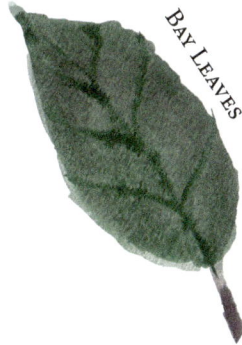

BAY LEAVES

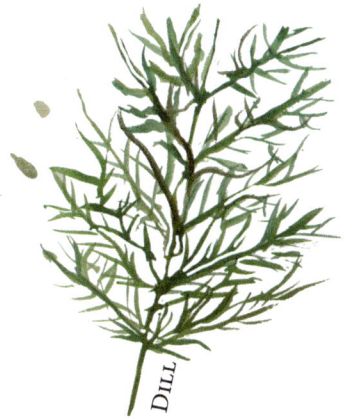

DILL

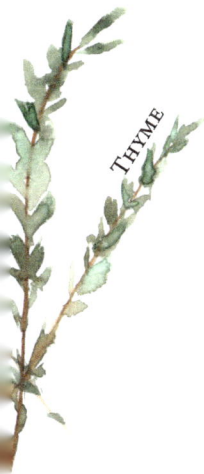

THYME

OREGANO

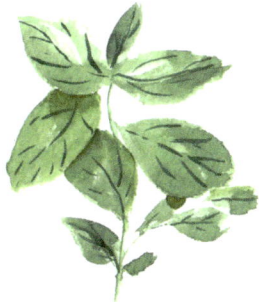

SORREL

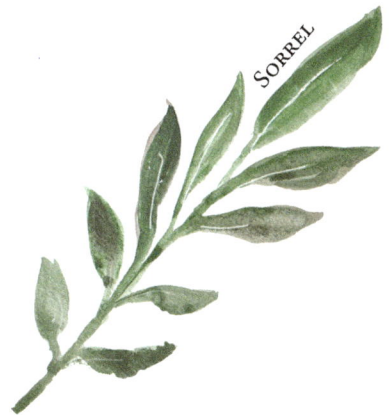

MINI EGG MUFFINS

SERVES 2 | ⏲ 20 MINS | GF V NF

"Mmmmmm muffins... A favourite breakfast, lunch or mini bite that packs a protein punch. Similar to a mini frittata, the filling possibilities are endless. Feel free to jazz these up with different veggies and cheese to suit."

It would be hard to find a healthier muffin as they include an array of green veg. These are packed with vitamins and minerals and plenty of protein from the eggs and cheese. Egg yolks in particular are known as one of the top ten highest nutrient dense foods on the planet.

Eggs are soo nutritious that they are actually known as "nature's multivitamin".

INGREDIENTS

25g	Tenderstem broccoli
½	Red onion *(small)*
1	Garlic clove
½	Celery stick
Handful of	Parsley
2 tsp	Coconut oil
3	Eggs
Handful of	Spinach
35g	Parmesan
Pinch of	Cayenne pepper
Crack of	Black pepper
Pinch of	Sea salt

EQUIPMENT

4 Mini, 2" cupcake moulds (silicone)

METHOD

1. Turn on the oven to 200°C.

2. Chop the broccoli, onion, garlic, celery and parsley fairly finely, and lightly fry with 2 tsp of coconut oil.

3. Crack the eggs into a mixing bowl and whisk, chop your spinach and stir in with the finely grated parmesan, cayenne pepper and the salt and back pepper. Oil the mini cupcake tray with the remaining coconut oil, and if silicone, place on a baking tray.

4. Once the fried vegetables and herbs have cooled, mix them into the mixing bowl and divide between 16 mini holders, and place in the oven for 10-12 minutes.

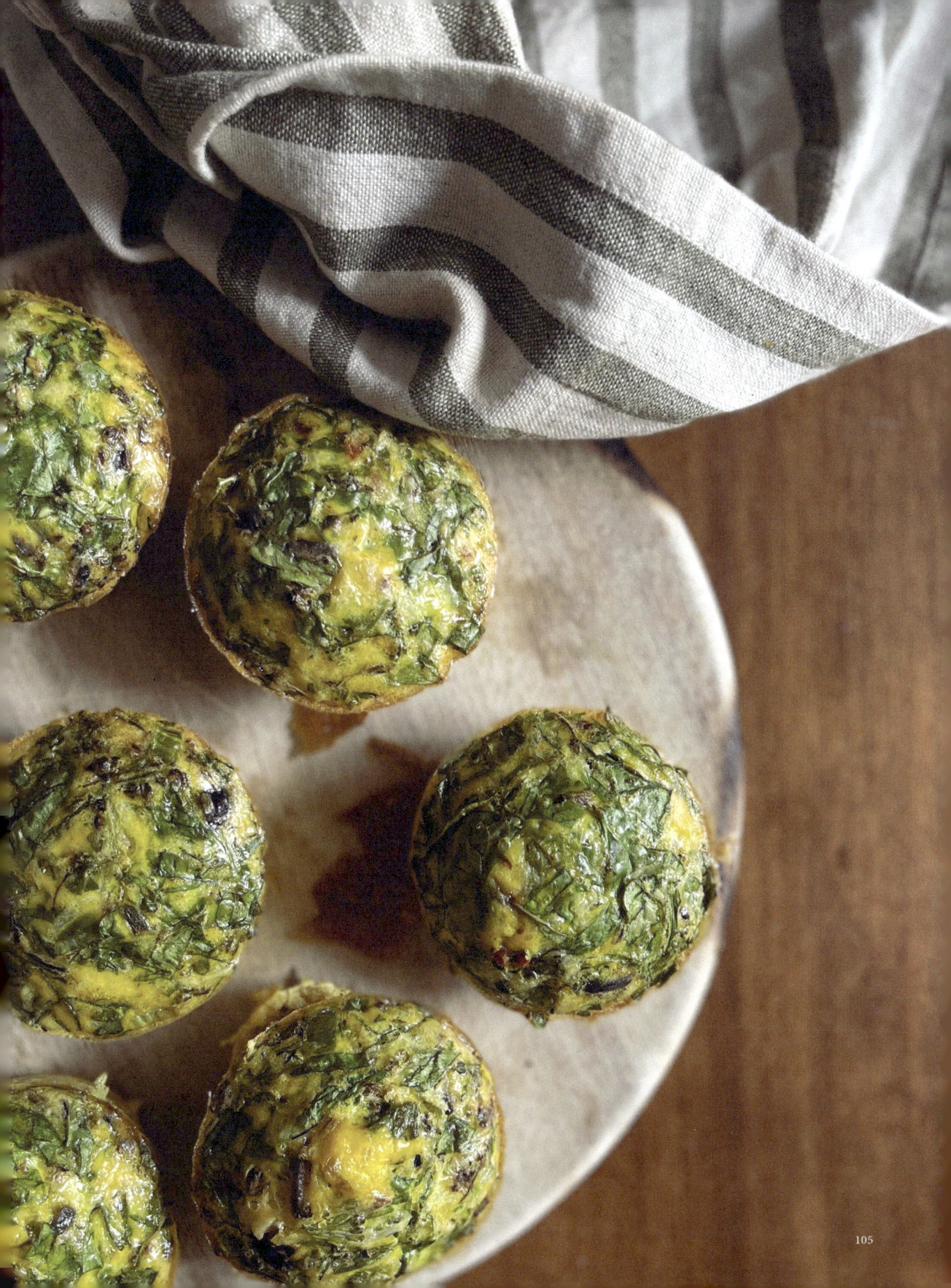

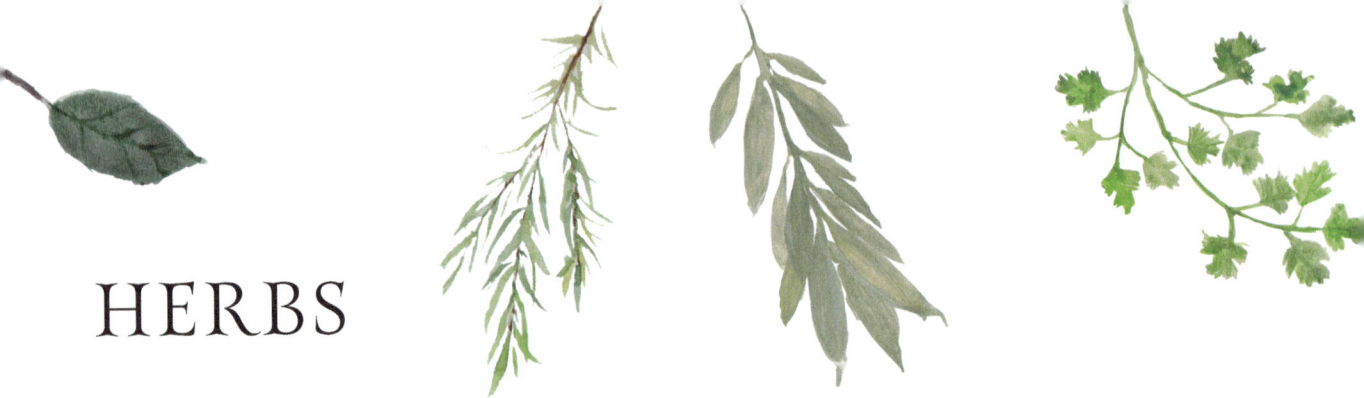

HERBS

Love life and your surroundings.

We may only use a small amount of culinary herbs in our food, but a little can go a long way therefore we should get into the habit of adding them wherever one can to a recipe.

Herbs are one of the light weight healthy vitamins and fuel which are easy to source, store and cook, let alone enhance our wellbeing. They are rich with iron, antioxidents, vitamins and those beautiful essential oils that strengthen us from the centre all the way out.

Herbs are generally anti-inflammatory and anti-bacterial and they also support digestion and detoxification. Some of our favourite herbs for Wholesome World recipes are coriander, parsley, basil, rosemary and mint.

Herbs: You only need a windowsill to grow a ready supply of herbs. If possible grow from seed as supermarket herbs are heavily sprayed. Fresh herbs are extremely nutritious and anti-inflammatory. Herbs also freeze well, so chop fresh herbs when you have them and freeze in small, labelled containers or bags.

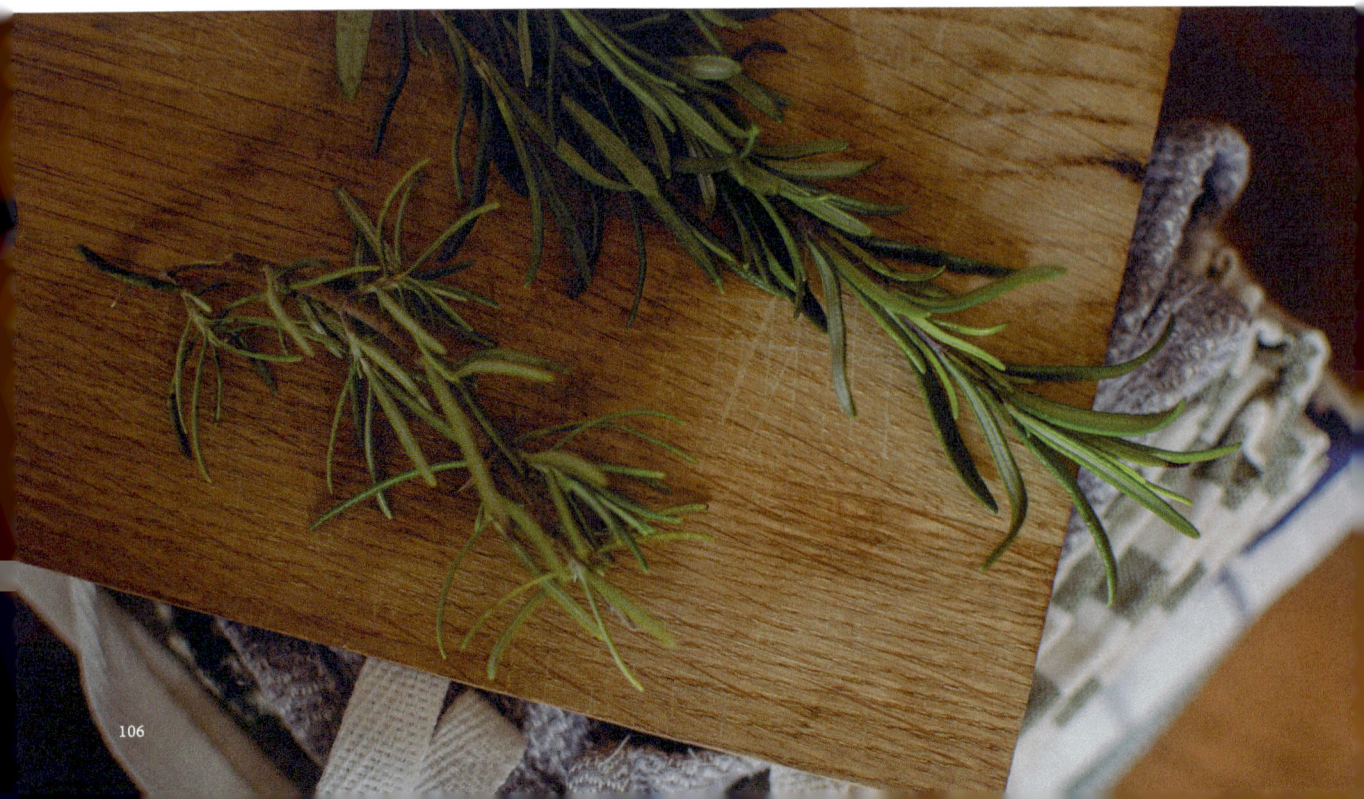

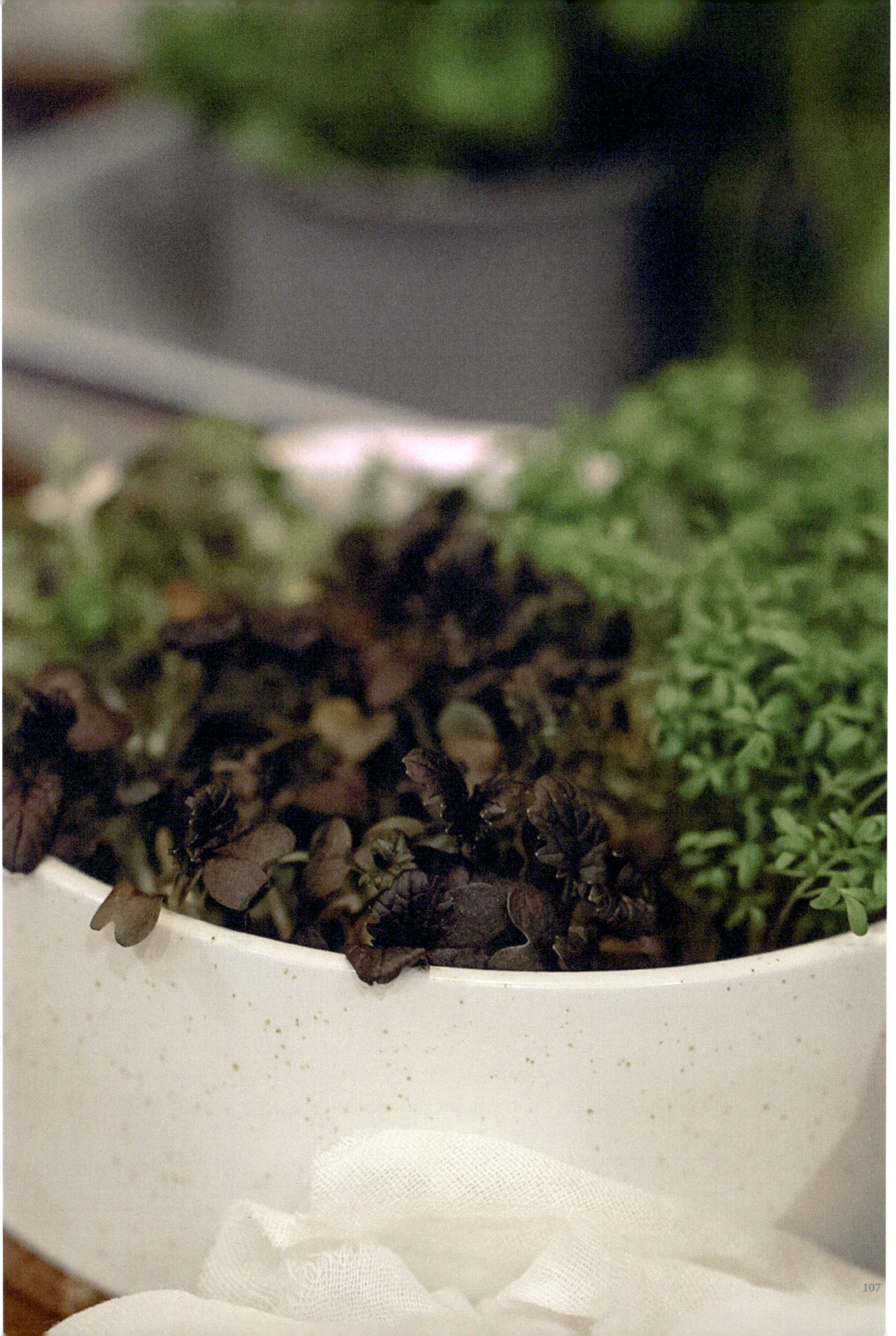

MY OMELETTE

SERVES 2 | ⏰ 10 MINS | GF V NF

"Eggs are not the demons we were once led to believe. Wahoo. An egg or two a day is absolutely fine and simple omelettes make a wonderful healthy lunch especially with four of your eight a day veg added."

Mushrooms are one of the top anticancer foods, as are red onions. Green leafy vegetables are always a healthy, nutrient dense choice, with spinach supplying iron and vitamin C in abundance, alongside important antioxidants and vitamin K.

INGREDIENTS

8	Eggs
8 tbsp	Milk
Crack of	Black pepper
Pinch of	Sea salt
12	White button mushrooms
1	Red onion
150g	Baby spinach
16	Cherry tomatoes
4 sprigs	Rosemary
4 dsp	Coconut oil
50g	Mature cheddar

METHOD

1. Crack eggs into a bowl, add the milk, lightly season with the salt and pepper, then beat well with a fork until blended.

2. Chunkily chop the mushrooms and finely slice the red onion.

3. Wash and dry the spinach, cut the cherry tomatoes in half, remove the rosemary leaves from the sprig and finely chop.

4. Melt half the coconut oil (2 tsp) in a heavy-duty frying pan, add the mushrooms and onions, cook for 2-3 minutes on a medium heat until just golden.

5. Add the spinach, tomatoes and rosemary and mix well and cook for a further 2 minutes. Remove the vegetables from the frying pan and place to one side.

6. Wipe out the pan with kitchen paper: on a medium heat add ½ remaining coconut oil (1 tsp), evenly spread over pan base, pour in ½ egg mix, spread until even and cook for 1-2 minutes.

7. Add ½ the pre cooked vegetables evenly across the omelette, grate ½ the cheddar over the top, add sea salt and freshly ground black pepper to taste.

8. When the omelette is just set carefully fold in half across the pan and roll out onto a plate. Repeat for more.

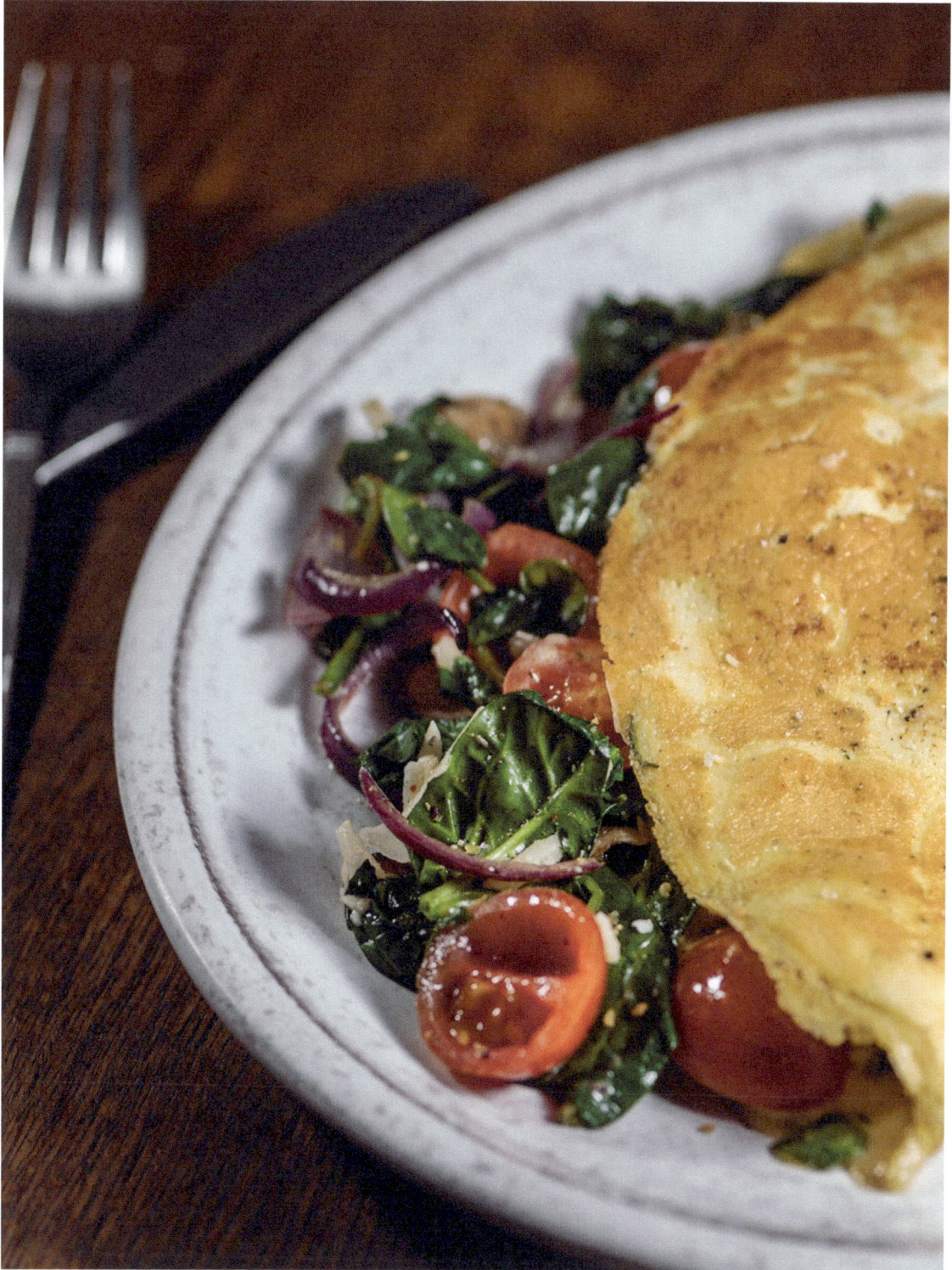

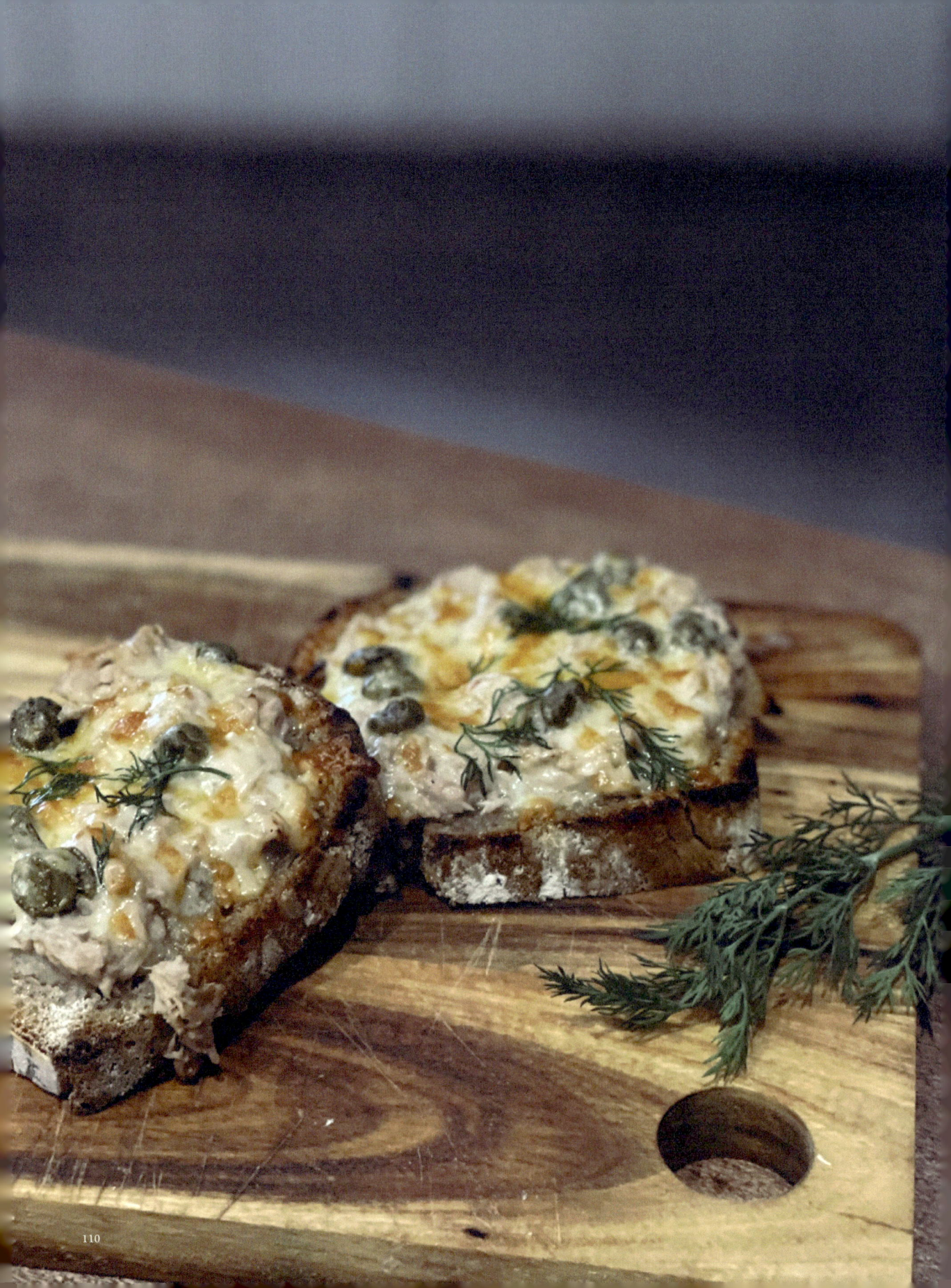

TUNA MELT

SERVES 2 | ⏱ 10 MINS | NF

"This reminds me of a teen film, Three to Tango, for which the dish looked so weird and new. I had to try it, and it was delicious, but is now updated to be made so so so much better. Here we are, the perfect morning fuel. Quick and easy is a needed boost too."

Albacore is my top tuna. Fish can contain high levels of dioxins and mercury, which can accumulate in our bodies and damage our organs, the brain being a the main issue. Large fish such as tuna or swordfish can absorb the ocean pollution, including microplastics.

Who would think of adding cloves to this dish but apart from adding flavour they are an excellent source of manganese, required for brain and nervous system function. Sourdough is the most digestable bread and provides plenty of fibre. Tuna and cheese will give a good boost to your protein requirements.

> "Albacore tuna are a little bit smaller than a yellow or blue tuna. The smaller size of the albacore means they are further down the food chain and have less bioaccumulation. This means that it takes only 1 week rather than 3 weeks for your body to to lose its contaminants."
>
> Beth Trevethnick
> Falmouth Marine College

INGREDIENTS

4 slices	Sourdough rye bread
1 can (160g)	Tuna
1 dsp	Mayonnaise
2 tsp	Cloves
20g	Cheddar
1 stem	Dill
Crack of	Black pepper

METHOD

1. Heat the grill to max temperature.

2. Cut 4 slices of bread and pop in the grill, for up to 1 min while it's heating.

3. Mix the tuna with the mayonnaise and cloves.

4. Grab the lightly crispy bread out and add the tuna mix to them.

5. Grate the cheddar, layer it on top, and put it into the grill for up to 5 mins. Rip the dill and throw on, crack the pepper and serve 2 per person.

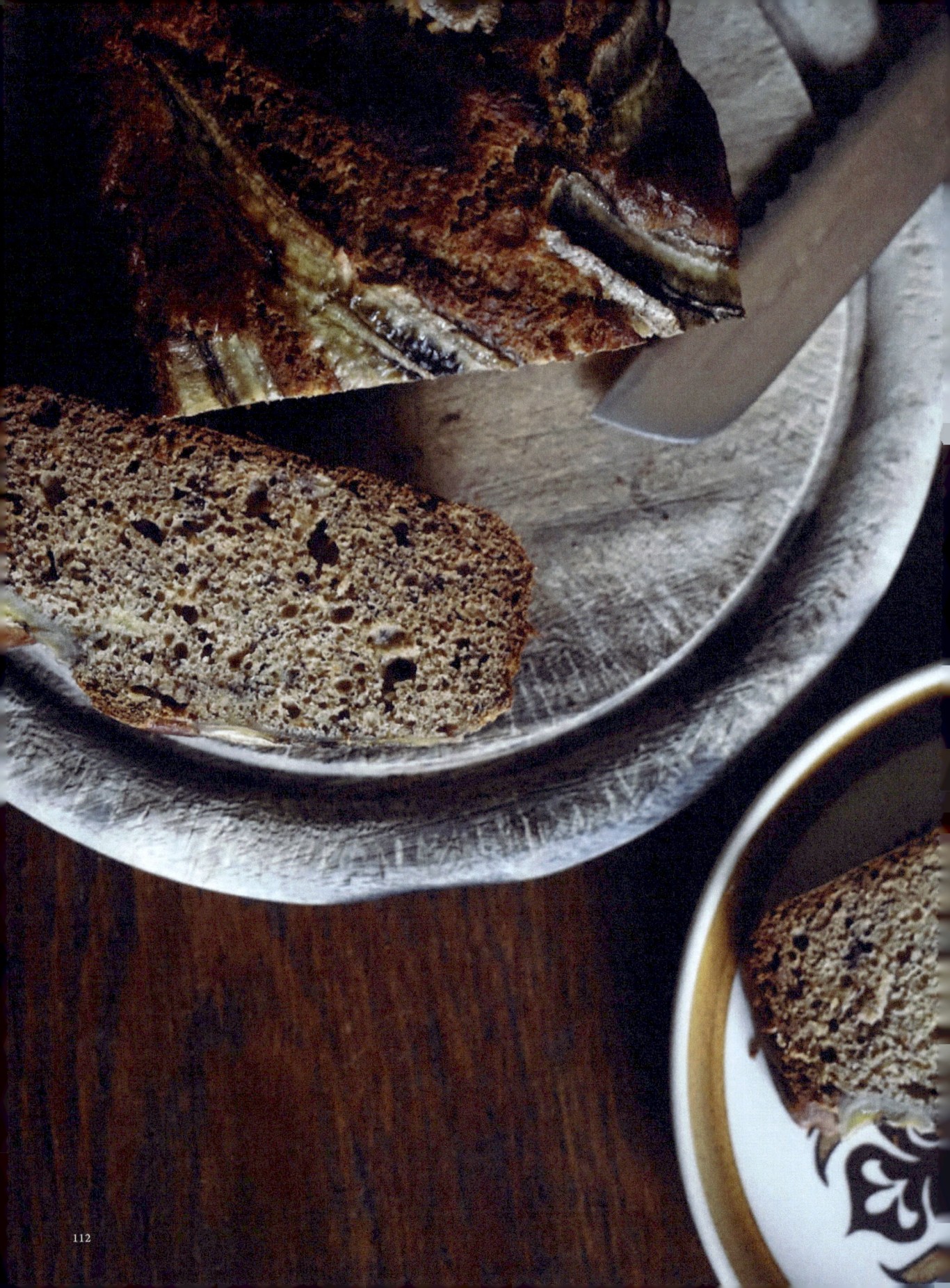

Banana Bread

SERVES 10 | ⏱ 1 HR | GF DF V

"This dish arose from my Australian days, and it is tastier and so so much healthier than the standard loaf. Officially, this is the most tried, tested, amended and eaten galore recipe to get it more healthy, nutritious and delicious."

Naturally it contains no refined sugars (choose unprocessed honey).

Bananas provide us with potassium and fibre. Eggs provide a super source of protein, helping to balance the blood sugar impact from fruits like bananas, for which the delicious cinnamon can help with too.

Walnuts are named in our top most healthy nuts category as they are rich in that all important anti-inflammatory Omega 3. You can treat yourself, safe in the knowledge that each mouthful is full of goodness.

INGREDIENTS

2	Bananas
60g	Soya mylk
2	Eggs
75g	Runny honey
1 tsp	Vanilla extract
75g	Walnuts
125g	Buckwheat flour
½ tsp	Salt
½ tsp	Ground cinnamon
1 tsp	Baking soda

EQUIPMENT

Loaf tin (silicone)
23.5cm x 13.5cm x 7cm

METHOD

1. Set the oven at 160°C.

2. Mash 1½ bananas using a fork.

3. Add the mylk, 2 eggs, runny honey and vanilla extract. Simply stir.

4. Blend or grind the walnuts, mix in with the wet ingredients alongside the buckwheat flour, salt, cinnamon and baking soda, and add the mixture to the loaf tin.

5. Thinly slice the last banana ½ for topping, decorate, and put in the oven.

6. Add to the oven, and cook for 45-60 mins.

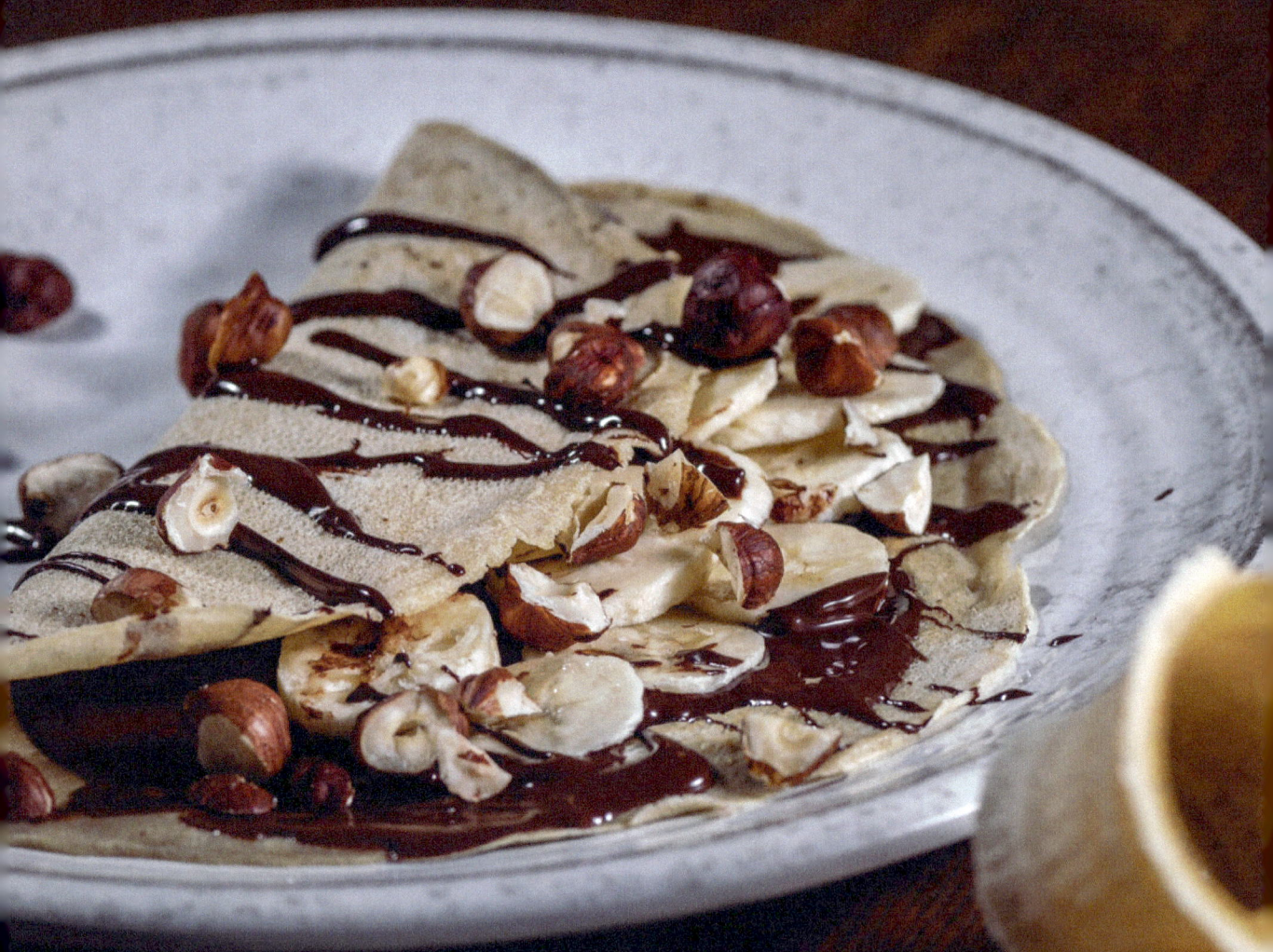
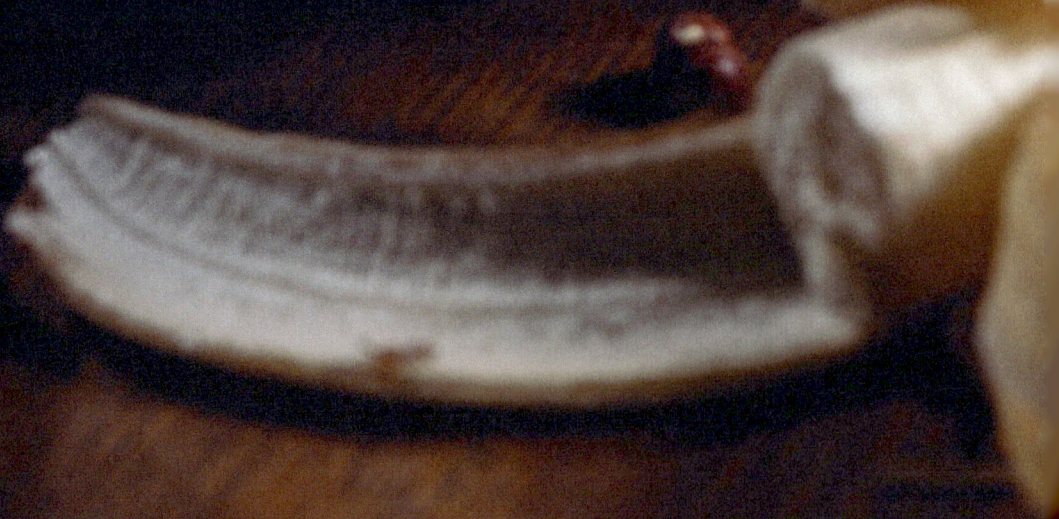

CRÊPES OF CHOCOLATE HEAVEN

SERVES 2 | 🕐 10 MINS | GF V

"My brother taught me this recipe after I got addicted to pancakes! I remember it being one of my Euro trip addictions when I would Eurotrain through France. Any really long train delays were made better by French crêpes on a beautiful long beach near the station. If you are cooking for more people than just yourself, I advise to turn on the oven - to a low temperature, to keep the made crêpes warm after they are being cooked."

Buckwheat flour really lends itself to pancakes and despite its name is not related to wheat. Nutritionally buckwheat is more replete than many other grains, providing carbohydrate, protein and numerous minerals and antioxidants. The sprinkle of hazelnuts top off the dish with a handful of healthy fats.

The more savoury choice use yoghurt, mint and a drizzle of honey. For a sweeter treat add chia blackberry jam to the seared banana slices. This makes a fairly low carb but energy dense breakfast.

INGREDIENTS

70g	Buckwheat flour
1	Egg
150ml	Almond mylk
20g	Coconut oil
-	-
1	Banana
10g	Hazelnuts
20g	70% Dark chocolate

METHOD

1. In a bowl place the buckwheat flour making a well in the middle. Whisk the egg in a jug and slowly whisk in the almond mylk until smooth, it should resemble single cream. Add more mylk if the batter is too thick.

2. On a medium heat add a small knob of coconut oil in a heavy-based frying pan, spread all over. When bubbling pour in just enough batter to thinly cover the pan base and then swirl around the batter quickly to get an even crêpe.

3. Cook for 1-2 minutes then flip and cook for a further 30 seconds. Remove and repeat until all the batter is used. This will depend on how thick/thin they are.

4. Lightly fry your banana once sliced, then lightly crush the hazelnuts and dry fry for 30 seconds and chunkily chop your chocolate to melt.

5. Serve the crêpes on a plate, and place a spoonful of the filling in one quarter. Fold in half and again in half; repeat until all the crêpes are filled.

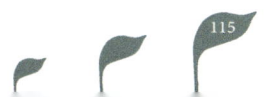

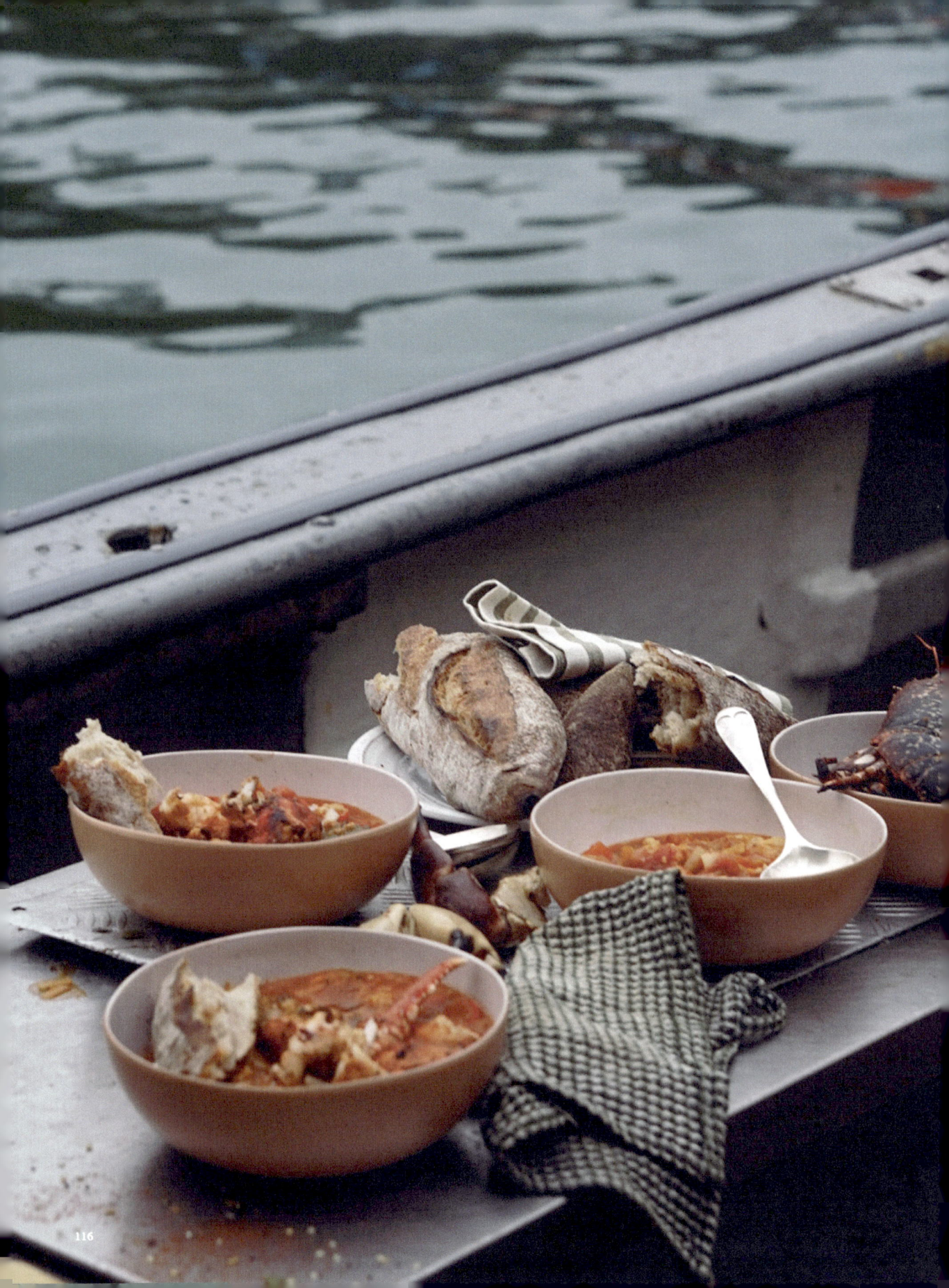

SOUPS

MUSHROOM SOUP

SERVES 4 | ⏱ 35 MINS | GF DF V VE NF SS

"I came across this dish near to the hospital during cancer days. I was with my father and it's one of those dishes that brings happiness and satisfaction as simply as can be. Freezable flavour and nutrition, for those tired moments in life."

Mushrooms are one of our top anticancer foods and mushroom soup is a simple but effective way of packing in an abundance of mushrooms. You could also use a variety of mushrooms in the soup to enhance the healthful properties.

A bowl of this each day may be very helpful during treatment to support your white immune cells. Garlic, onion and thyme add some super antioxidants to make this soup an all round comforter and healer.

INGREDIENTS

½ tbsp	Coconut oil
2	Celery sticks
1	Red onion
450g	Brown mushrooms
4	Garlic cloves
4	Thyme sprigs
400ml	Vegetable stock
400ml	Coconut milk
Crack of	Black pepper
Pinch of	Sea salt

EQUIPMENT

Blender

METHOD

1. Warm the coconut oil in a large pan, finely dice the celery and onion add and cook for 10 minutes on medium, low heat until soft, do not allow to brown.

2. Slice the mushrooms and add to the soft onions, finely chop the garlic and also add along with the thyme sprigs, cook for a further 5-8 minutes stirring frequently.

3. Pour in the vegetable stock, bring to a boil and simmer for 15 minutes. Pick out the 4 thyme sprigs the leaves should have come off their woody stalks.

4. Add the coconut milk, and stir until evenly blended.

5. Using a slotted spoon lift out ⅔ of the mushroom mix into 4 warm soup bowls.

6. Blend the remaining mushroom mix until smooth and blended.

7. Pour into the soup bowls and simply add black pepper and salt to taste.

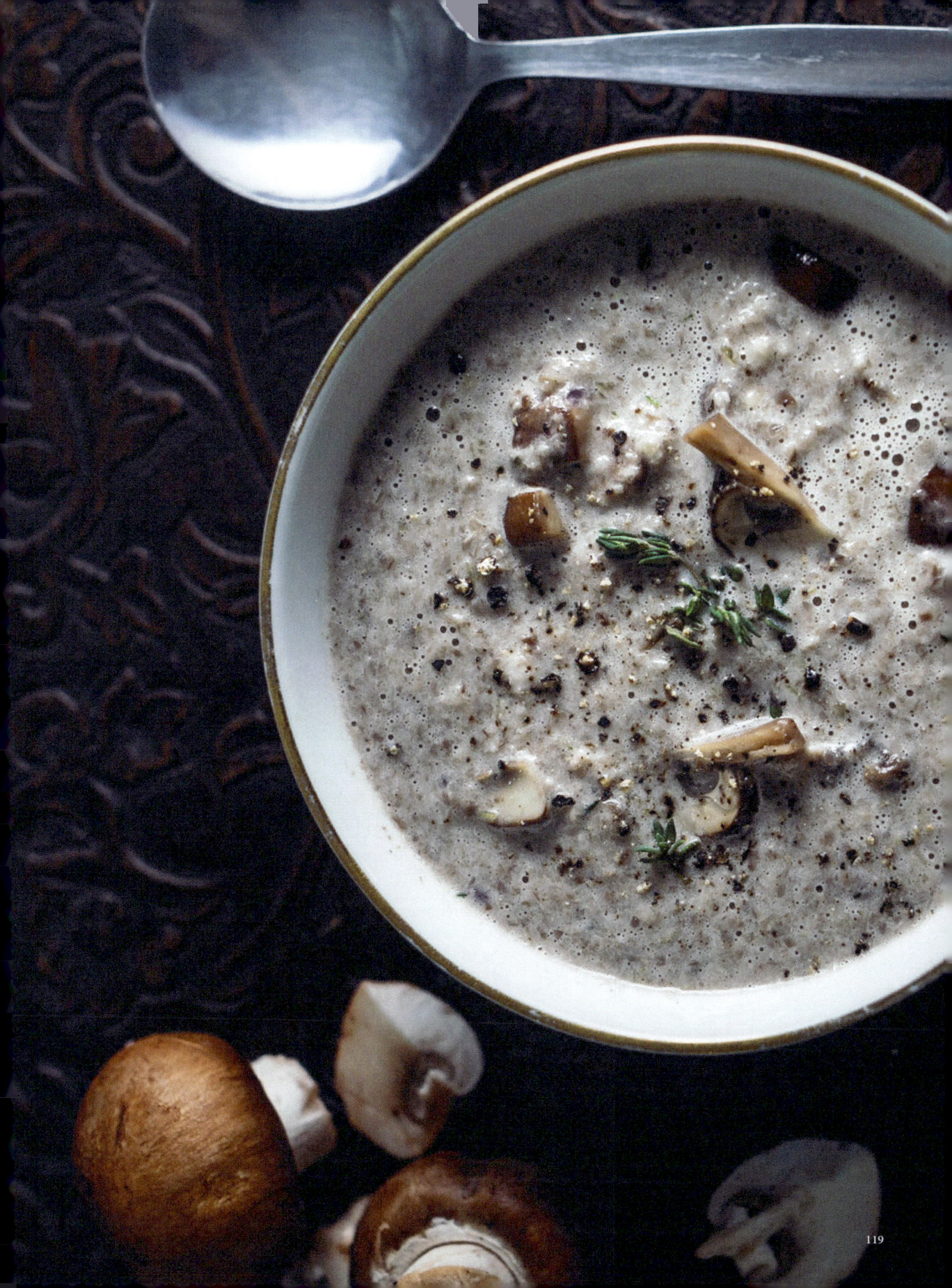

PEA & COCONUT SOUP

SERVES 4 | 🕐 20 MINS | GF DF V Ve NF SS

"Peas enjoy this. I think that it reminds me of the gazpacho in the Caribbean hot aura. But in the classic GB, warm it, and indulge in it as much as possible.

Did you know... Peas are known as edible legume and are in the same group as even peanuts, lentils, chickpeas and beans."

Peas are legumes and are actually considered a starchy vegetable like potatoes and corn. This does not however mean that they do not provide us with some impressive nutrients. They are high in protein and contain vitamins A, B1, K and C along with a decent amount of the minerals magnesium, potassium and calcium. Despite their high starch content they are actually considered a low glycaemic food due to the fibre and protein. Plant chemicals known as saponins may also make peas effective at inhibiting cancer cell growth and the polyphenol called coumestrol in peas has been shown to protect against stomach cancer.

This is created for complete ease of speed and nutrition.

INGREDIENTS

60g	Spring onion
1 tbsp	Coconut oil
500g	Peas (frozen)
500ml	Vegetable stock
660ml	Coconut milk
Sprig of	Mint
Pinch of	Sea salt
Twist of	Black pepper

EQUIPMENT

Blender

METHOD

1. Chunkily chop and sauté the spring onions in the oil on a medium heat until seared and set aside.

2. Meanwhile, boil some water for the peas and simmer for 3-4 mins.

3. Drain the peas and add the stock and coconut milk to the spring onions and almost all the mint. Simmer and then turn off the heat until it is cool enough to blend (a heat safe blender or hand blender).

4. Finish with salt and pepper to taste and remaining mint to garnish.

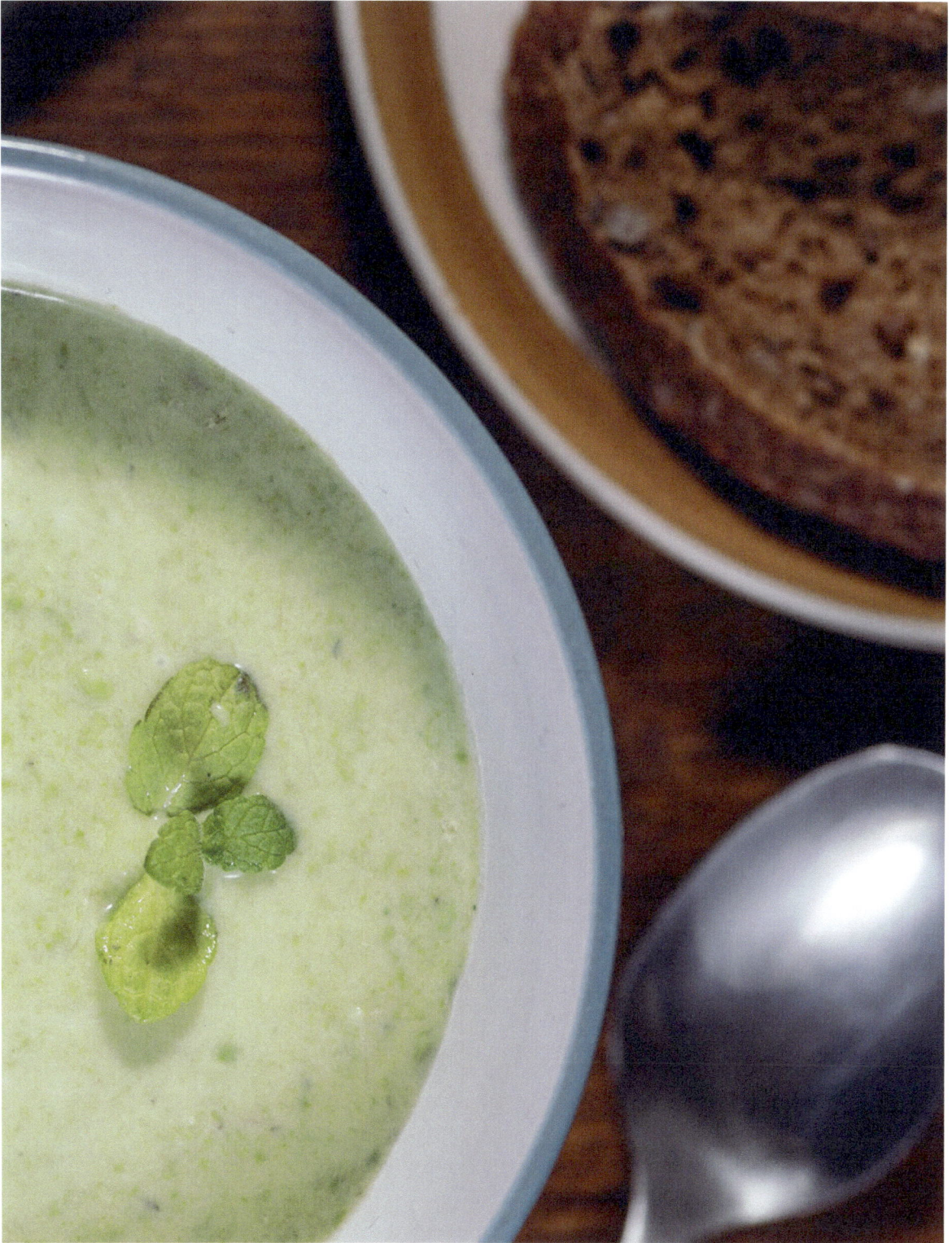

ROASTED BUTTERNUT SQUASH SOUP

SERVES 4 | ⏱ 55 MINS | GF DF V Ve SS

"Hearty, warming and delicious. I love these soft and warm flavours, easily thrown together loosely and quickly."

Soups, just like smoothies, are a useful way to pack in lots of veg. They are also perfect for adding in some health enhancing spices such as turmeric, ginger, cumin, chilli and some garlic cloves.

Red onions are a more nutritious choice than white or brown onions as they have higher levels of antioxidants. Coconut milk adds some healthy fat for energy and brain function and the red lentils provide fibre for healthy gut function.

INGREDIENTS

1kg	Butternut squash *(deseeded & skinned)*
1 tbsp	Coconut oil
Pinch of	Sea salt
Crack of	Black pepper
1 tsp	Chilli flakes
3	Garlic cloves
1	Red onion
5 cm	Ginger knob
250g	Red lentils
1 tsp	Cumin
1 tsp	Turmeric
1 litre	Vegetable stock
400ml	Coconut milk
Handful of	Pumpkin seeds

METHOD

1. Heat the oven to 180°C.

2. Chop up the butternut squash into roughly 1cm chunks.

3. Place the coconut oil in a large roasting pan and heat in the oven. Then, when melted, add the butternut to the roasting pan, season with salt and pepper and sprinkle with chilli flakes and roast for 25 minutes.

4. Roughly chop the garlic, onion and ginger add to the butternut squash after 25 minutes, mix well and roast for a further 10 minutes.

5. Whilst the vegetables are roasting, In a large pan of water cook the lentils for 15 minutes until tender.

6. Remove vegetables from the oven and add them to the pan with the cooked lentils and water. Add the cumin, turmeric, vegetable stock, coconut milk and seasoning mix well and bring to the boil.

7. Simmer for approx 10 mins, then remove from the heat and blend mix until until smooth. Garnish with the pumkin seeds.

I would season with salt and pepper before roasting to help bring out the flavours, as there are a lot of lentils and liquid so it's important to season everything well.

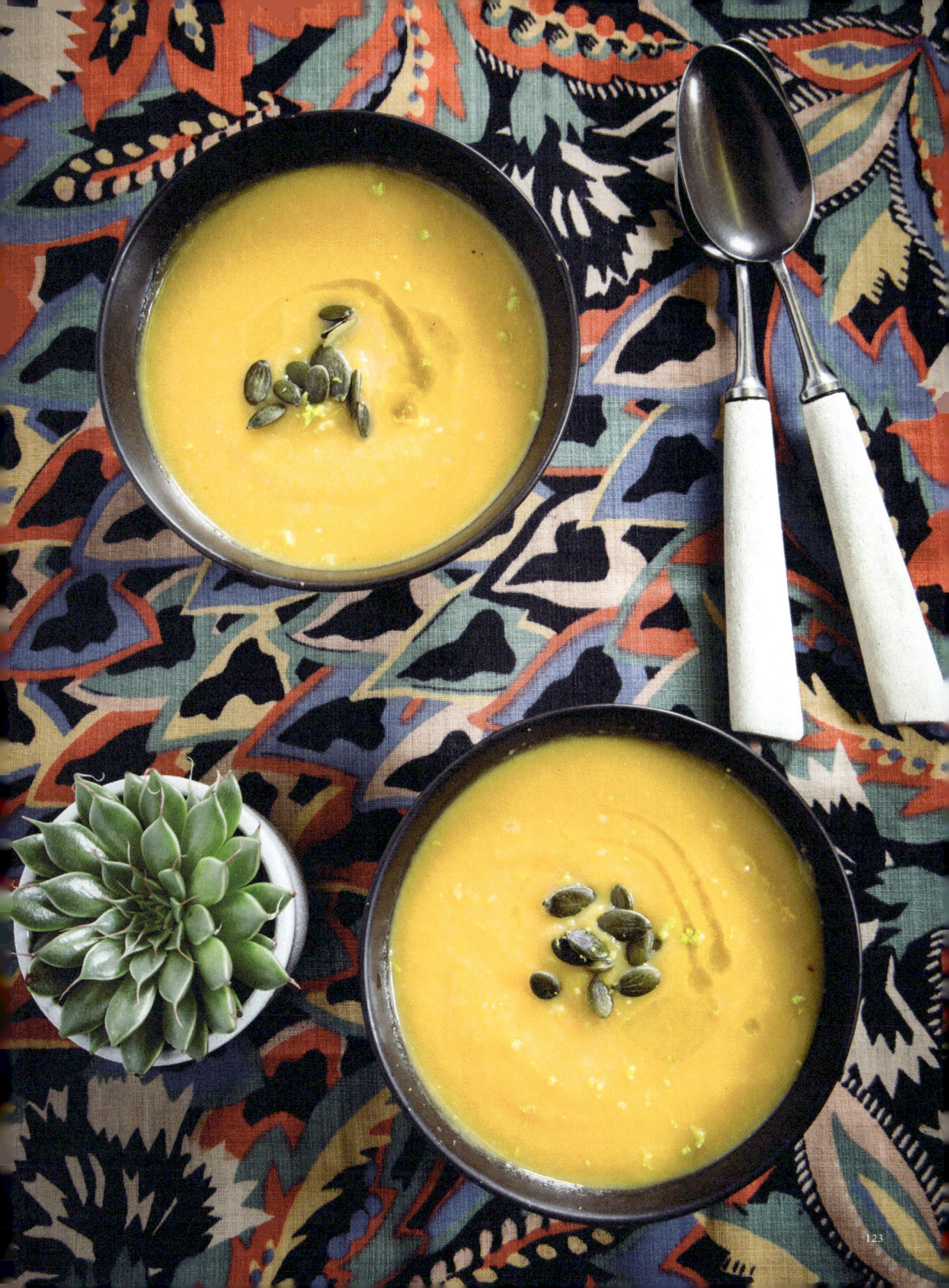

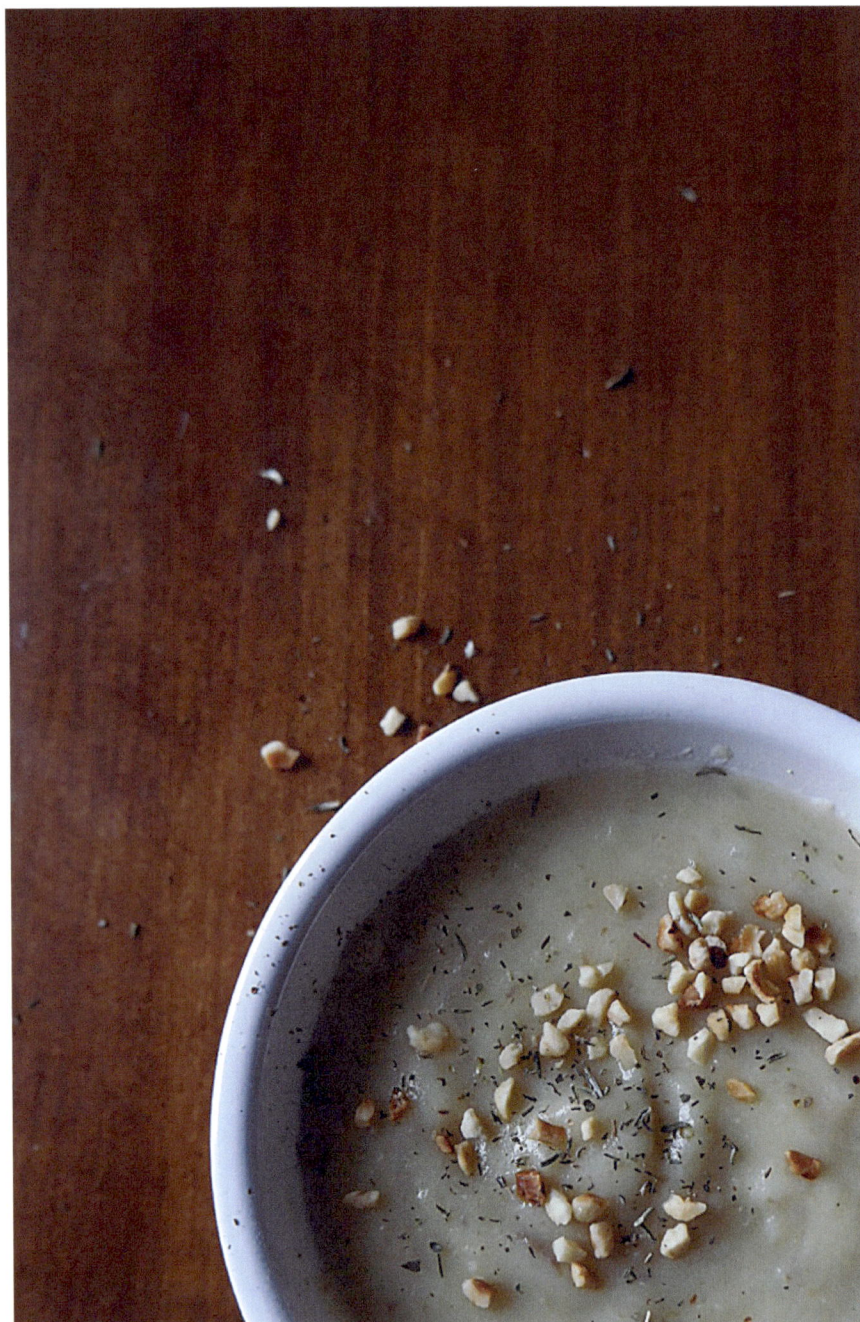

CELERIAC SOUP

SERVES 6 | ⏱ 10 MINS | GF DF V VE SS

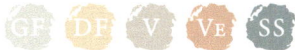

"Celeriac. What is 'celeriac?' A root veg which is rough, solid, and one of the toughest ingredients to understand. I think it is most easily seen as a de-sweetened husky parsnip. Perfect with the savoury soft and crunchy flavourful additions. A little bonus is enjoying it with a drizzle of truffle oil."

Celeriac is a very underrated vegetable, maybe not surprisingly as it isn't the most attractive of vegetables. But once you can get past that it is a great low carb alternative to potatoes and gives a fresh but mild celery taste to many dishes. It is in fact a type of celery which is purely grown for its root. Despite its lack of colour it does pack a punch when it comes to nutrients providing vitamins B6, C and K, and minerals such as phosphorus, potassium and manganese.

The soup is also an excellent source of fibre so good for gut health along with those benefits of onions and garlic.

Hazelnuts and almonds are rich in healthy fats and provide protein adding a balance of macronutrients to this dish.

INGREDIENTS

1	White onion
1 (500g)	Celeriac
2	Potatoes
3 cloves	Roast garlic
Sprig of	Thyme
100ml	Olive oil
Pinch of	Salt
Crack of	Black pepper
1 litre	Vegetable stock
350 ml	Almond mylk
-	-
50g	Toasted hazelnuts
1 pinch of	Parsley

METHOD

1. Dice the onion, celeriac and potatoes. Finely chop the garlic and thyme.

2. Heat the olive oil at a low heat in a thick based pan, add the onion, celeriac, potatoes, garlic, thyme and salt and pepper seasoning.

3. Cook for 10 minutes, then add the vegetable stock and simmer for 30 minutes. Add the almond mylk, and cook for a further 10 minutes.

4. Purée the liquid in a food blender until smooth. Check the seasoning and dilute, by adding water to thin the soup to your preferred texture while heating before you serve.

5. Chunkily chop the toasted hazelnuts and parsley and use them to garnish the soup when served.

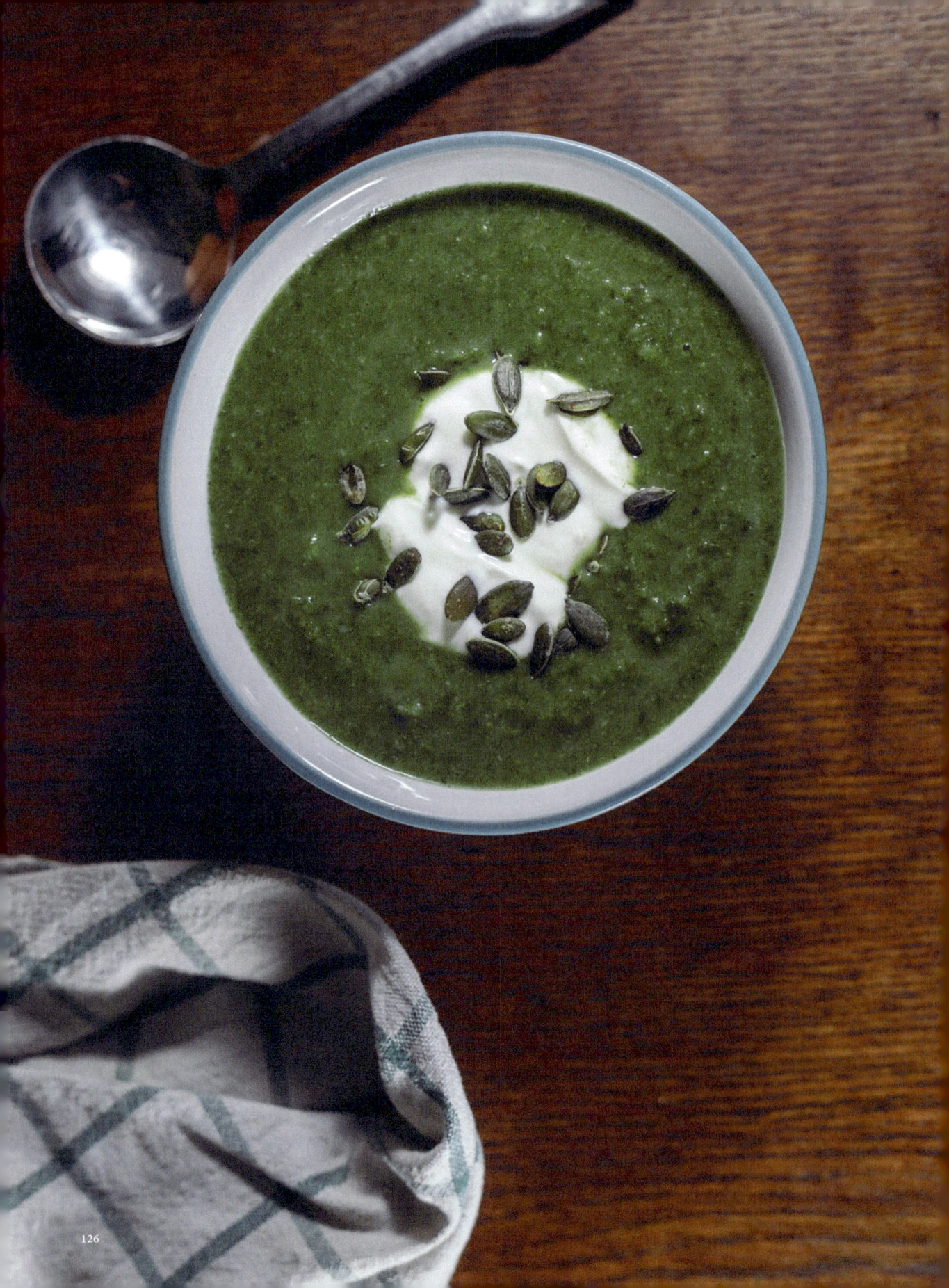

GREEN SOUP

SERVES 4 | ⏱ 30 MINS | GF DF V VE NF SS

"Green green green galore through your mouth, your oral door. I do genuinely call this the green machine diet. Lightweight, so if you are ravenous, have it with a doorstep of bread if you need an extra fill."

This is packed with nutrient dense green leafy veg, which are top of our list of anticancer foods. Green leafy veg provide an abundance of vitamins and minerals, some super fibre and are low in sugars, so a useful low carb recipe to keep our blood glucose levels in check.

Green peppers contain more vitamin C than an orange which will help the body to absorb the iron in the spinach.

Spinach is also an excellent source of vitamin A, C, K, folic acid and calcium.

Watercress is a member the Brassica or Cruciferous vegetable family and as such contains some amazing anticancer compounds. It is very high in vitamin K which is a key component of healthy bones.

INGREDIENTS

1 tbsp	Coconut oil
1	Red onion
1	Celery stick
½	Green pepper
100g	Courgette
1	Garlic clove
500ml	Vegetable stock
120g	Broccoli
40g	Watercress
100g	Spinach
Handful of	Toasted pumpkin seeds
Pinch of	Sea salt
Crack of	Black pepper

add a dollop of coconut or greek yoghurt to weight out the dish if wanted

METHOD

1. Heat up a medium to large pan with the coconut oil.

2. Finely chop and fry the onion and celery, then add the chunkily chopped green pepper and courgette. Fry for up to 10 mins, with a stir here and there. Chop and add the garlic for the last couple of minutes.

3. Make 250ml of stock in a jug and add to the pan.

4. Chop the broccoli stalks and add to the pan. Let them simmer for 5 minutes and save the florets to simmer for the last 2 mins.

5. Add the watercress and spinach. Cover and boil for just a minute 'til soft.

6. Let cool slightly, and then blend with a hand blender. Top up with water, approximately 400ml, to thin out the soup.

7. Add a pinch of sea salt and a good grind of black pepper. Stir. Keep going until it tastes good for you.

8. Scatter with toasted pumpkin seeds to serve. Eat as soon as possible to enjoy the beautiful bright green colour.

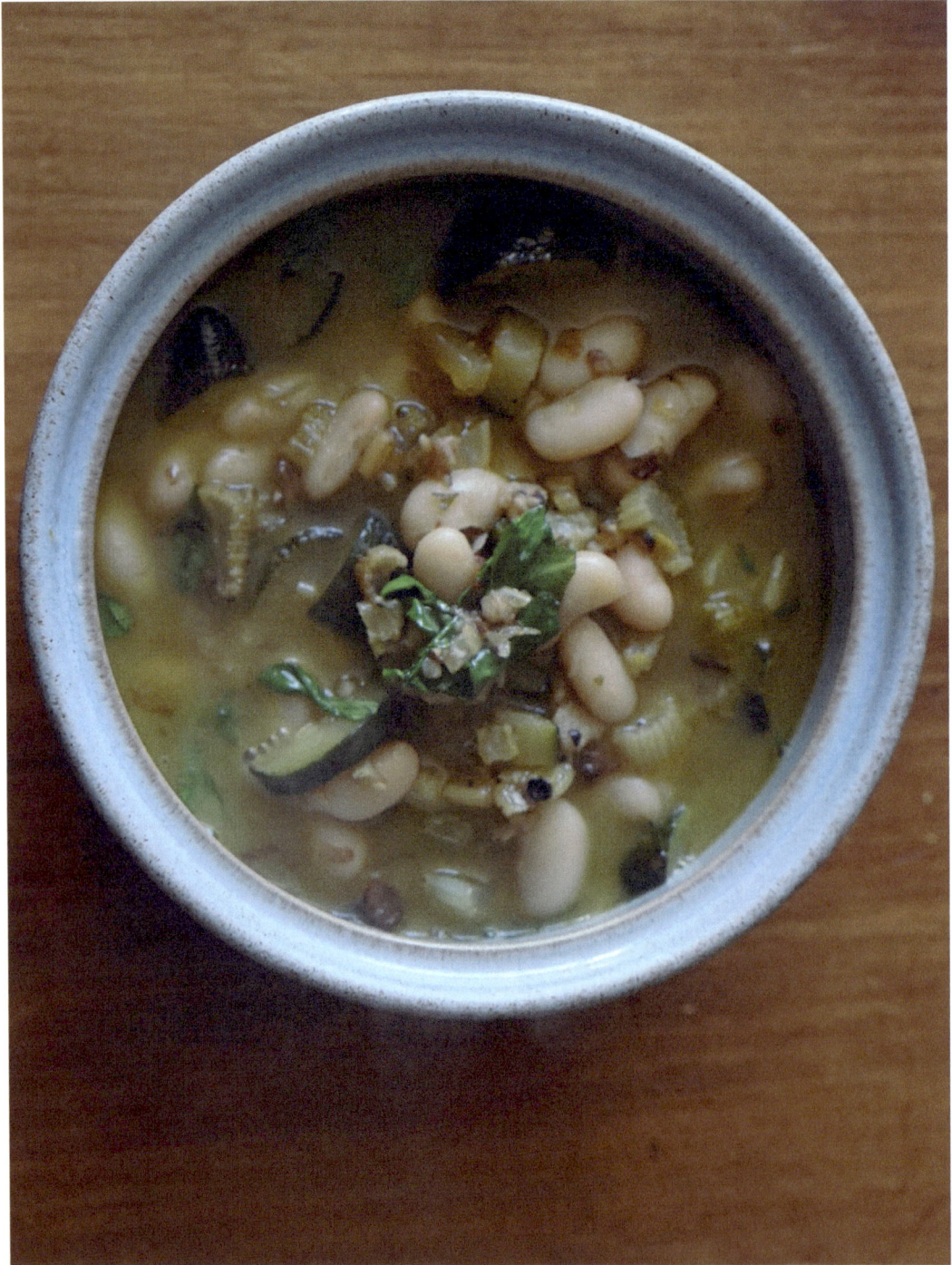

White Bean & Courgette Broth

SERVES 4 | ⏱ 30 MINS | GF DF V Ve NF

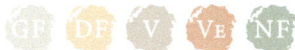

"Souper soups. Luckily there is a never ending world of these in life. This is a broth or simply blended soup, a good flexible dish. I think I prefer the chunky broth version, but the decisions never stop changing!"

Courgettes, being part of the squash family, contain a good amount of vitamin A and carotenoids but are low in carbohydrates. This dish provides a very good level of both soluble and insoluble fibre from the courgettes and the beans which is extremely beneficial to the health of our gut. It can help to reduce inflammation and reduce heart disease and diabetes.

White beans are high in potassium but also contain good amounts of thiamine, iron, folate, magnesium and manganese. Added to this is a good helping of garlic. Chop the garlic 10 minutes before using to allow the therapeutic properties to develop and cook very gently so that the benefits are preserved as much as possible. Garlic is one of our top anticancer foods.

INGREDIENTS

4 tbsp	Coconut oil
1kg	Courgettes (x6)
2	Celery sticks
6 cloves	Garlic
480ml	Vegetable stock
800g	Cannellini beans (cooked)
Big pinch	Sea salt
Big crack of	Black pepper
Splash of	Extra virgin olive oil
40g	Basil

METHOD

1. Heat the coconut oil in a saucepan.

2. Chunkily chop up the courgettes and finely slice the celery, and add to the frying pan.

3. Chop up the garlic cloves fairly finely and fry lightly.

4. Just 5 minutes will soften and start to darken the courgette and celery. When it starts to colour, then add 300ml of water, And leave the courgette to soften for another (up to) 5 minutes occasionally stirring.

5. Create your stock, and once the courgette has softened, add the stock and the beans, season with a big pinch of salt and crack in black pepper to taste – and bring to a simmer to blend the flavours for about 5 minutes, add more water if needed.

6. Lightly chop up the basil and stir in (save a couple of leaves to decorate each bowl). Turn off the heat and serve alongside salt and pepper, the last basil leaves and a drizzle of olive oil.

WOLF'S FISH BOWL

SERVES 4 | ⏱ 45 MINS | GF DF NF

"This delightful dish was uncovered in SE Germany through my 'uncle' ... possibly once removed or whichever path I can name him alongside friend. It is delicious. Though similar to the classic boullaibaisse, it's significantly different and worth adding to the Wholesome World cookbook. A warm and hearty dish."

Packed with protein and healthy fats from the fish and enough veg to give a good helping hand towards your quota of eight a day, this is a truly nutrient dense meal. The tomatoes, pepper and orange also provide carotenoids which are extremely healing for the gut and appear to block tumour progression in some cancers. Garlic, onions and leeks may equally lower cancer risk as they are rich in sulphur compounds.

INGREDIENTS

2	Onions
1	Celery stick
2	Garlic cloves
1	Leek
2 tbsp	Rapeseed oil
1 tsp	Thyme
4	Bay leaves
600g	Tomatoes *(fresh & small)*
1 tbsp	Tomato paste
1	Red pepper
1	Orange
Tsp	Saffron
½ litre	Fish stock
200g	Monkfish
200g	Salmon fillet
200g	Sea Bass
150g	Shrimps *(peeled)*

METHOD

1. Roughly chop the onions, celery stick, garlic cloves and leek.

2. Add the rapeseed oil to the cooking pot and set to a medium heat.

3. Add the chopped ingredients to lightly sear. Add the de-stemmed thyme and loose bay leaves and leave in for 10 mins while stirring and simmering.

4. Lightly chop the tomatoes, and add to the pot alongside the tomato paste and loosely chopped red pepper.

5. Finely grate the orange to add to the mix and then juice it and add to the pan, alongside the saffron.

6. Add the stock and simmer for 20 mins. Chunkily chop the fish, and add with the shrimps to the pan and allow to cook for 8-10 mins.

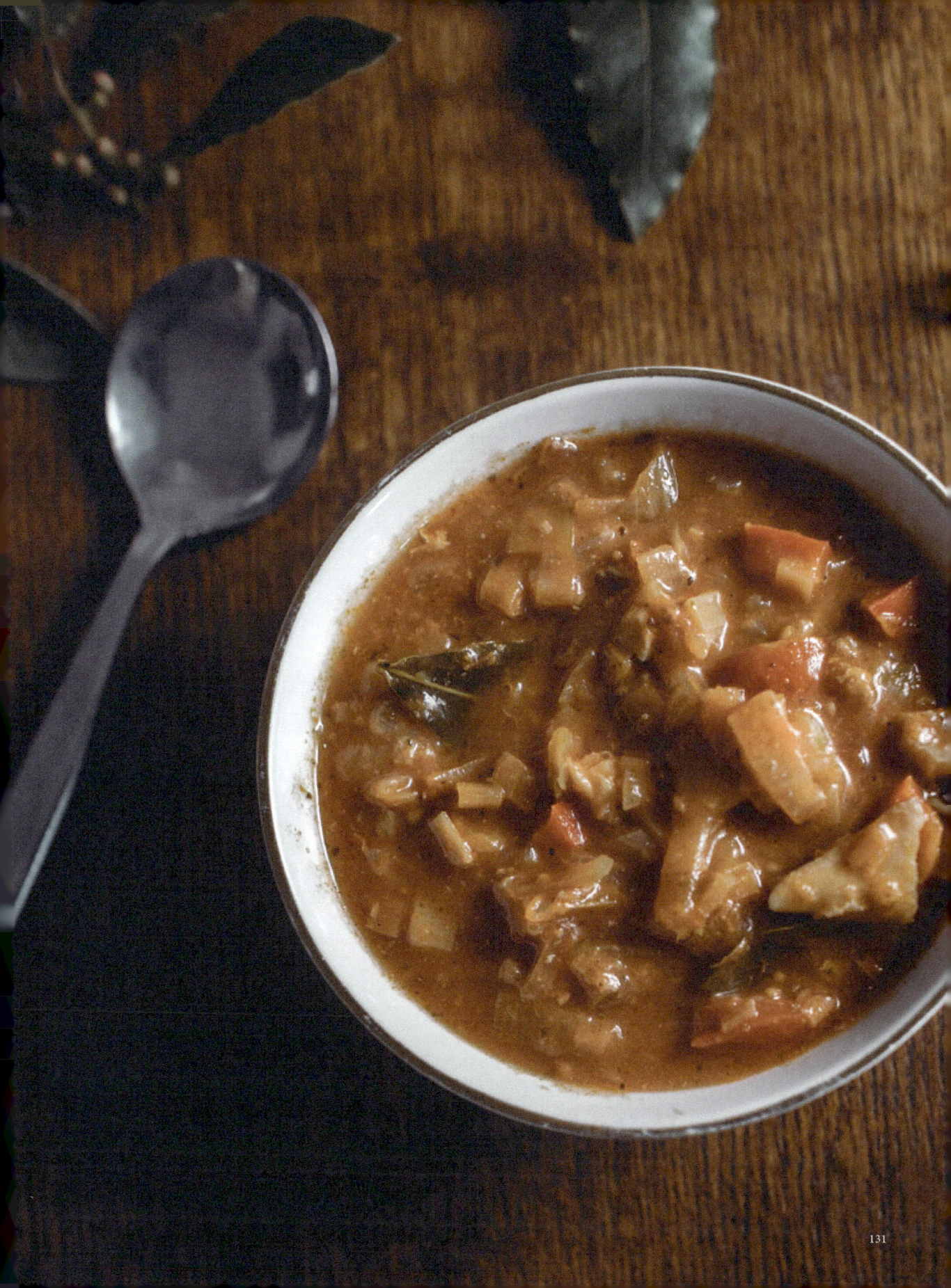

COASTAL CHOWDER

SERVES 6 | ⏲ 55 MINS | GF NF

"This Chowder is the ultimate comfort food and extremely tasty, the perfect balance of smokiness and texture from chunky potatoes and flakey haddock. I like to serve it with fresh warm rye or sourdough bread and ladle it into bowls for an easy delicious wholesome meal."

Fish is often referred to as brain food, especially salmon as it contains the fat omega 3. It is recommended that we eat fish 2-3 times a week. It provides good quality protein and high levels of vitamins and minerals, particularly vitamin B12 and iodine.

Leeks and onions are part of the allium family and contain highly anticancer sulphurous compounds. Celery contains numerous antioxidants and phytonutrients, all of which are anti-inflammatory and thus anticancer. It is also rich in vitamins A, C & K and minerals galore.

INGREDIENTS

1 tbsp	Rapeseed oil
3	Celery sticks
1	Onion
1	Leek *(large)*
1	Potato *(large)*
1	Butternut squash
2	Corn cobs
3	Garlic cloves
400g	Haddock fillet
200g	Salmon fillet
3	Bay leaves *(fresh)*
3 sprigs	Thyme *(fresh)*
1 litre	Fish stock
150ml	Single cream

METHOD

1. Heat the oil in a large saucepan over a medium heat. Trim and finely slice the leek, onion and celery, add to the pan and stir.

2. Scrub the potato, chop into 2cm chunks and run under a tap until the water runs clear to de-starch them. Chop the squash to a matching size and add both to the pan when the onions are golden in colour, and the leeks are touching brown. Mix well to stop things from sticking. Keep an eye on the pan, stirring often for around 8-10 mins.

3. Add the sweetcorn, by slicing it raw from the cob, to the pan and mix through. Finely chop and add in the garlic too.

4. Chunkily chop the fish to approx 2cm.

5. Make a little space in the middle of the pan for the fish. Add the haddock and salmon with 3 bay leaves and the leaves from 3 sprigs of thyme.

6. Make the stock, add to the pan, stir and then put the lid on to cook for 15 mins on a medium heat (to reduce a little).

7. Check on the chowder, give it a good stir and season to taste — at this point the fish should be flaking and smelling delicious.

8. Turn off the heat and add the cream and stir well just before serving. Check the temperature and warm if needed, you also have the option to blend lightly with a fork or masher, or keep it deliciously chunky.

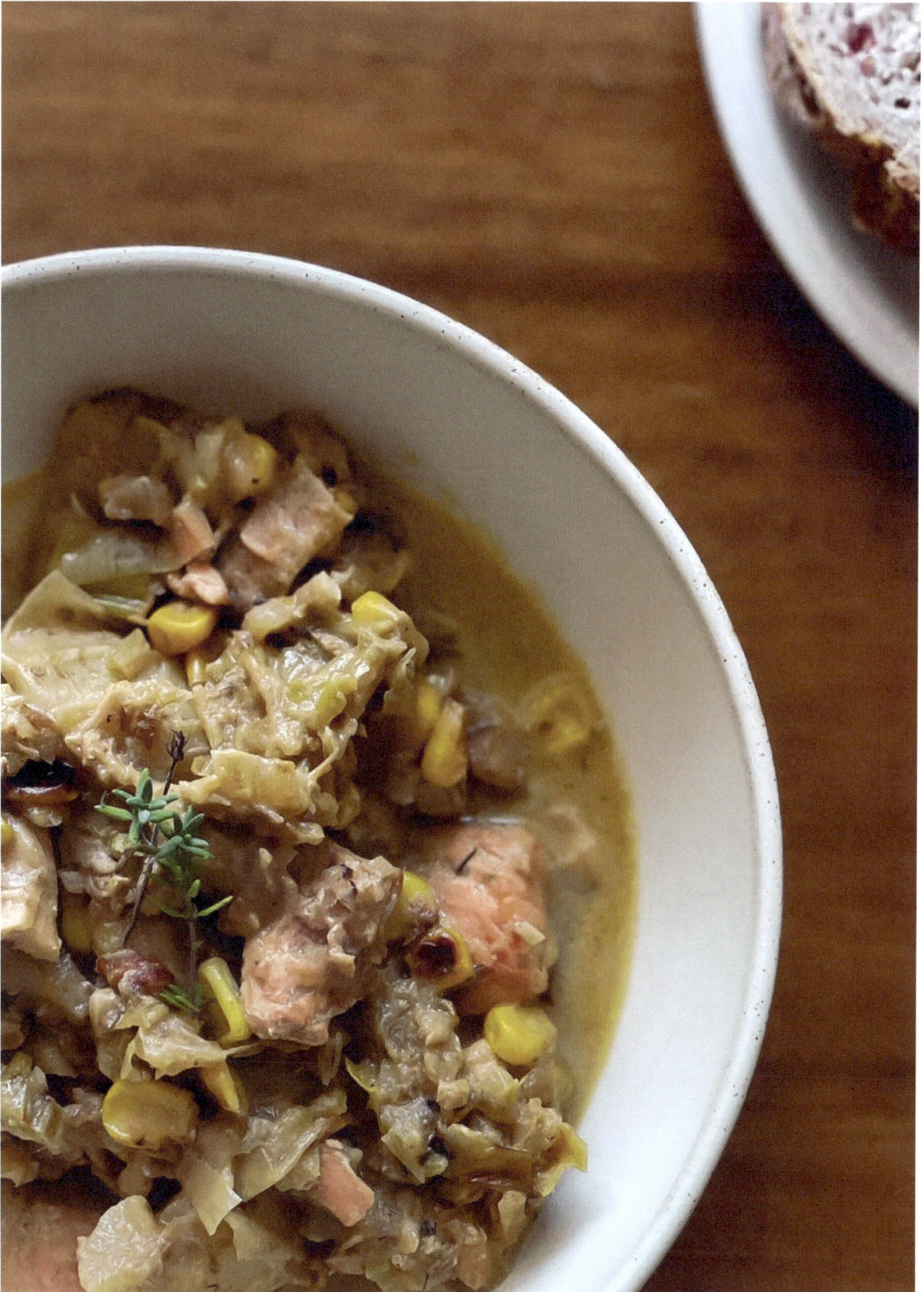

Ocean Bouillabaisse

SERVES 6 | 🕐 55 MINS | GF DF NF

"Cod, snapper or monkfish. Sustainable fishing in your area is so important, be it liaising with the local fisherman or the shops that know and support the sources.

I do love a simply seared lobster, when you find a good local source, just grilled or bbq'd and thrown in chunks on top of this dish. Twist it with whatever you stumble upon, I see foraged mussels as nutrition halos if you get them within the season during low tide."

A hearty one-pot meal, high in protein, vitamins and minerals from the fish. Fennel contains some exceptional antioxidants and acts as a digestive aid. It also provides vitamin C, as does the red pepper.

Celery is great added to any dish that will take it. It has some very special pectin-based polysaccharides which are protective of the stomach and its lining. Add a good handful of parsley to support the liver too as this aids detoxification.

INGREDIENTS

1 tbsp	Coconut oil
1	Onion *(large)*
4	Celery legs
2	Leeks *(large)*
1	Fennel
4 cloves	Garlic
1	Red pepper
125ml	Dry white wine
400g	Large tomatoes
½ litre	Fish stock
150 ml	Tomato purée
600g	Cod
Pinch of	Sea salt
Crack of	Black pepper
Handful	Curly parsley

METHOD

1. Turn on the heat, low, and add the coconut oil to large saucepan to melt.

2. Chop the onion, celery, leeks and fennel into thin slices alongside finely chopping the garlic. Fry the chopped ingredients, cover and cook for 10 minutes, on a low heat stirring occasionally.

3. Whilst frying, chop the red pepper into slim strips, chunkily chop your tomatoes, then add all to the pan with the wine, stir together and cook for a further 10 minutes at low temperature.

4. While this is cooking, set up your fish stock, so it is ready to add. After the 10 mins is up; add the purée, fish stock and bring to a boil stirring well. Simmer uncovered for 15 minutes, to get the right saucy thickness.

5. Chop the fish into chunky bite size pieces and add to the pan; cover and cook for 10 minutes until tender.

6. Add salt and pepper to taste, followed by the parsley, which you can rip up and stir in; you can save some parsley and sprinkle some to garnish individual servings.

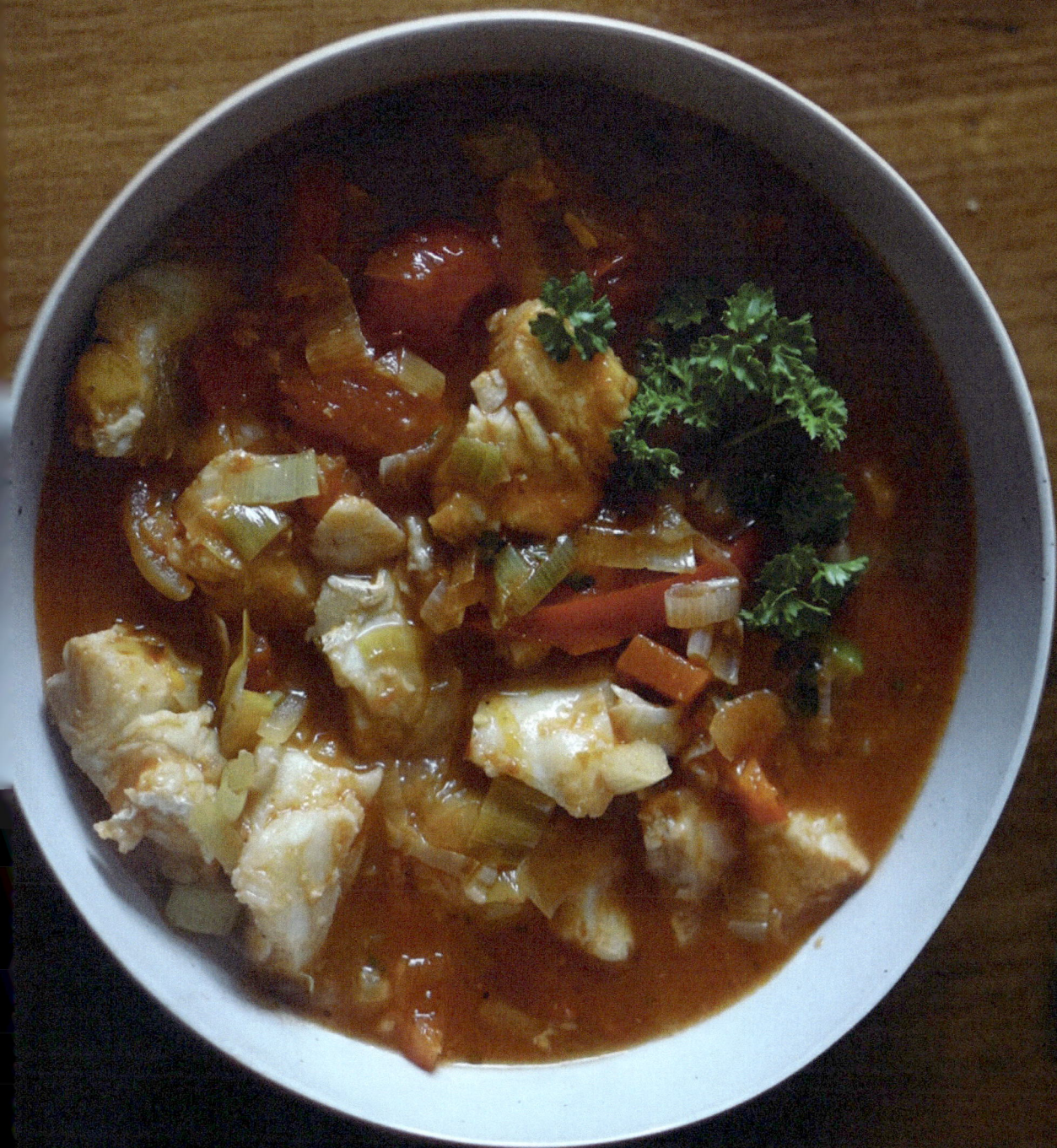

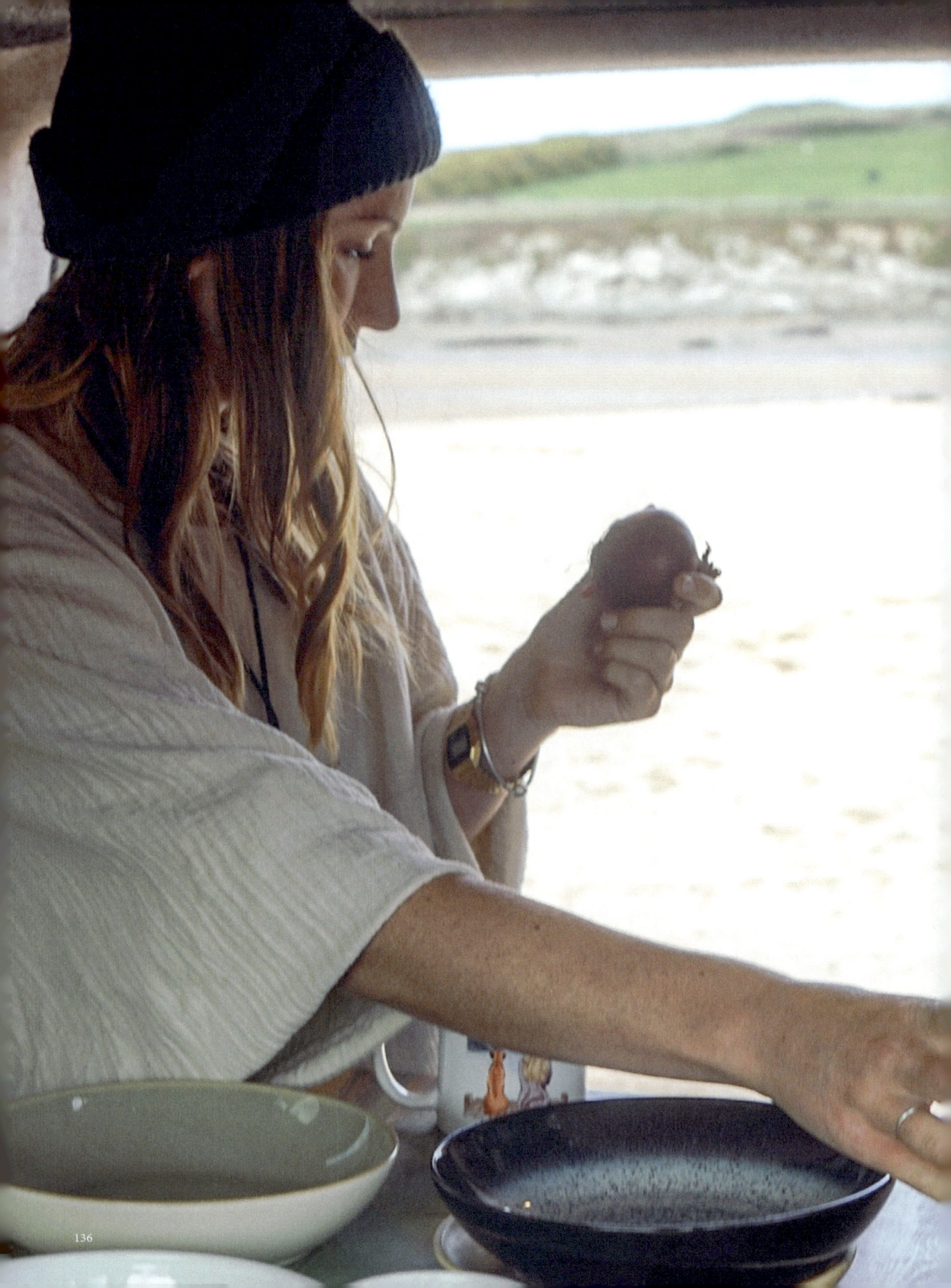

MAINS

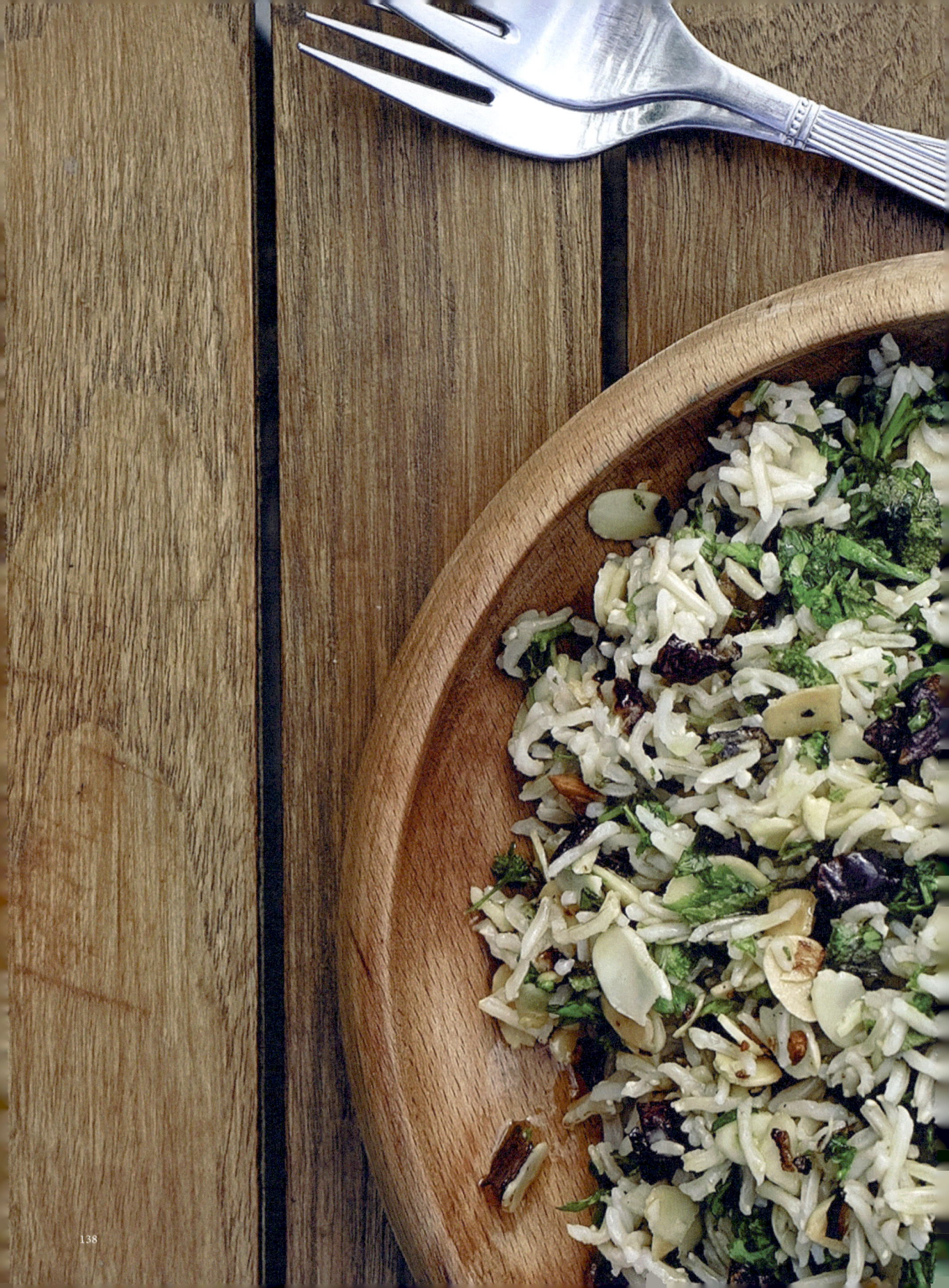

RICE, ALMOND & HERB SALAD

SERVES 4 | 🕒 45 MINS | GF DF V VE

"A tasty rice salad that is so good due to the large amount of herbs used making this a satisfyingly green dish."

Use brown rice for added fibre and B vitamins. Almonds will provide healthy fats and vitamin E which may reduce blood pressure and help blood sugar control. Onions are one of our top anticancer foods and using red ones adds to its antioxidant profile. Adding plenty of herbs always ups the healthfulness of a dish by providing an array of antioxidants, vitamins and minerals. Parsley is known for its detoxifying properties so supports liver health but any of those herbs provide amazing health benefits.

INGREDIENTS

200g	Brown rice
2 tbsp	Olive oil
1	Red onion
1	Clove garlic
100g	Sliced almonds
Pinch of	Sea salt
Crack of	Black pepper
100g	Herbs
	parsley, coriander, dill, basil, sage, mint, tarragon or use a mixture
1	Lemon

METHOD

1. Wash the rice well by rinsing and draining repeatedly in cold water.

2. Heat a pan of water with 450ml water, add the rice and bring to a gentle rolling boil, before reducing it to simmer and cook for 25 minutes.

3. Turn the heat off, place a lid on and leave to sit and absorb the excess water for 10 minutes.

4. Turn out into a shallow large dish, spread the rice and leave to cool. This can all be done a few hours before.

5. Gently heat the oil, dice the red onions and add to the pan to cook for 5 minutes, constantly mixing so that they do not brown, add the garlic, almonds and seasoning and cook for a further 5 minutes until golden.

6. Add to the cooled cooked rice and mix well.

7. Finely chop your chosen herbs finely, mix in with the rice, check seasoning, and adjust if needed. Finish by juicing the lemon, adding to taste and adding a little more olive oil.

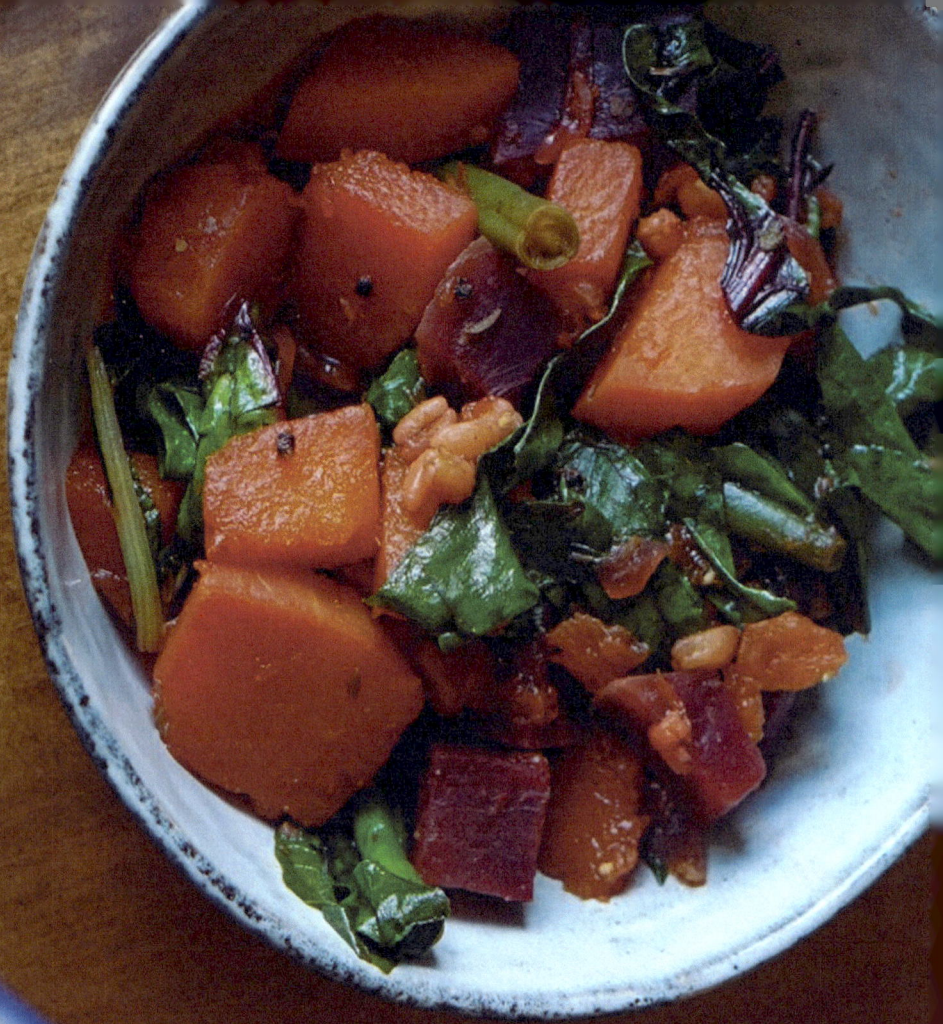

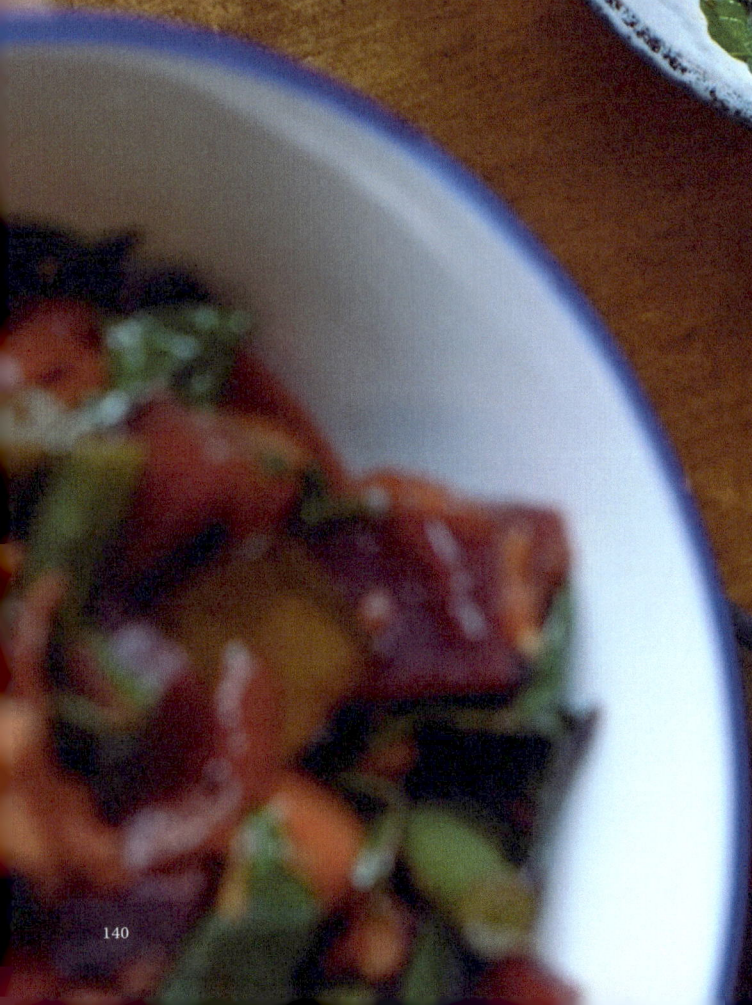

MIXED BEANS BUTTERNUT POT

SERVES 4 | 🕐 30 MINS | GF DF V Ve NF

"A warm filling dish, perfect for a post-surf filler. Warms you up through and through. Also good on a cliff walk or sunny beach flop picnic. It's just good to have the 'leftovers' with you to re-fuel or pick at! Gorgeous in both flavour and looks."

This is a dish high in beta-carotenes from the apricots and butternut squash. Beta-carotenes are antioxidants known particularly for their anticancer properties.

The beans add some super fibre which our beneficial gut bacteria love to feed on.

The spices aid our digestion.

INGREDIENTS

1 tbsp	Olive oil
1	Onion
2	Garlic cloves
2 tsp	Ground cumin
2 tsp	Ground coriander
3 tsp	Harissa
Pinch of	Sea salt
Crack of	Black pepper
500ml	Vegetable stock
400g	Butternut squash
100g	Dried apricots
200g	Mixed beans *(tin)*
Bunch of	Coriander chopped

METHOD

1. Heat the olive oil in a medium add the sliced onion and chopped garlic, cook for 5 minutes over a medium heat until soft and lightly golden,

2. Add the cloves, cumin, coriander, harissa, seasoning and stock and bring to a gentle simmer.

3. Peel and chop the butternut into dice sized cubes, add to the mix along with the apricots (chunkily chopped), stir well and then simmer for 10 minutes.

4. Drain the mixed beans and add to the pan cook for a further 8 minutes.

5. Chop the coriander and scatter it to serve the dish.

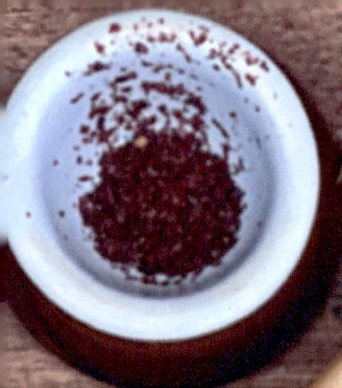
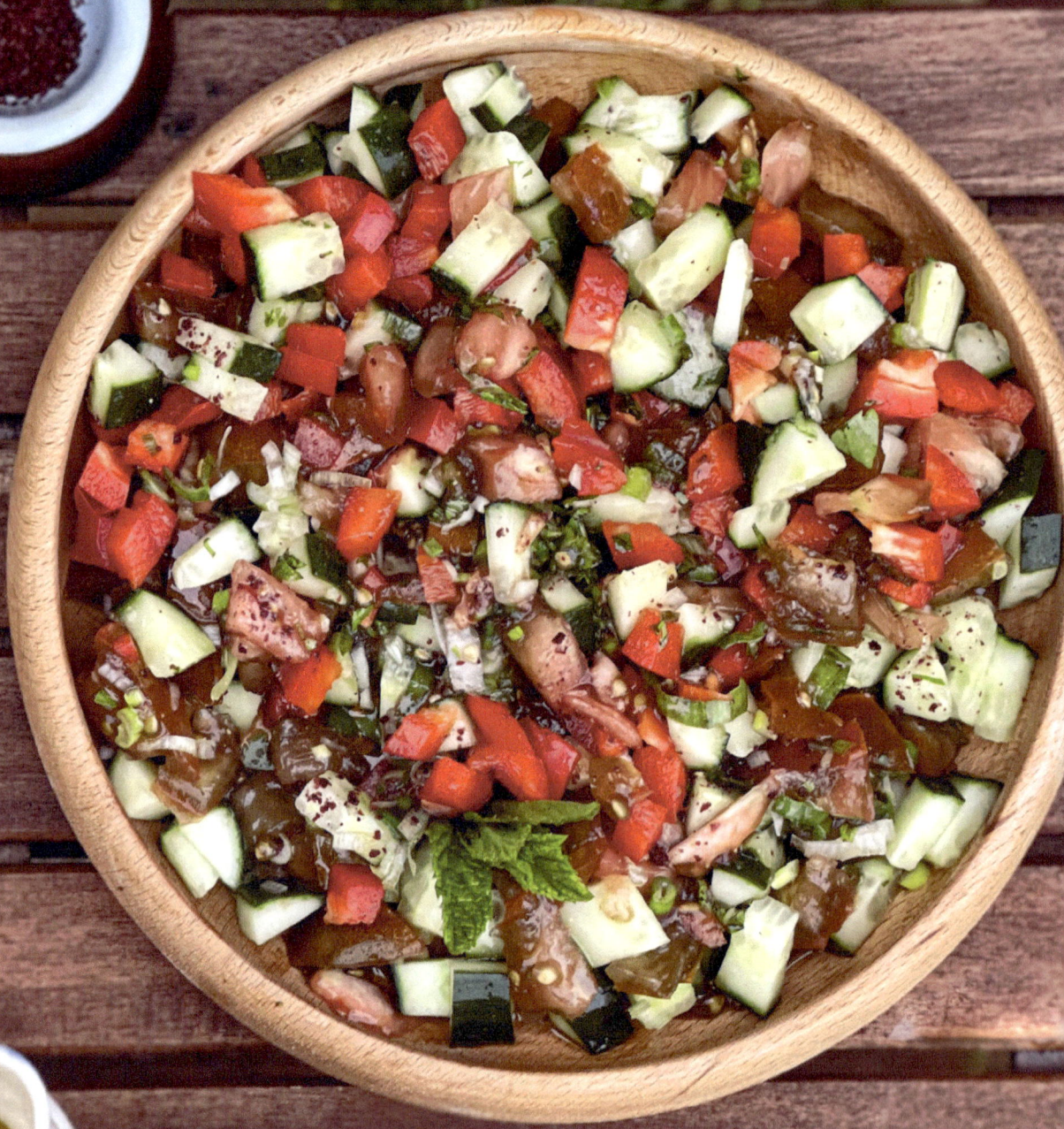
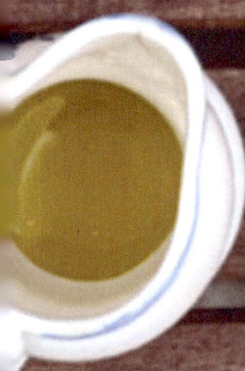
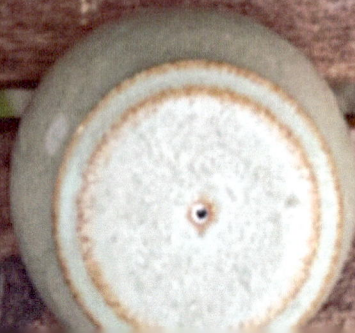

Cucumber, Mint & Sumac

SERVES 4 | ⏱ 25 MINS | GF DF V VE NF

"A fresh light and simple salad that will give your taste buds a blast."

A healthy mix of reds and greens means a plentiful supply of vitamins and antioxidants.

Red peppers are one of the richest sources of vitamin C and the tomatoes will top this up considerably along with vitamin K1, for healthy bones, and folate for healthy cell functioning.

Peppers also contain vitamin B6 which plays a role in keeping the brain healthy, improving mood and preventing anaemia. Beta carotene is found at high levels in the peppers and tomatoes and is converted into vitamin A, a very important vitamin for eye health.

Spring onions provide more vitamin K which contributes to healthy blood clotting. Cucumbers are composed of 96% water and so promote hydration... they also contain vitamins, minerals and antioxidants. To gain the most benefits from cucumber eat unpeeled.

INGREDIENTS

25g	Large cucumber
1	Red pepper
2	Large tomatoes
4	Spring onions
Bunch of	Mint
Bunch of	Flat leaf parsley
4 tbsp	Olive oil
2 tbsp	White wine vinegar
1½ tsp	Sumac
Pinch of	Sea salt

METHOD

1. Cut the cucumber in half, then into batons and finely dice, cut the red pepper and tomatoes into similar sizes.

2. Finely dice the spring onions.

3. Pick the mint leaves and parsley off their stalks and chop.

4. Place in a bowl, drizzle with the olive oil, vinegar, then sprinkle with the sumac and salt and toss well to coat the whole salad with dressing.

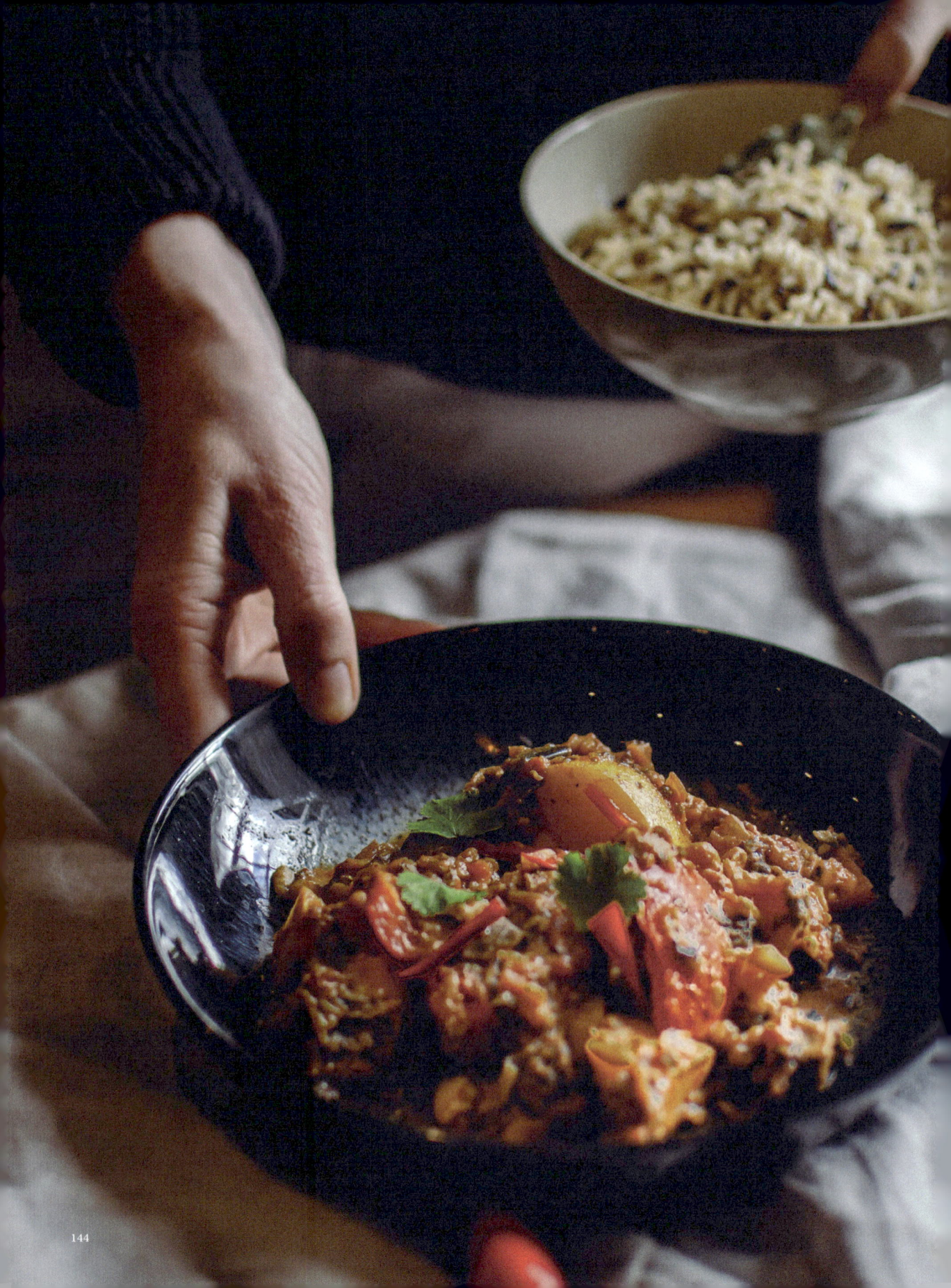

Aubergine & Potato Curry

SERVES 4 | 🕐 40 MINS | GF DF V VE NF

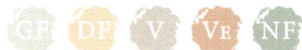

"Grated aubergine is one of the best bases of a vegetable based curry. Enhances the look, taste and weight of the dish, and when smothered with spices, herbs and local tomatoes, it is perfection for a mindful meal."

Aubergines have an excellent antioxidant profile including lutein and zeaxanthin which is important in preventing age-related macular degeneration. Other antioxidants have an anti-inflammatory effect which protects against cancer, heart disease and cognitive decline.

Spinach is an excellent source of iron which helps create haemoglobin for oxygenising our cells.

Further anti-inflammatory effects are found in the spices and herbs.

INGREDIENTS

500g	Frozen chopped spinach
1 tbsp	Coconut oil
1	Onion
2	Garlic cloves
2	Aubergine
½ tsp	Cumin seeds
½ tsp	Ground turmeric
½ tsp	Ground chilli
½ tsp	Ground coriander
2	Potatoes
400g	Chopped tomatoes *(tinned)*
1	Red pepper
Pinch of	Sea salt
Crack of	Black pepper
Handful of	Coriander *(fresh)*
1	Green chilli

METHOD

1. Pull out your frozen spinach to defrost. Heat up the pan with 1 tbsp coconut oil.
2. Crush the garlic, chop with the onion fairly finely and add them to the pan.
3. Chunkily chop the aubergine, add to the pan and stir until lightly bronzed.
4. Add the spices, chunkily chop the potatoes and add alongside the tin of chopped tomatoes, and cook for 20+ mins (to taste) on low heat. Then slice up your red pepper to throw in and leave it to simmer for 2 mins, before adding the spinach, to cook for just 5 more mins to finish the dish.
5. Taste and add salt and pepper. Chunkily chop and garnish with fresh coriander and finely sliced green chilli to taste.

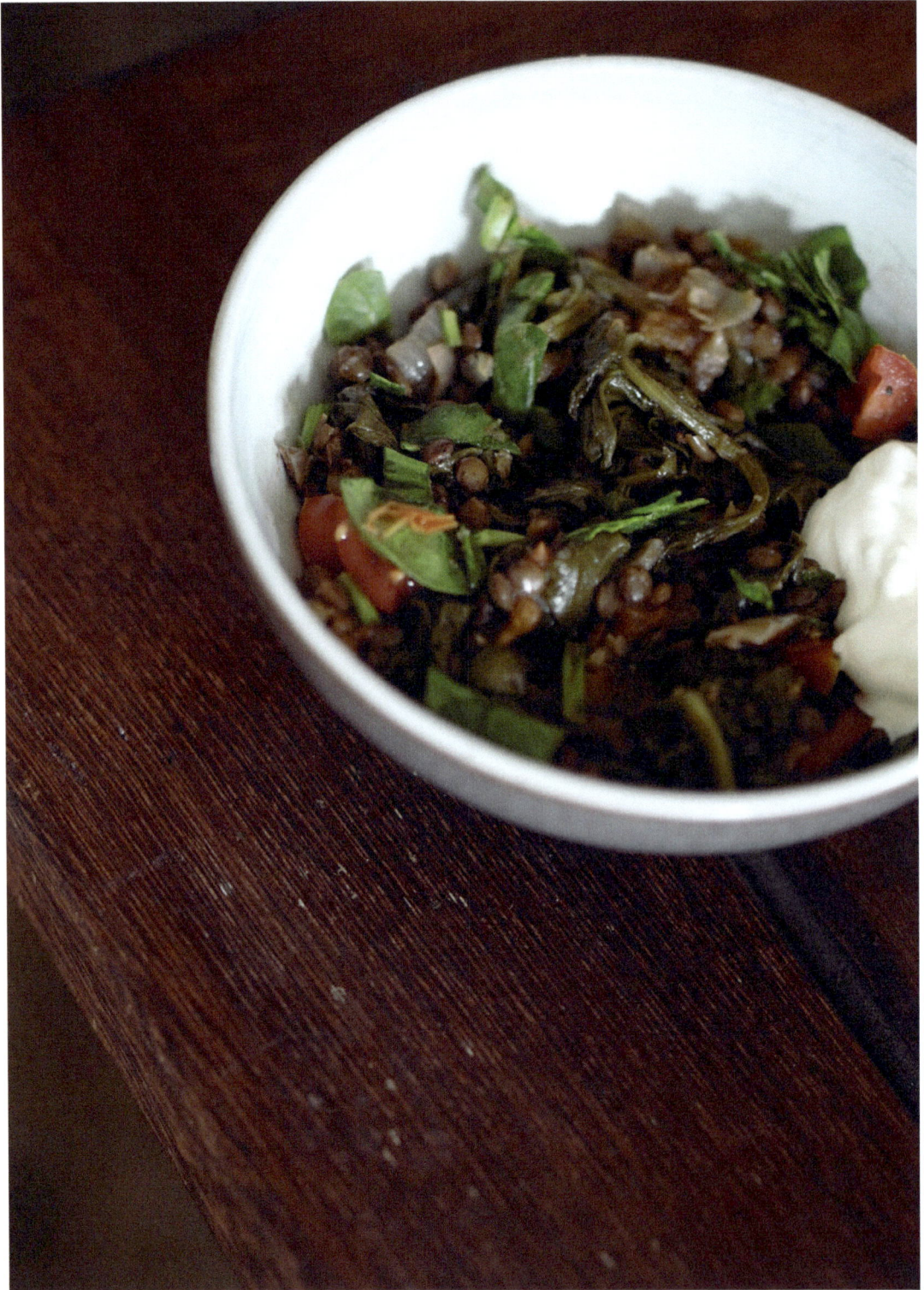

Garam Masala Lentils & Spinach

SERVES 4 | 🕐 40 MINS | GF DF V Ve NF

"Garam masala is an Indian blend which consists of ground spices like cinnamon, cumin, mace (a cumin sister spice), coriander, cardamom, nutmeg, bay leaves, cloves and black pepper. It's perfect with the tomato and lemon. Then throw in a yoghurt to calm it down spice-wise if needed."

Lentils are a classic ingredient to make a quick protein rich vegetarian meal. They are also packed with fibre, folate and iron.

Coconut oil is a healthy fat to cook with, made up of saturated fats of which 65% are medium chain triglycerides (MCT's). These fats, specifically lauric acid, have health benefits and are a good source of energy for the body.

Tomatoes and spinach, due to their bright colour, are full of healthy anticancer compounds, vitamins and minerals. Zesting a lemon into a recipe adds some healthful antioxidants such as D-limonene and vitamin C. Be sure to use unwaxed, and if possible, organic lemons.

INGREDIENTS

4 tbsp	Coconut oil
1	Onion
2	Garlic cloves
1 tsp	Garam masala
1 tsp	Curry powder *(medium hot)*
4	Cardamom pods
250g	Brown lentils
4	Tomatoes *(large)*
200g	Spinach
1	Unwaxed lemon
Pinch of	Sea salt
Crack of	Black pepper
-	
4 dsp	Coconut yoghurt

METHOD

1. Heat the oil in a medium saucepan, dice the onion, add to the pan, and cook for 5 minutes.

2. Finely chop and add the garlic, garam masala, curry powder and crushed cardamom pods, mix well, then cook for 3 minutes.

3. Add the brown lentils with 500ml water bring to the boil, then reduce the heat and simmer for 20 minutes, stirring frequently.

4. When the lentils are soft add the tomatoes, spinach, lemon zest, juice and seasoning, stir well and serve topped with a spoonful of yoghurt.

Warm Quinoa Salad

SERVES 4 | 🕐 35 MINS | GF DF V VE NF

"It's a soft dish, something filling that's warm, full of texture, and not difficult to digest. Quinoa is one of the grains that is delightfully quick to cook, fills you up and keeps well if you cook for double the table."

A dish that provides the colour, taste and nutrients of much that is good about the Mediterranean diet — thought to be the most healthy choice of diet.

Packing in 6 of your '8' veg and fruit a day, this dish is high in fibre especially if you don't peel your sweet potatoes. Remembering that, in general, the darker the colour of our fruit and veg the healthier it is. Aubergine is a great example as the wonderful purple skin contains some super antioxidants in the form of anthocyanins.

Sweet potatoes being more colourful than ordinary potatoes contain many more nutrients including important beta carotenes which support the immune system.

INGREDIENTS

1 tbsp	Coconut oil
2	Sweet potatoes
1	Courgette
1	Aubergine
¼	Red onion
4	Garlic cloves
400g	Red quinoa
1 tsp	Chilli flakes
50g	Tomato
100g	Spinach
Pinch of	Sea salt
Crack of	Black pepper
½	Lemon

METHOD

1. Heat the oven to 180°C fan. Warm the coconut oil in the oven as it heats to melt it.

2. Peel the sweet potatoes and 1cm dice them; slice courgette and the aubergine. Thinly slice the red onion. Crush, and chunkily chop the garlic.

3. Once the oil has melted, add the chopped vegetables to the baking tray to coat them. Sprinkle with the chilli flakes, then cook for about 10 mins.

4. Rinse the quinoa in a fine sieve under cold running water, then boil it with double the amount of water, sprinkle with salt and leave it for 10-15 minutes, before draining, and adding to the salad bowl to lightly cool.

5. Roughly chop the tomatoes and spinach and toss them into the vegetable mix. Leave for another 10 minutes.

6. When roasting is done, mix all the ingredients together, including the raw spinach (which will need a rinse).

7. Finally add sea salt, cracked pepper and lightly squeeze half a lemon over to taste.

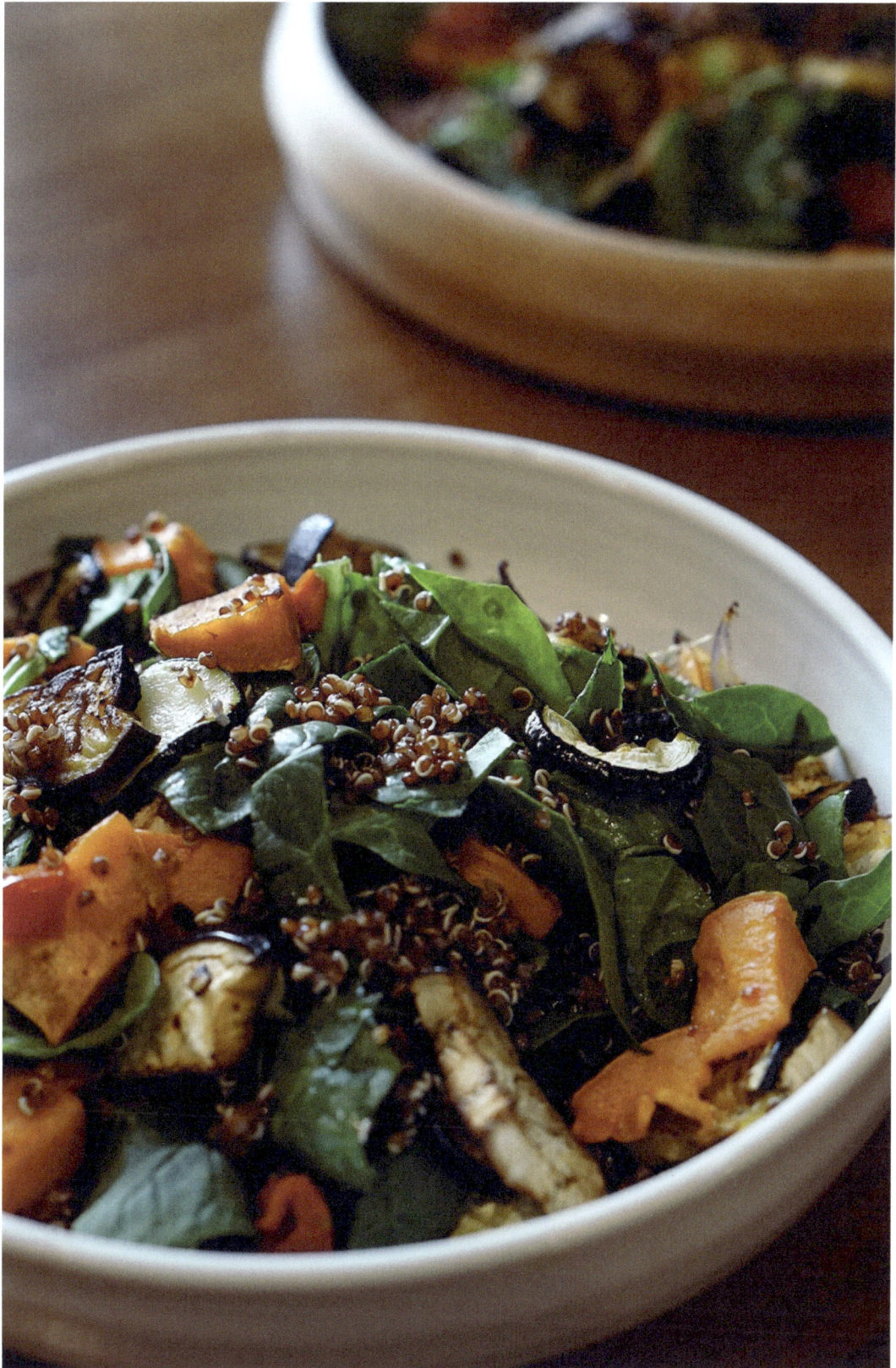

SPROUTING HEALTH AT HOME

Sprouts: Germinating or sprouting increases the nutrition content of the seeds and legumes (Mung beans, broccoli, alfalfa and so many more!)

They reduce anti-nutritional compounds such as lectins, which makes them much more easily digestible.

Sprouts are readily available in supermarkets and health food shops but it is easy to sprout your own.

To sprout your own seeds, rinse them and then place them in a large jar with water (ratio 1 part seeds to 3 parts water).

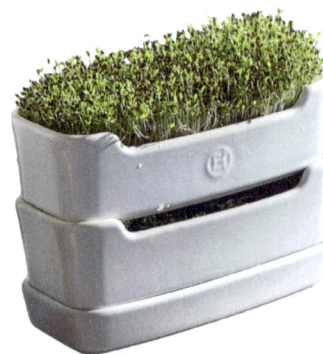

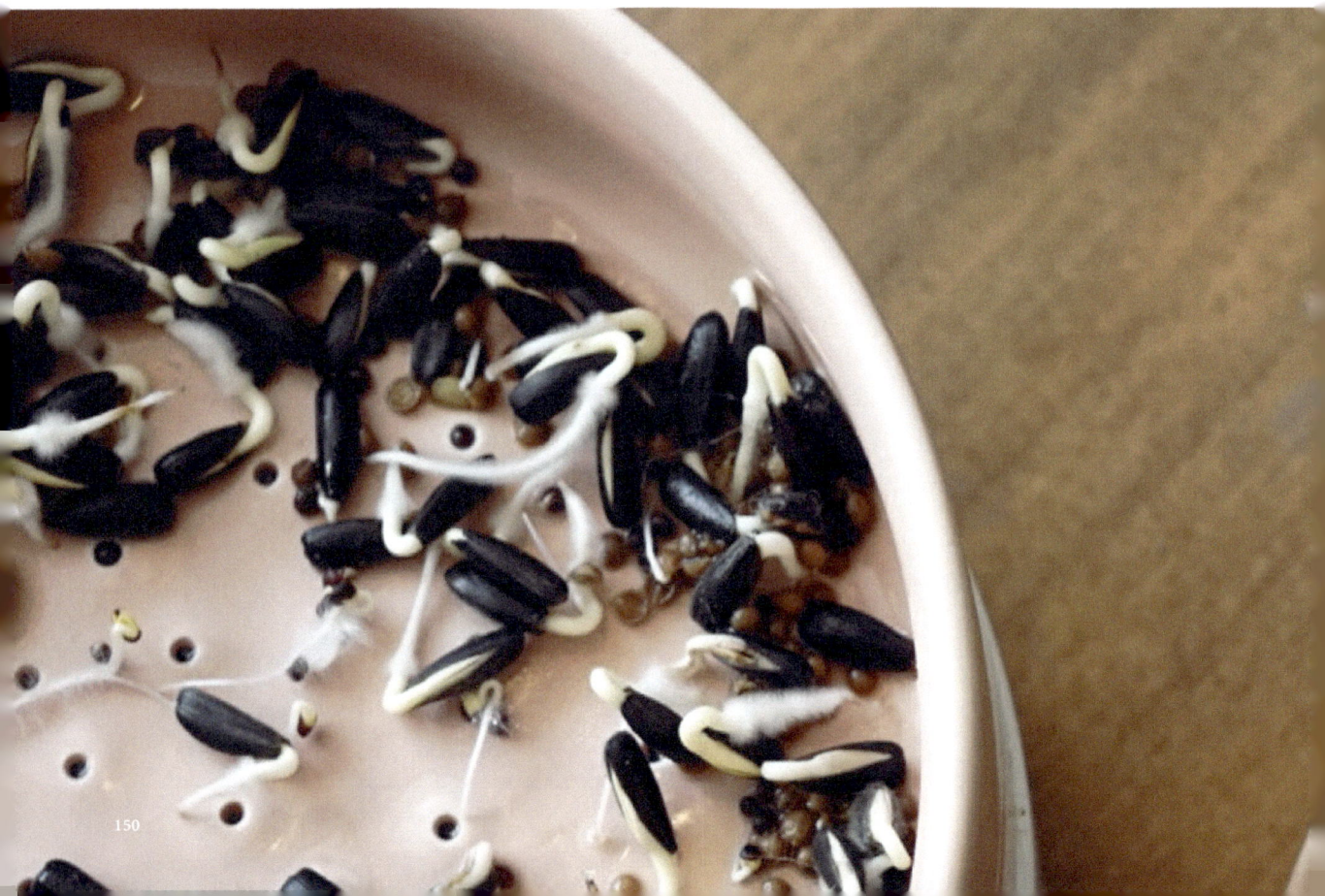

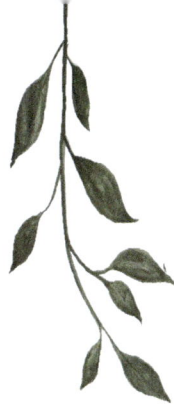

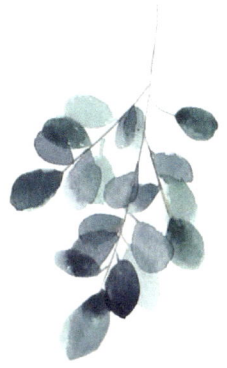

Leave to soak for 12–24 hours until they have started to sprout. Drain and rinse them and then return to the jar. Lay the jar on its side and spread the seeds out.

Leave the sprouts in a light position but out of direct sunlight.

Rinse the seeds at least 3 times a day. The rinsing is most important to prevent the seeds going mouldy and bacteria forming. The sprouts should be ready to eat in 2-3 days.

Always rinse sprouted seeds well before eating.

They can be stored in an airtight container in the fridge for up to 2 days.

OR use the seed sprouter kits, which have multiple layers with draining holes that just need a daily rinse.

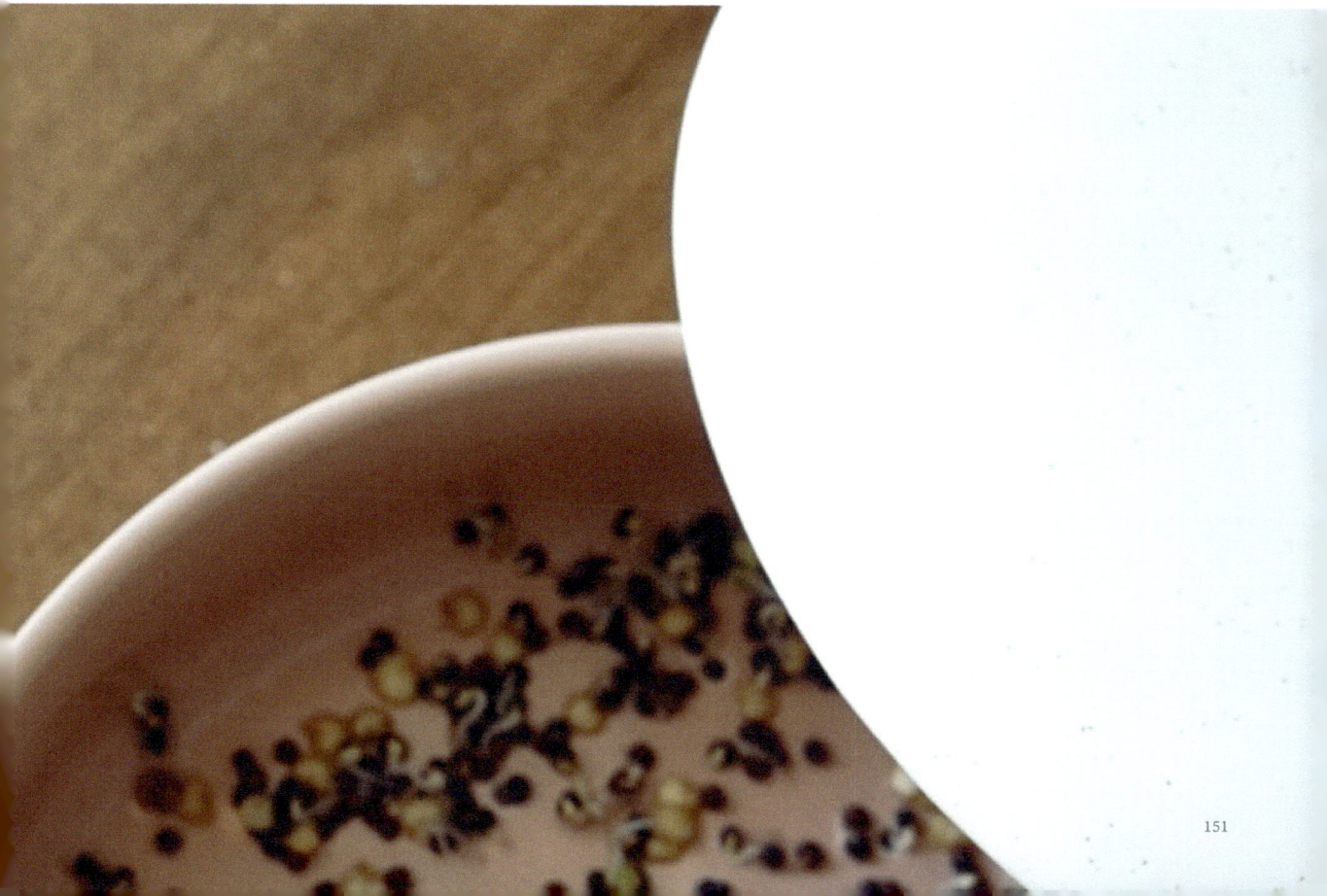

SQUASH & BEETROOT SALAD

SERVES 4 | 🕐 45 MINS | GF V

"A warm, hearty, wholesome salad — what more could one want? Especially when it has a beautiful soulful aura and is laden with benefits, from the ultra speedy digestion and the long slothic de-amalgumation from the root vegetables."

Squash and beetroot are a wonderful combination and along with the spinach and rocket leaves almost provide the colours of the rainbow and therefore a whole host of antioxidants.

Beetroot is great for enhancing the liver's detoxification powers. If you use sprouted broccoli seeds, these contain high levels of sulforaphane which has been shown to be protective (particularly in hormonally related cancers).

Hazelnuts are rich in healthy fats, calcium, magnesium, B vitamins and vitamin E.

Adding the crumbly feta cheese provides the protein and a change in texture to entice the taste buds. Feta is a healthy choice of cheese which is easily digested by humans.

INGREDIENTS

800g	Butternut squash
200g	Raw beetroot
3 tbsp	Olive oil
50g	Hazelnuts
100g	Rocket
100g	Spinach
100g	Feta cheese
½	Lemon
Handful	Sprouted seeds
Pinch of	Sea salt
Crack of	Black pepper

METHOD

1. Heat the oven to 180°C. Peel and cut the butternut into 2cm chunks, so it cooks more quickly. Wash the beetroot and cut them into wedges.

2. Add the prepared vegetables to a baking tray and the olive oil season with salt and pepper, toss in the oil. (TIP: keep the beetroot to one end of the tray to avoid bleeding its colour into the squash). Cook for 20 minutes.

3. Check and turn to get an even colouring and cook for a further 20 minutes, until soft and starting to char on the edges.

4. Roughly chop the hazelnuts and place on a baking tray to toast in the oven for the last 5 minutes, until golden. Once the vegetables and nuts are cooked, remove and place to one side to cool a little.

5. Wash the salad leaves and place in a serving bowl, crumble over the feta, squeeze the lemon and season. Top with the roasted vegetables and hazelnuts, and drizzle over any extra olive oil from the roasting tray.

6. Finally sprinkle the mixed sprouted seeds — done.

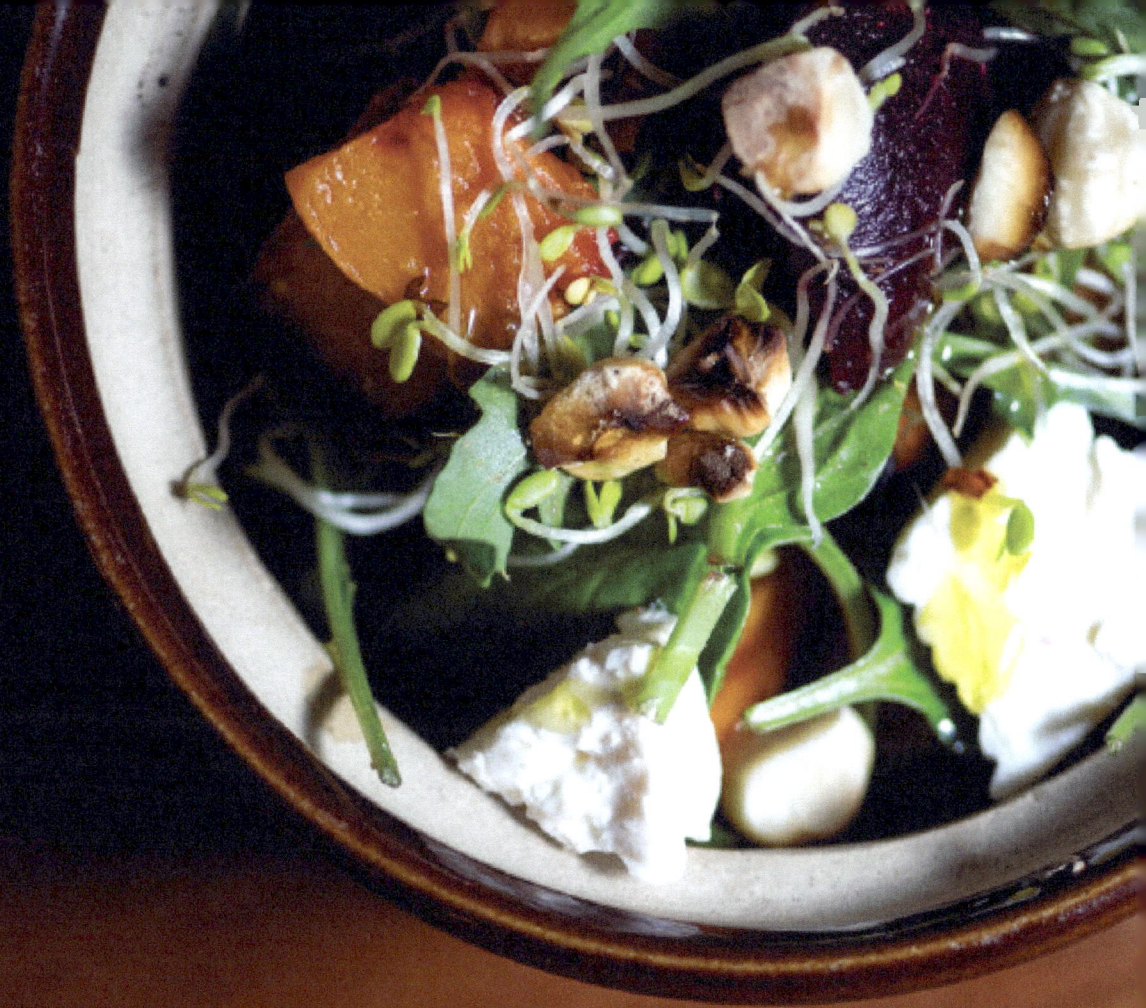

SIMPLY FUSILLI

SERVES 4 | 🕐 30 MINS | Ⓥ ⓃⒻ

"This is one of the ingredients that was my sole ingredient in my younger years... Pasta. I think that it is impossible to give up, yet simple to switch to wholegrain so that our energy levels don't spike and immediately dissipate."

Use wholewheat fusilli to reduce the effect of blood glucose spikes. Spinach is an excellent source of iron which will be more easily absorbed by the vitamin C in the lemon juice and zest. Spinach is also high in vitamins A, C, K, folic acid and calcium. It has good levels of B6, B9 and vitamin E.

INGREDIENTS

300g	Wholemeal fusilli
2	Garlic cloves
2	Unwaxed lemons
2 tbsp	Olive oil
4 tbsp	Crème fraîche
200g	Baby spinach
50g	Parmesan

METHOD

1. Heat a large pan of water and when boiling add the pasta, reduce the heat and simmer for 12 minutes.

2. While waiting, crush and dice the garlic cloves, then zest and juice the lemon.

3. Drain the pasta when cooked, add then add the olive oil, garlic, lemon juice, zest, creme fraîche and seasoning to the pan. Return the pasta back to the pan and mix well with two wooden spoons.

4. Once evenly mixed return to a low heat, with a lid on for 3 minutes. Rip the spinach and stir in.

5. Serve with the freshly grated Parmesan on top.

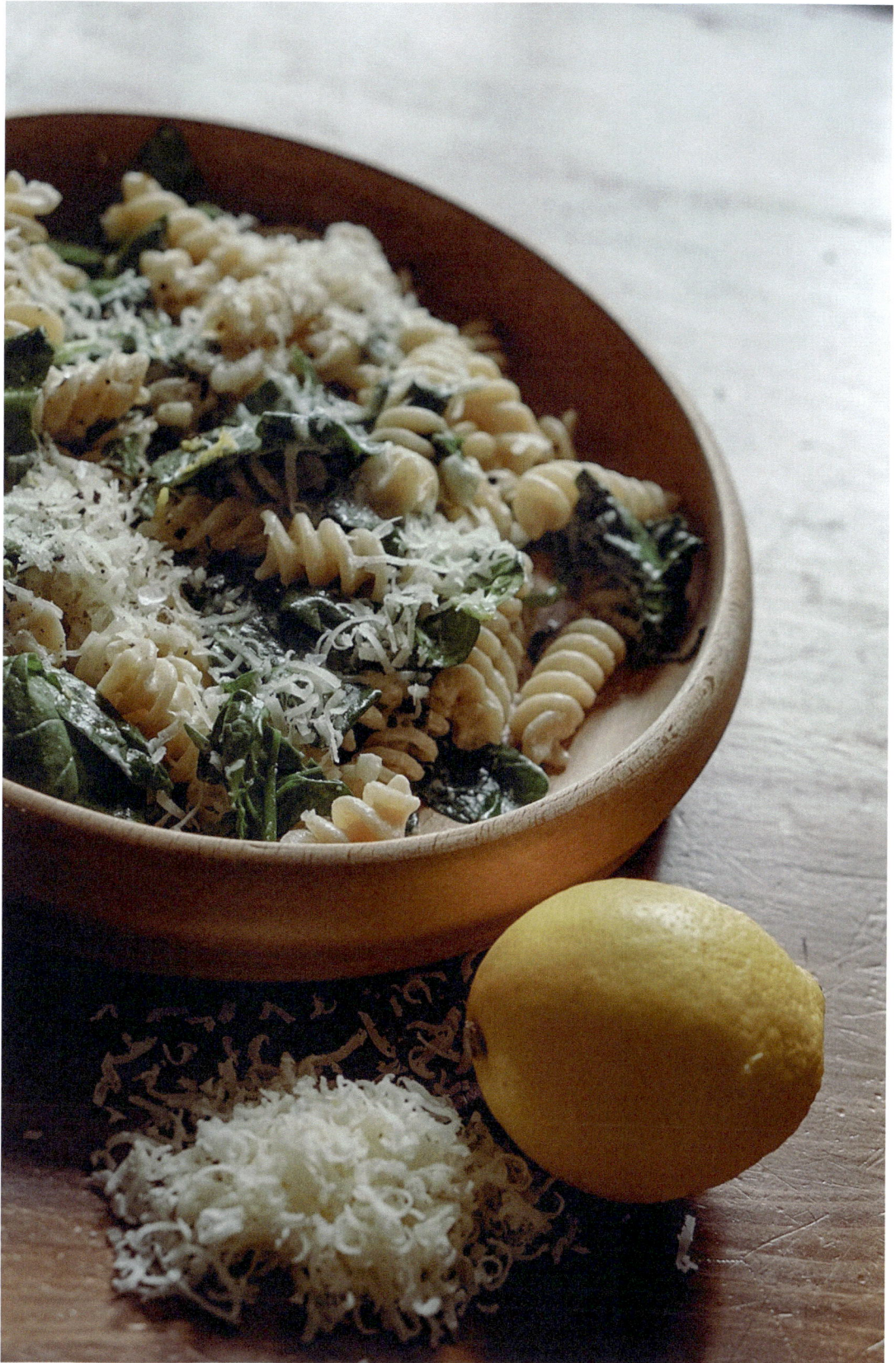

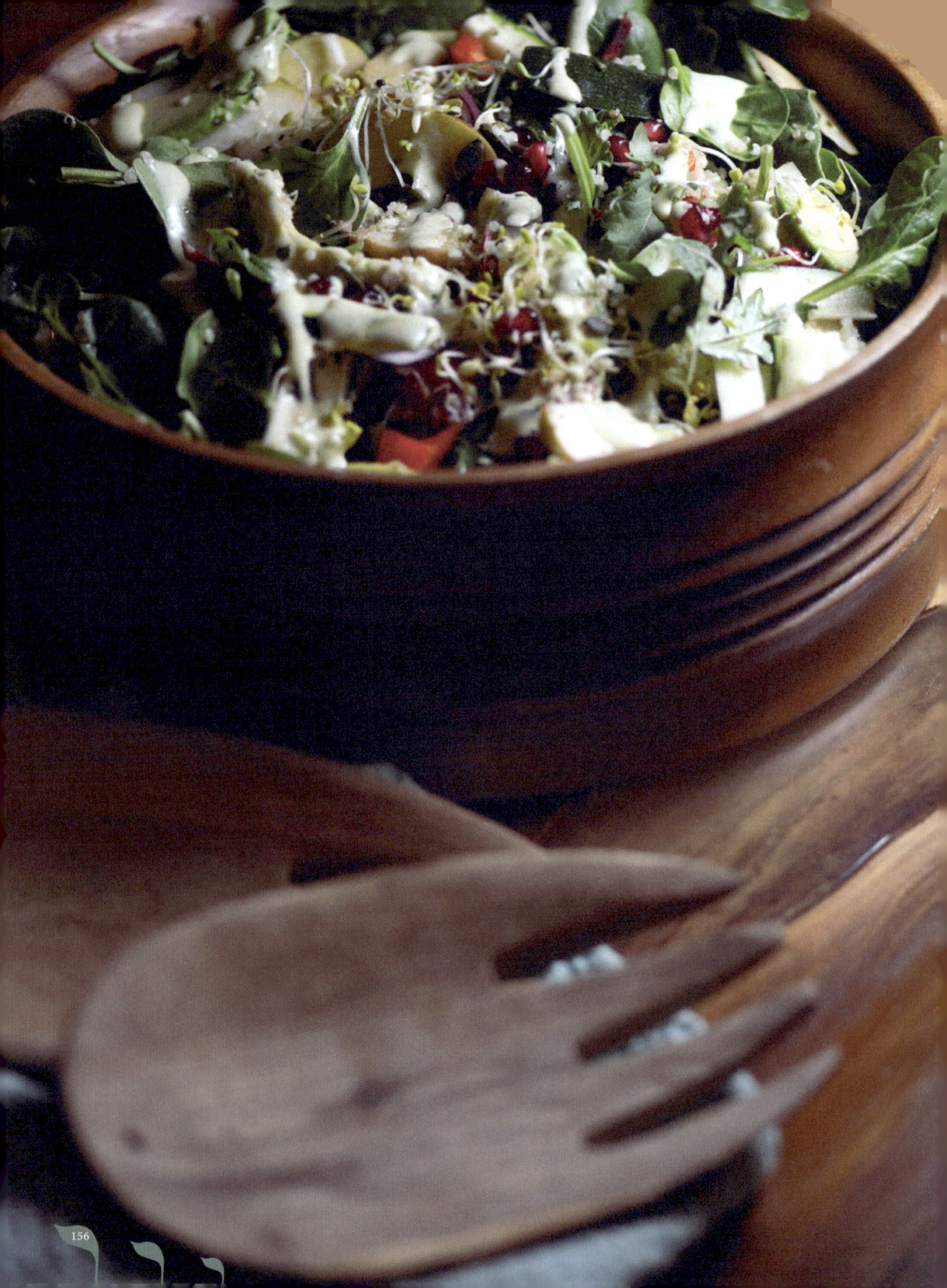

SUPER WORLD SALAD

SERVES 4 | ⏱ 35 MINS | GF DF V NF

"To start with, this serves 4 as a main course, but is the perfect dish as a heavenly side with simplistic roast potatoes or wholegrain pasta if your group size suddenly grows. Delicioso. See the WW Sauerkraut recipe on p213."

This salad truly encompasses the 'eat a rainbow a day' ethos; lots of colourful fruits and vegetables providing an amazing array of plant nutrients.

Red pepper, the brightest of all, contains beta carotenes which are anticancer nutrients and good for eye health too. Did you know though, that a green pepper has a higher concentration of vitamin C than an orange?

Healthy dressings can really pep up a salad and this is no exception.

Alfalfa sprouts are a great addition to any salad as they have very high levels of calcium. Any 'living foods' such as sprouted seeds will have higher concentrations of vitamins and minerals.

INGREDIENTS

SALAD
120g	Quinoa
150g	Baby leaf greens
150g	Spinach
1	Red pepper
½	Red onion
½	Courgette
100g	Pomegranate
1	Pear
1	Apple
1	Avocado
25g	Hemp seeds
20g	Pumpkin seeds
½ Handful	Alfalfa sprouts

DRESSING
80ml	Extra virgin olive oil
2 tbsp	Lemon juice
1 tsp	Runny honey
2 tbsp	Coconut yoghurt
1	Garlic clove
Handful	Fresh basil
Crack of	Black pepper

METHOD

1. Rinse the quinoa with fresh water, place in a pan of boiling water and simmer and for 15-18 mins. Once cooked, drain any excess water and allow to cool.

2. Wash the salad leaves and spinach, roughly chop and place in a large salad bowl with the quinoa.

3. Deseed the pepper and cut into thin strips. Peel and finely slice the red onion and finely slice the courgette.

4. Cut the pomegranate in half and hold over a large bowl, with a wooden spoon bash to knock the seeds out, pick out any bitter yellow membrane. Add the above prepared vegetables to the bowl and mix well.

5. Cut the pear and apple in halves and remove the cores, slice into slim wedges and add to the bowl.

6. Peel, destone the avocado and slice. Add to the salad along with the hemp and pumpkin seeds, alfalfa sprouts.

7. In a blender make the salad dressing. Finely chop the garlic add lemon juice, honey, coconut yoghurt, olive oil, basil and seasoning and blend until smooth. Drizzle over the salad and toss well.

*Sauerkraut recipe p213
A good side dish for this salad.

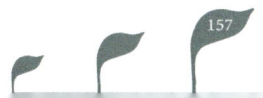

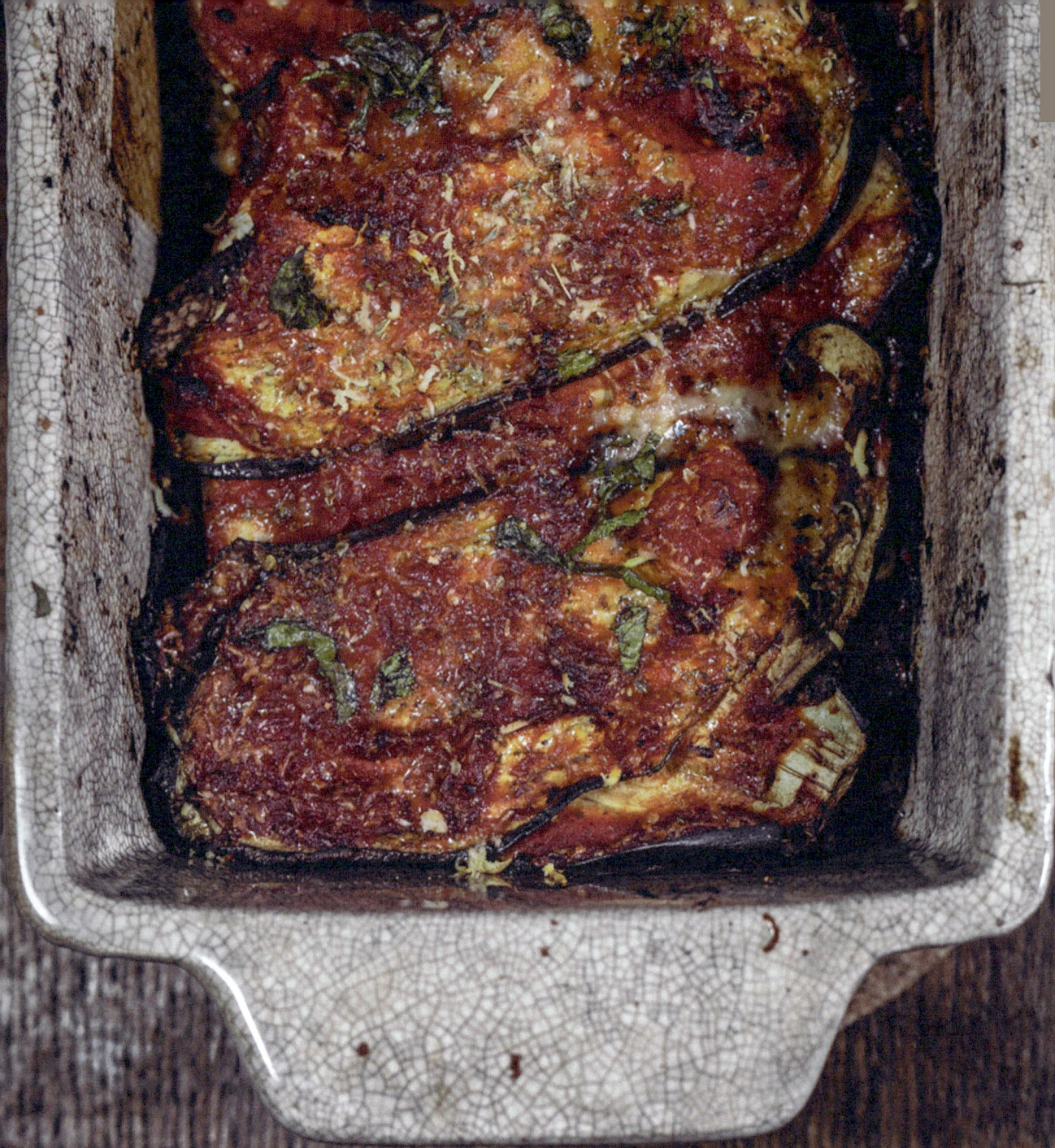

AUBERGINE LASAGNE

SERVES 4 | ⏱ 40 MINS | GF V NF

"Love love love love love. I see this as a vitamin laden version of lasagne, and perfect to cook for one or two with the same number of ingredients as eating the next day, I think grows the flavour."

A tasty twist on a pasta lasagne and full of exceptional antioxidants, such as anthocyanins and lycopene, which are due to the vibrant pigment of these vegetables.

Aubergines contain a particularly potent anticancer compound called solasodine rhamnosyl glycoside. They are also very rich in fibre and so beneficial to gut bacteria.

The egg and cheese provides some good quality protein. Add plenty of fresh basil as this will contribute to the nutrient density of the dish and aid digestion. The cheese also adds a good tasty crisp to the top of the dish. Texture is so important to me, it almost beats flavour.

The volatile oils in basil help to relax the smooth muscle of the digestive tract and dilate small blood vessels, making it a good antispasmodic.

It is also a good option to try it with extra cheese on top. Mozzarella is a recommended addition.

INGREDIENTS

4	Aubergines
6 tbsp	Olive oil
2	Garlic cloves
400g	Chopped tomatoes *(tinned)*
2 tsp	Tomato purée
2 tsp	Oregano
Pinch of	Sea salt
Crack of	Black pepper
100g	Parmesan
1	Egg
1 tbsp	Milk
handful	Basil

METHOD

1. Slice the aubergines lengthways into ½ cm thickness and brush with olive oil.

2. Heat the grill and in a single layer grill them on each side for 3-5 minutes until just golden.

3. Once all the aubergines are cooked, crush and chop up the garlic, add to a pan with a little coconut oil and gently cook for a couple of minutes, then add the chopped tomatoes, and simmer for 10 minutes.

4. Add the tomato purée and lightly chopped oregano and keep simmering for a further 5-10 min, season with salt and pepper, then turn off the heat.

5. Heat the oven to 180°C. In an oven proof dish place a layer of aubergines, top with a thin layer of tomato mix and a sprinkle of finely grated parmesan, repeating until all the ingredients are used.

6. Chop the basil leaves, whisk the egg with the milk, add the basil, remaining parmesan and a little seasoning and pour over the top of the spreading evenly. Place in the oven and bake for 30 minutes until golden.

Coconut Dhal with Spinach & Cumin

SERVES 4 | 🕐 50 MINS | GF V NF SS

"This is a heart and belly warming dish. Anyone who knows me, knows my mantra on green leafy veg, and this number is the king of greens. It enshines some of the most nutrient dense foods and can be used to jazz up many a dish. Retain their colour and vitamins by cooking for the briefest of moments and bulking them up with lentils, spices and cooling to taste with coconut.

I'd also say that the 'SS - Simply Smooth' choice is mine, soft enough for my body to handle back in the chemo days, and easy to digest."

This dish is packed with fibre and anti-inflammatory ingredients. Take a look at our list of healthy herbs and spices and you will see this recipe includes many of them. The fat in coconut milk can be easily converted in the body for energy. The lentils provide carbohydrate and protein, and along with the vegetables this makes for a very well balanced meal.

INGREDIENTS

4	Onions *(m)*
50g	Butter
3	Cloves of garlic
1 tsp	Cumin seeds
1 tsp	Whole black mustard seeds
3	Garlic cloves
2 tsp	Tumeric
½ tsp	Chilli powder
200g	Split red lentils
400ml	Coconut milk
4	Ginger slices
1 tin	Chopped tomatoes
250g	Baby spinach
Crack of	Black pepper
1	Lime
Handful of	Coriander

METHOD

1. Peel and slice the onions very finely, melt the butter in a large pan at a low heat, then add the onions and cook gently for 8 minutes until soft. Do not allow to brown.

2. Crush and chop the garlic cloves and add to the pan with the cumin and mustard seeds. Mix well and cook for a further 5 minutes.

3. Add the tumeric and chilli. Cook for 3 minutes.

4. Add the lentils, coconut milk, 400ml water, ginger, tinned tomatoes and lightly torn spinach. Mix well and then reduce to a gentle simmer to cook for 30 minutes until tender.

5. Finally crack the black pepper over the dish, squeeze the lime, chop the coriander and add to garnish to serve.

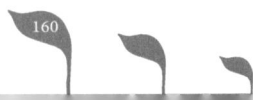

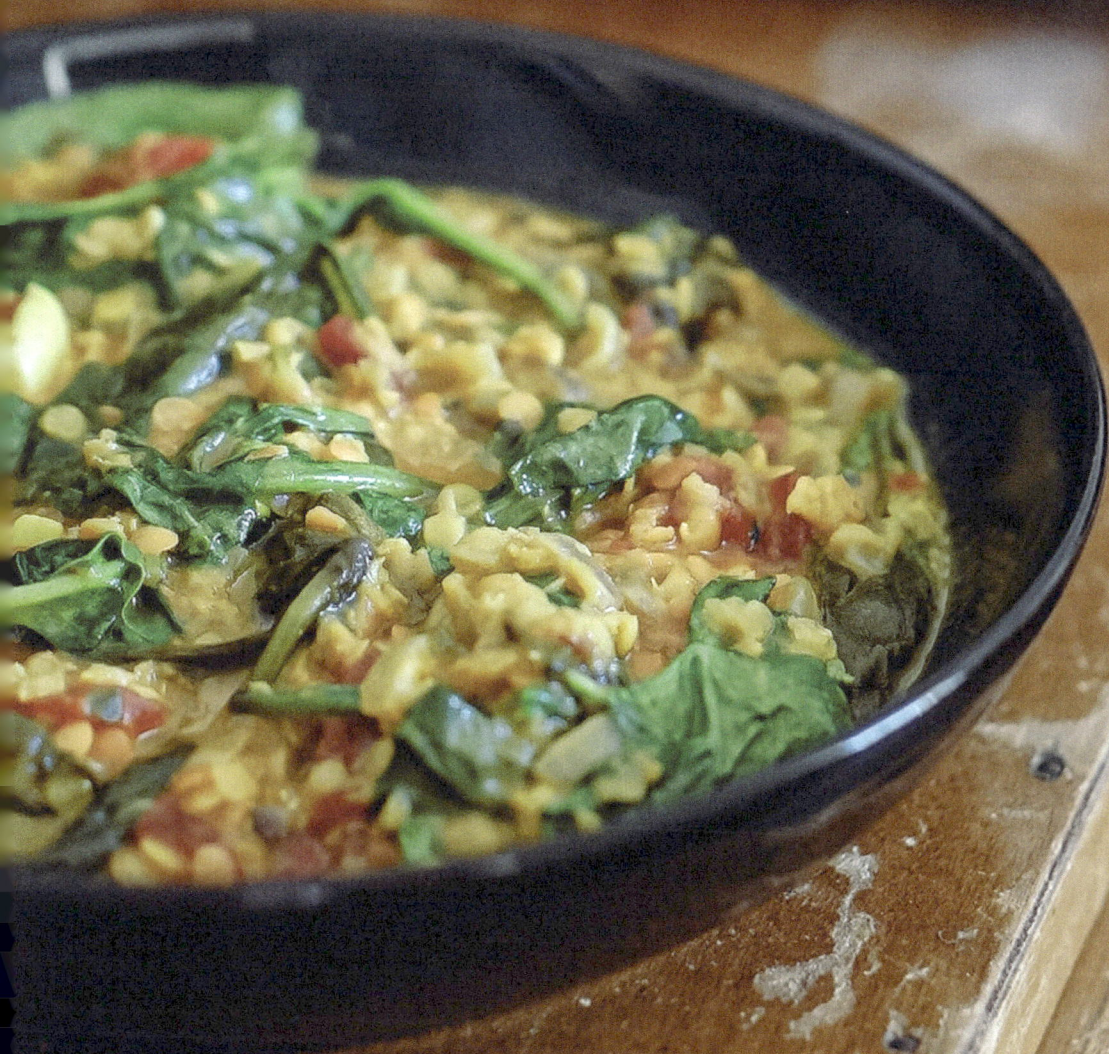

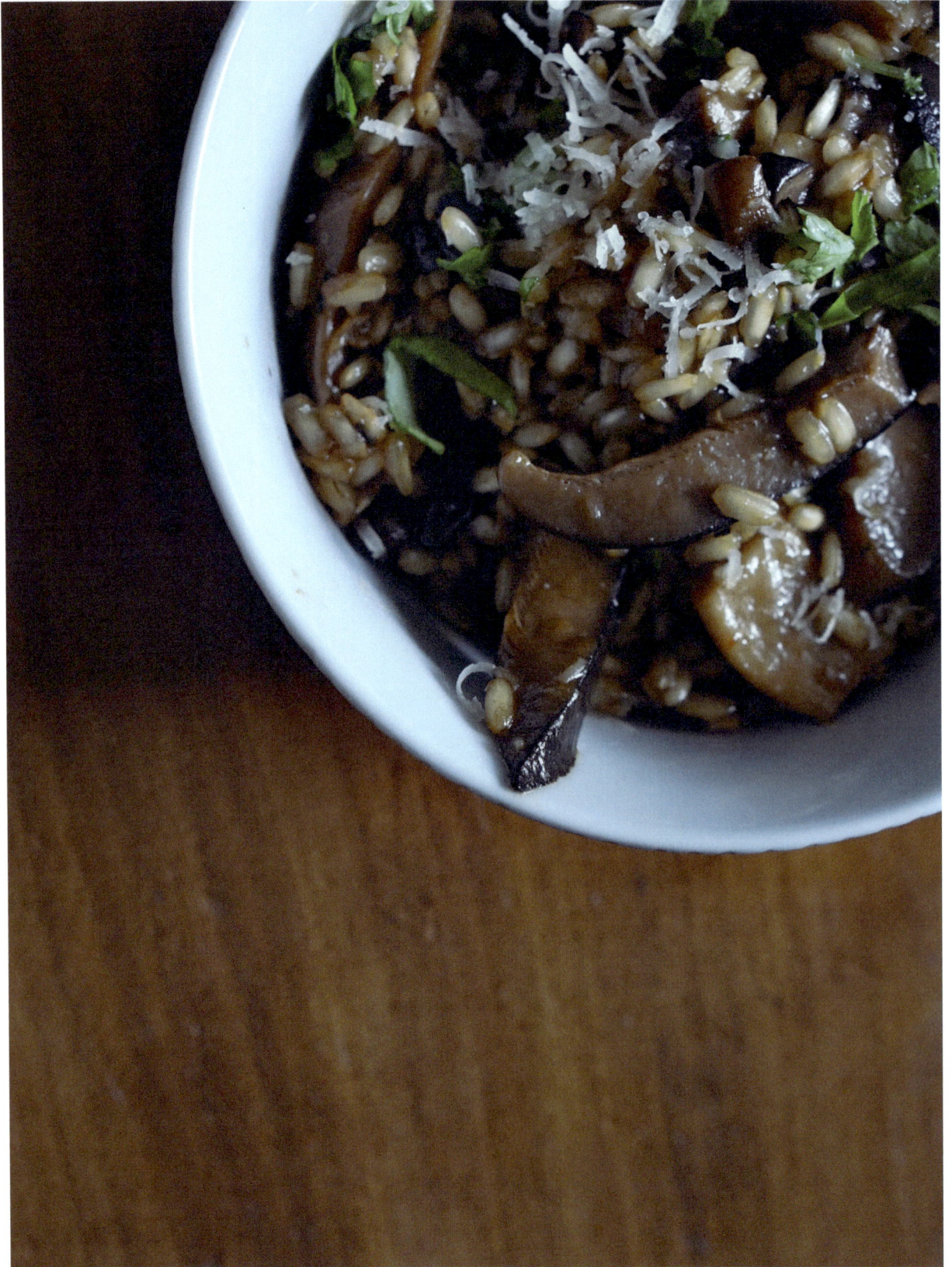

MUSHROOM RISOTTO

SERVES 4 | 🕐 1 HR 20 MINS | GF V NF

"This is a classic staple. But with a hint of extra health. The consistency is strengthened by the wholegrain risotto rice, which adds to the bite and texture, and enhances the amount of fibre in the dish."

The use of wholegrain risotto rice helps to lower the glycaemic effect of this dish, meaning it will have less impact on blood glucose levels. The flavour of a risotto is dependent on the quality of the stock. Use homemade stock for flavour and nutrient value. Mushrooms contain compounds which help support a healthy immune system along with protein, iron, B vitamins and anticancer minerals such as selenium. Add in plenty of parsley for its excellent nutrient profile which earns it a reputation as an efficient detoxifier.

INGREDIENTS

200g	Mushrooms
25g	Butter
1 tbsp	Olive oil
2 cloves	Garlic crushed
1	Shallot
300g	Wholegrain risotto rice
1.5 litres	Vegetable stock
75ml	Dry white wine
75g	Parmesan
Pinch of	Sea salt
Crack of	Black pepper
Handful of	Parsley

METHOD

1. Take your mushrooms, slice them, and fry them off in a small chunk of butter and drizzle of olive oil until just golden. Set aside for later, in a bowl.

2. Crush the garlic and finely chop the shallot. Melt half the remaining butter with the oil in the saucepan, add the garlic and shallot, and gently cook for 5 minutes over a low to medium heat. Do not allow to brown.

3. Add the rice to the pan and mix well, coating the grains in the oil and butter.

4. Heat the stock, add a ladle of the hot stock to the rice and mix well, over a medium heat. When the rice has absorbed the stock, add another ladle and stir well.

5. Repeat the above process with the remaining stock. This should take approx 40 minutes in total when the rice should also be perfectly cooked.

6. Add the mushrooms to the rice along with the wine, seasoning, chopped parsley, remaining butter and almost all the freshly grated parmesan cheese and mix well for 2 minutes on a low to medium heat.

7. Serve with a a crack of black pepper, pinch of salt and a little extra fresh Parmesan to add at the table.

8. Chop the parsley and scatter over the dish to serve.

You can switch the wine for vermouth, or use extra stock if you prefer..

1 If using dried mushrooms (chop into even sized pieces) add to the stock and gently bring to a simmer with a lid on for 15 minutes.*

4 Add a ladle of the hot stock and mushrooms and mix well, over a medium heat, when the rice has absorbed the stock add another ladle and stir well.*

163

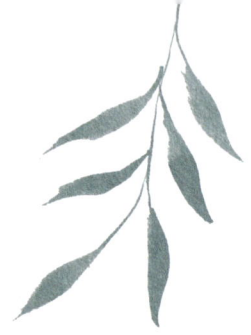

FUNGI

There is so so mush-room in our bodies and mind to accept these lovely land souls. Our world holds over 10,000 fungi species that create our delicious and nutritious mushrooms.

They are divided into three categories:
- edible mushrooms
- poisonous mushrooms
- magic mushrooms

The edible mushrooms are good sources of protein, vitamins (particularly B vitamins), minerals, antioxidants and fibre. They are also one of the few foods to contain some vitamin D. This amount can be boosted by putting your mushrooms in direct sunlight for 10-15 minutes, as their skin responds in the same way as humans to produce vitamin D.

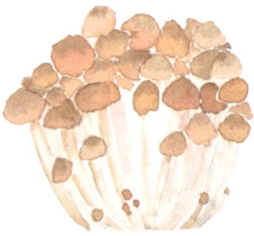

There has been a significant amount of research on mushrooms, particularly in Asia where medicinal varieties such as shitake, reishi and maitake are used in oncology to treat cancer, improve the effectiveness of chemotherapy and reduce its side effects.

Mushrooms contain compounds known as polysaccharides, which have been found to stimulate white cell count and dampen down inflammation. They are therefore considered excellent for supporting the immune system.

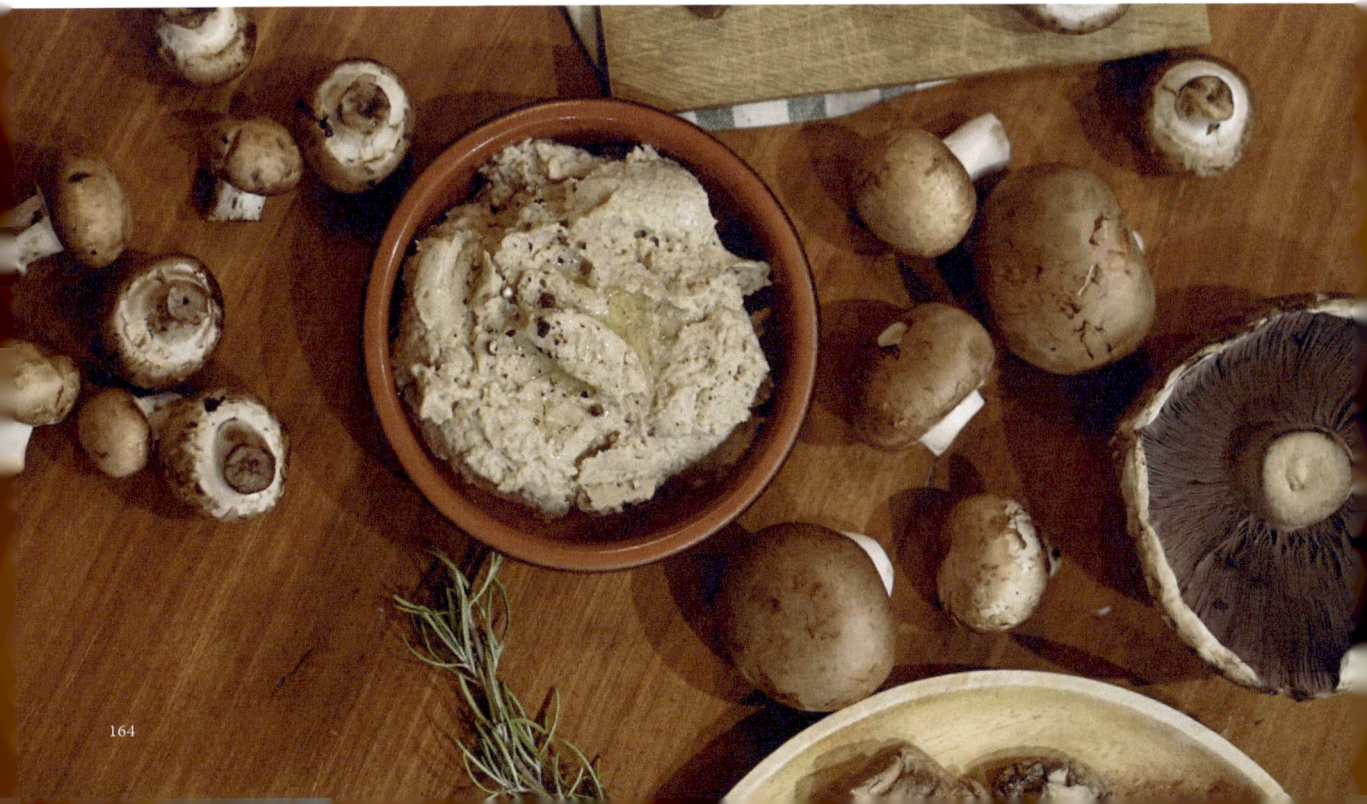

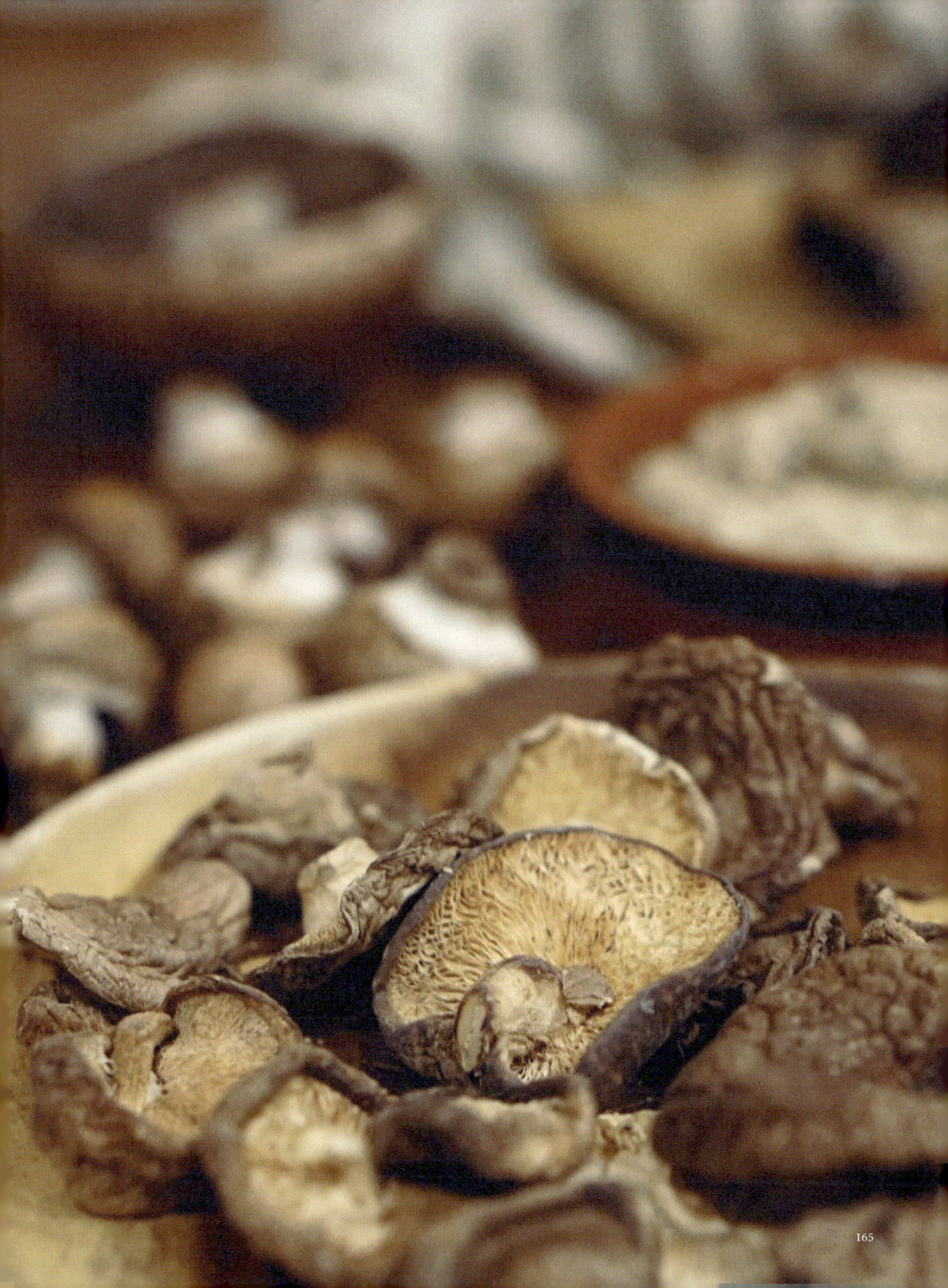

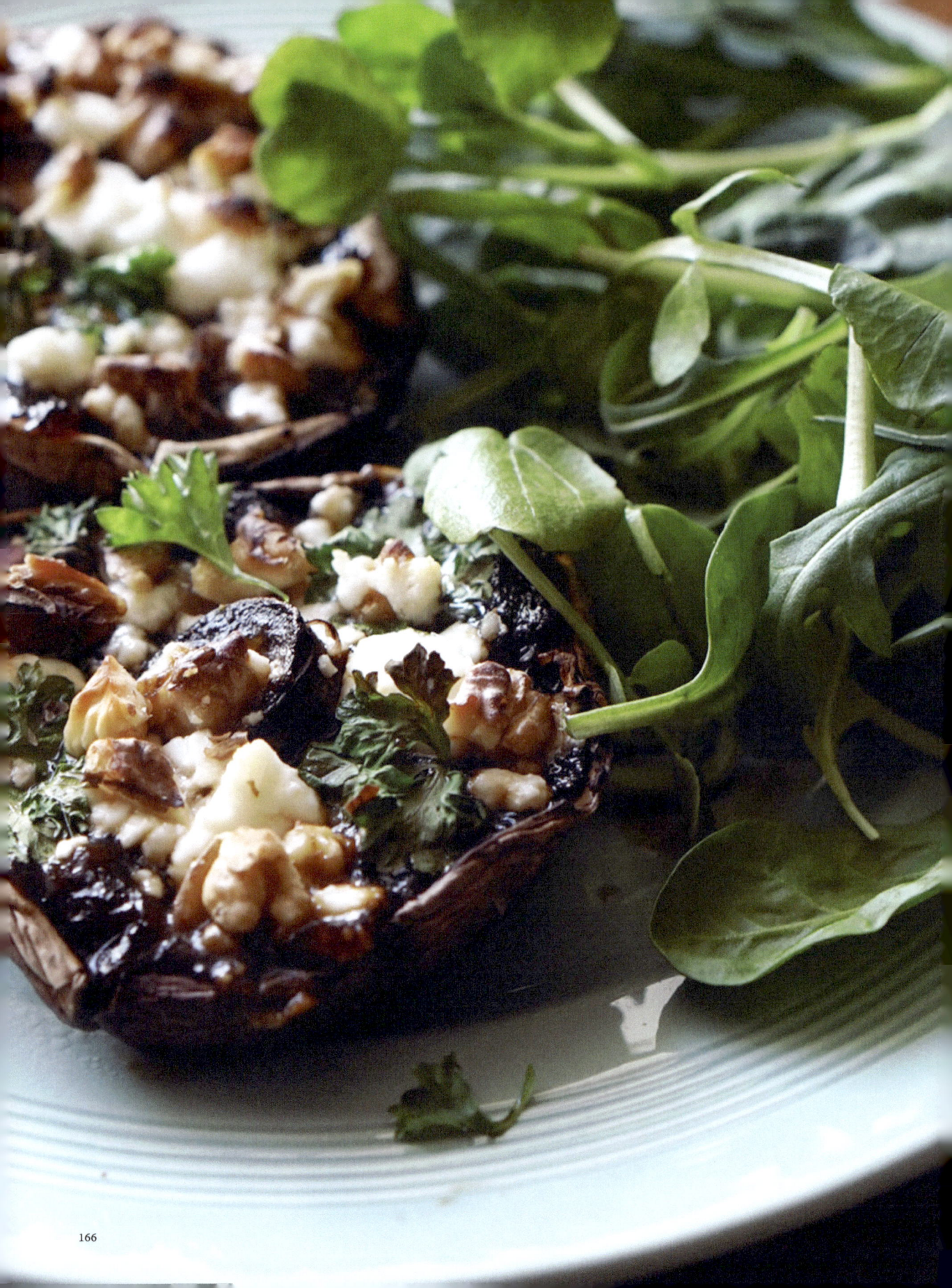

Roasted Feta & Nut Flat Mushrooms

SERVES 4 | 🕒 10 MINS | **GF** **V**

"I normally put these delicious flavours with a light set of greens, or maybe dauphinoise potatoes, depending on one's hunger!"

Mushrooms provide us with protein and compounds, known as beta glucans, which help to support our immune cells.

Feta adds to the protein intake — choose an authentic sheeps milk feta if possible.

Walnuts contain higher levels of antioxidants than any other nut and are a rich source of the anti-inflammatory omega 3 fatty acid, so are good for heart and brain health.

INGREDIENTS

8	Flat Mushrooms
8 tsp	Onion Chutney
	(see recipe p225)
4 sprigs	Parsley
60g	Feta
16	Walnuts

METHOD

1. Turn on the oven to 180°C.

2. Place the mushrooms on a tray with parchment and put in the oven to sweat for 10 minutes.

3. Take the mushrooms out, add the onion chutney, followed by the ripped parsley. Crumble on the feta, followed by the walnuts, which need a light chop or crush to sprinkle.

4. Switch the oven to a full temperature grill, and put back in for approximately 5 minutes, until it just starts to brown.

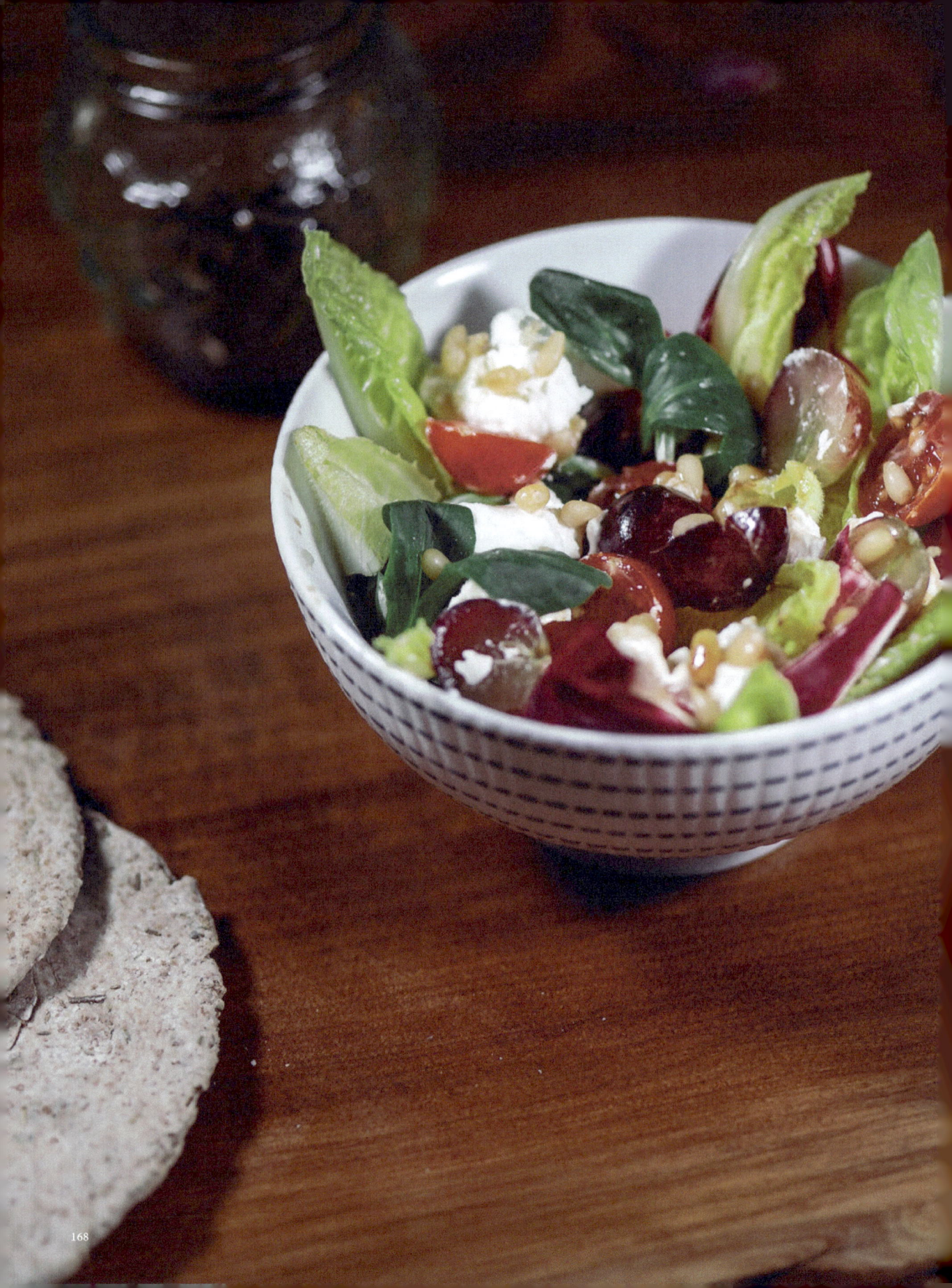

Goats Cheese Salad

"Found in semi-German notes by my man, so, though we used to make it together, pulling together old scribbled notes, rather than just making it from scratch was a little more effort for me and my friend, Jani. Especially after the brain op; as I was so forgetful, I made her translate it twice, but can now enjoy in galore during the warm months of the year."

Eating sheep or goats cheese can be a healthier option than cows as humans are able to digest the proteins more easily. You can now often buy raw sheep or goats cheese which contain probiotics meaning that it will be good for your gut too. However if your immune system is compromised then you need to be cautious.

Grapes are a lovely addition to a salad — the darker the grape colour the more antioxidants they contain. Black grapes would be a good choice. A good mix of leaves including some of the more bitter leaves such as raddichio and chicory are good choices as bitter leaves assist digestion.

INGREDIENTS

2 tsp	Dijon mustard
2	Garlic cloves
Pinch of	Sea salt
Crack of	Black pepper
1 tsp	Balsamic vinegar
½	Lemon
3	Olive oil
60g	Pine nuts
240g	Mixed lettuce
	romain, chicory
	radicchio, lambs tongue
100g	Cherry tomatoes
100g	Seedless red grapes
200g	Goats cheese

METHOD

1. Make the dressing in a jam jar or in the serving salad bowl: 1 tsp dijon mustard, garlic cloves crushed and finely chopped, a pinch of sea salt, and a twist of black pepper.

2. Mix well until blended. Add the balsamic vinegar and squeeze of lemon and mix, finally drizzle in the olive oil and whisk vigorously, taste and adjust if needed.

3. In a pan gently toast the pine nuts until golden.

4. Wash and dry the salad, place in a serving bowl, cut the tomatoes and grapes in half and scatter over the salad.

5. Crumble over the goats cheese. Drizzle the dressing when serving.

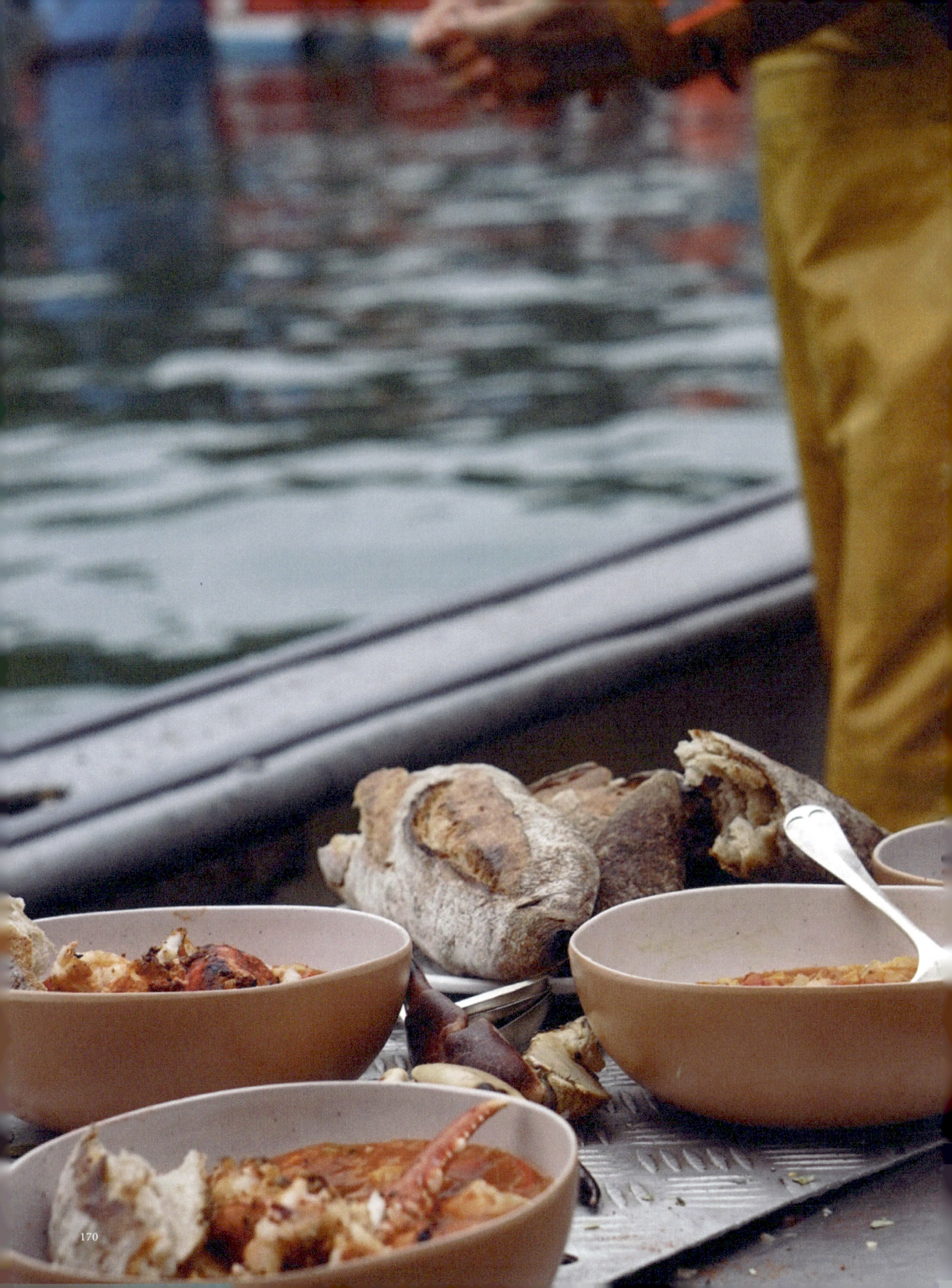

SOMETHING MORE OCEAN?

With much of our soil depleted of various minerals especially zinc, selenium and iodine... A good way to combat this deficiency is by eating seafood and sea vegetables which are bathed in the abundant minerals in the sea.

Zinc, selenium and iodine, are particularly important for immune support, reducing cancer risk and supporting detoxification.

Seaweed is also a great option for vegans and vegetarians as it has good levels of protein and vitamin B12.

---

*Tissues of the breast and prostate appear to have a high affinity to iodine and a deficiency may be linked to an increased risk for these cancers.
Sea vegetables are an excellent way to increase iodine intake.

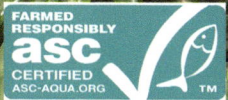

Fish can be an excellent protein source. Often referred to as brain food, it is nutrient dense and can include high levels of the very important brain nutrient Omega 3. It is also one of the few foods which can contain vitamin D. Fatty fish such as salmon, sardines, mackerel, and herrings are considered the healthiest options.

However, fish can also contain high levels of dioxins and mercury. These toxins can accumulate in our body and may damage organs — especially the brain. Microplastics have also been found to accumulate in fish. It's important to have large fish varieties such as tuna and swordfish with time for your body to refresh inbetween dishes, as they have been living in the ocean longer so they have absorbed more toxic products. Most bodies can handle them if regulated. Just don't eat them too often!

We should think responsibly when buying fish and choose local, trusted suppliers who can guide us on the most sustainable varieties. Ideally this should be non-trawler catch as this method of fishing is the most destructive for marine life and the ocean floor.

Some responsibly farmed fish may be a good choice. Eat organically farmed to avoid antibiotic issues and look for 'Aquaculture Stewardship Council' certification to help inform you of best practice.

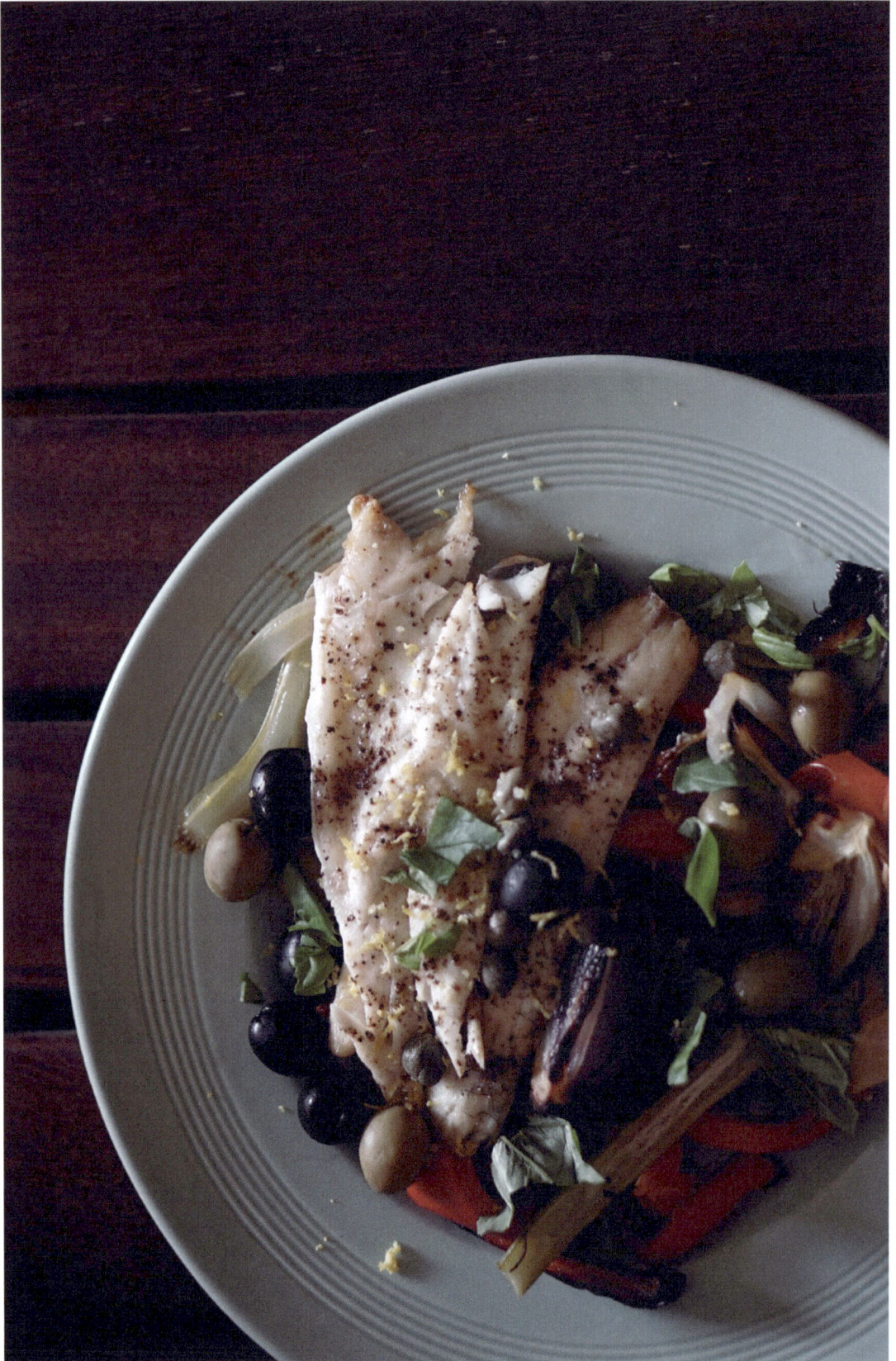

Mediterranean Roasted Cod, Fennel & Olive

SERVES 4 | 🕐 35 MINS | GF DF NF

"It's very easy to make a dish that goes really well with warm focaccia bread or brown rice; the fish can be changed for whatever is available or looks best at your fish counter, think salmon, mackerel, haddock, trout or tuna."

Fish is a great source of protein and has a reputation for being 'brain food'. It is rich in iodine, vitamin B12, niacin, phosphorus, selenium and a good source of anti-inflammatory omega 3.

This dish is also packed with vitamins, minerals and antioxidants from the peppers, tomatoes, fennel and red onions. Adding olives, capers, lemon and the herbs increases the nutrient profile of this dish considerably.

Olives and capers are good sources of calcium and iron. Basil helps to aid digestion.

INGREDIENTS

2	Red peppers
6	Tomatoes
1	Red onion
1	Fennel bulb
2	Garlic cloves
3 tbsp	Olive oil
4 x 200g	Cod loins *(skinned)*
75g	Black olives *(pitted)*
75g	Green olives *(pitted)*
25g	Capers
1	Unwaxed lemon
Pinch of	Sea salt
Crack of	Black pepper
Handful of	Fresh basil

METHOD

1. Heat the oven to 200°C Gas 6.

2. Cut the peppers into strips, halve the tomatoes, quarter the onion, finely slice the fennel and finely chop the garlic. Then place the vegetables into a roasting pan, add olive oil and toss well to coat

3. Place in the oven and cook for 15 minutes.

4. Remove and add the 4 pieces of portioned cod, season well and return to the oven. Cook for a further 12 minutes until the cod is done.

5. Add the olives, capers, lemon zest and juice then return to the oven for a couple of minutes to warm.

6. Serve garnished with fresh torn basil.

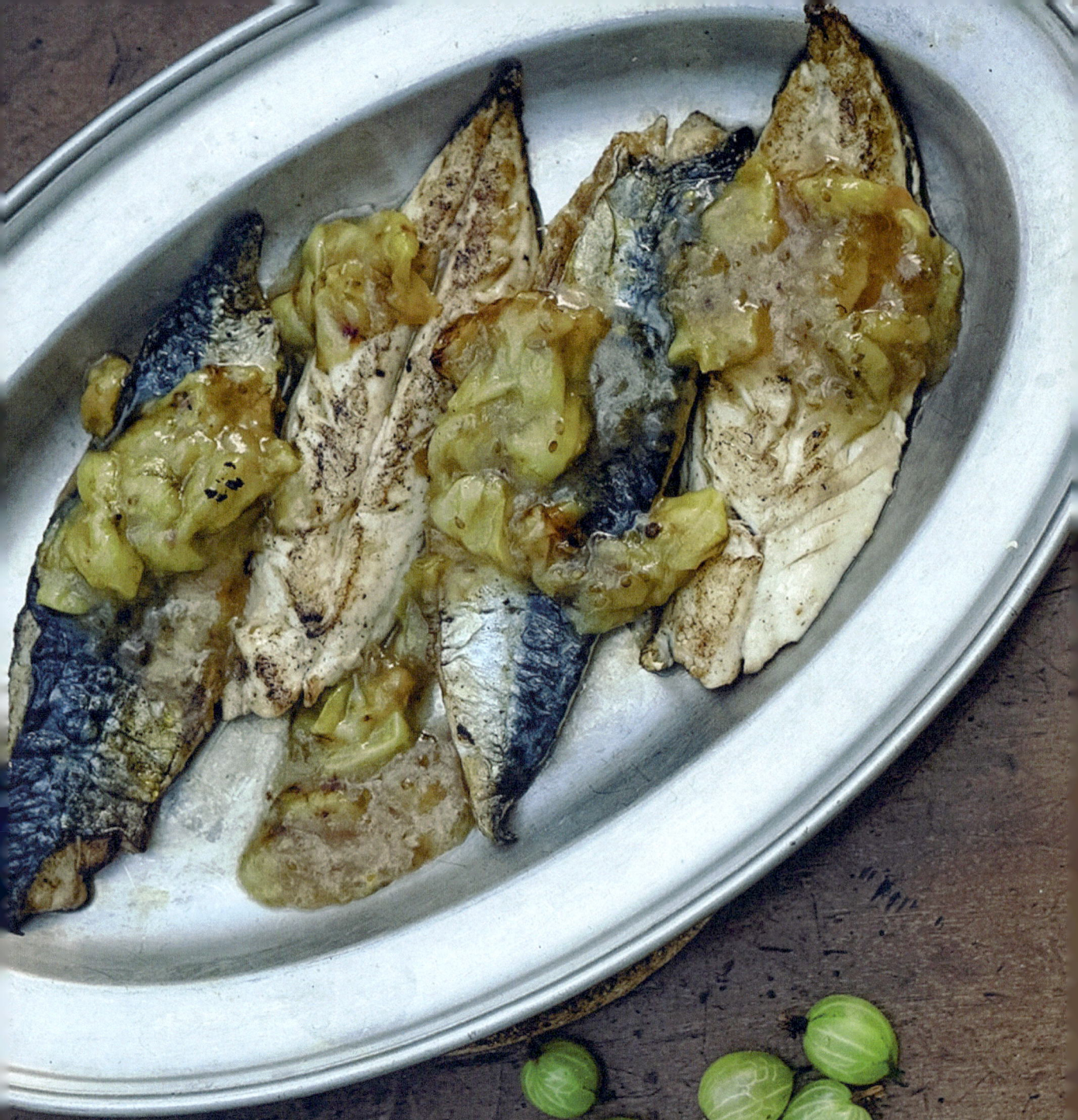
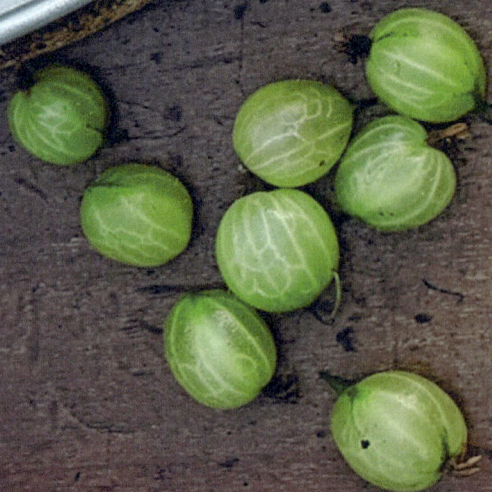

174

MACKEREL WITH GOOSEBERRIES

SERVES 4 | ⏱ 30 MINS | GF NF

"Tart gooseberries cut through the richness of this superb oily mackerel fish, making a good balance of flavours. If you are by the sea and lucky enough to have caught your own, after gutting they can be cooked and served whole (they will just need a little longer cooking). This is a great dish as a light but nutritious meal or as a larger meal add new potatoes and a salad. "

Gooseberries, being a tart fruit, contain very little sugar and are therefore low in calories and have little effect on blood glucose levels.

They are an excellent source of fibre, along with vitamin C, copper and other antioxidants which provide potential anticancer effects and immune support.

Adding to the healthy profile of gooseberries is the oily fish mackerel. Mackerel is rich in omega 3 and is one of the best sustainable fish.

INGREDIENTS

300g	Gooseberries
15g	Butter
2 tbsp	Honey
2 tbsp	Rapeseed oil
4	Mackerel fillets

METHOD

1. Trim the gooseberries, add to a small pan with melted butter and gently simmer on a low heat with a lid on for 10 minutes, stirring from time to time. Add the honey, slightly increase the heat and cook until reduced and a nice coating consistency. Cover the pan and turn the heat off.

2. Gently heat a large pan with the rapeseed oil, score the skin side of the mackerel, place skin side down and cook for 3-4 minutes. Quickly flip over with a pallet knife and cook for 2 minutes.

3. Serve with the gooseberry sauce.

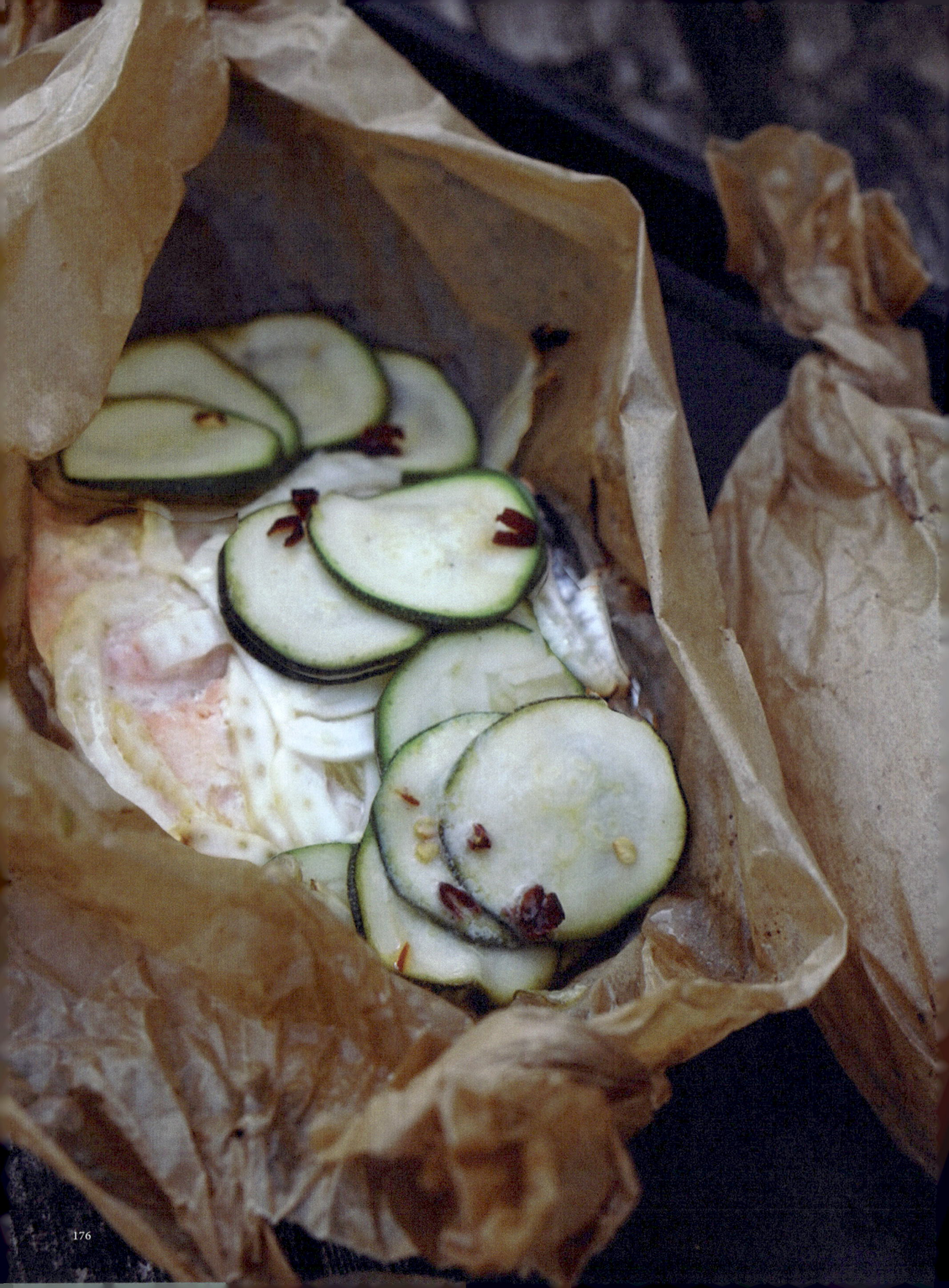

Spiced Steamed Salmon Parcels

SERVES 4 | ⏱ 30 MINS | GF DF V NF

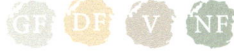

"Easily made dairy free by switching the butter to coconut oil for a light flavour twist. A good and easy one for a home dinner event, and I generally serve it with a seasonal salad, and wholegrain rice, brown or black for the texture."

Cooking this way is a perfect method for retaining all the cooking juices, nutrition and flavour. Fennel is a healthy, healing vegetable and good for bone health too, providing vitamin C, manganese, calcium, potassium and magnesium. Salmon is classed as an oily fish and so contains the anti-inflammatory fat omega 3 which is so important for brain and general health.

INGREDIENTS

4	Salmon fillets
1	Fennel bulb
1	Courgette
1	Red chilli
½	Lemon
Pinch of	Sea salt
Grind of	Black pepper
40g	Butter / Olive oil

METHOD

1. Heat the oven to 180°C. Take 4 large sheets of baking parchment. To wrap the salmon and veg, fold each sheet in half and reopen. In the middle, toward the folded seam place the salmon skin side down.

2. Finely slice the fennel and courgette (a mandolin is really good for this) divide and arrange on top of the salmon, repeat with the courgette, add some chopped chilli, a squeeze of lemon, seasoning and 10g butter/olive oil per portion.

3. Fold the paper over the ingredients and roll all the edges inwards towards the ingredients sealing it and making a parcel. Another way is to double fold in and then use a stapler to secure, but this is not the traditional way and dose not look as nice at the table.

4. Place the parcels on a couple of baking sheets and put in the oven, cook for 6 minutes, then rotate in the oven and cook for a further 5 minutes.

5. Remove from the oven, use a spatula to lift onto dinner plates. Allow each parcel to be opened on by those at the table to release the delicious aroma and steam.

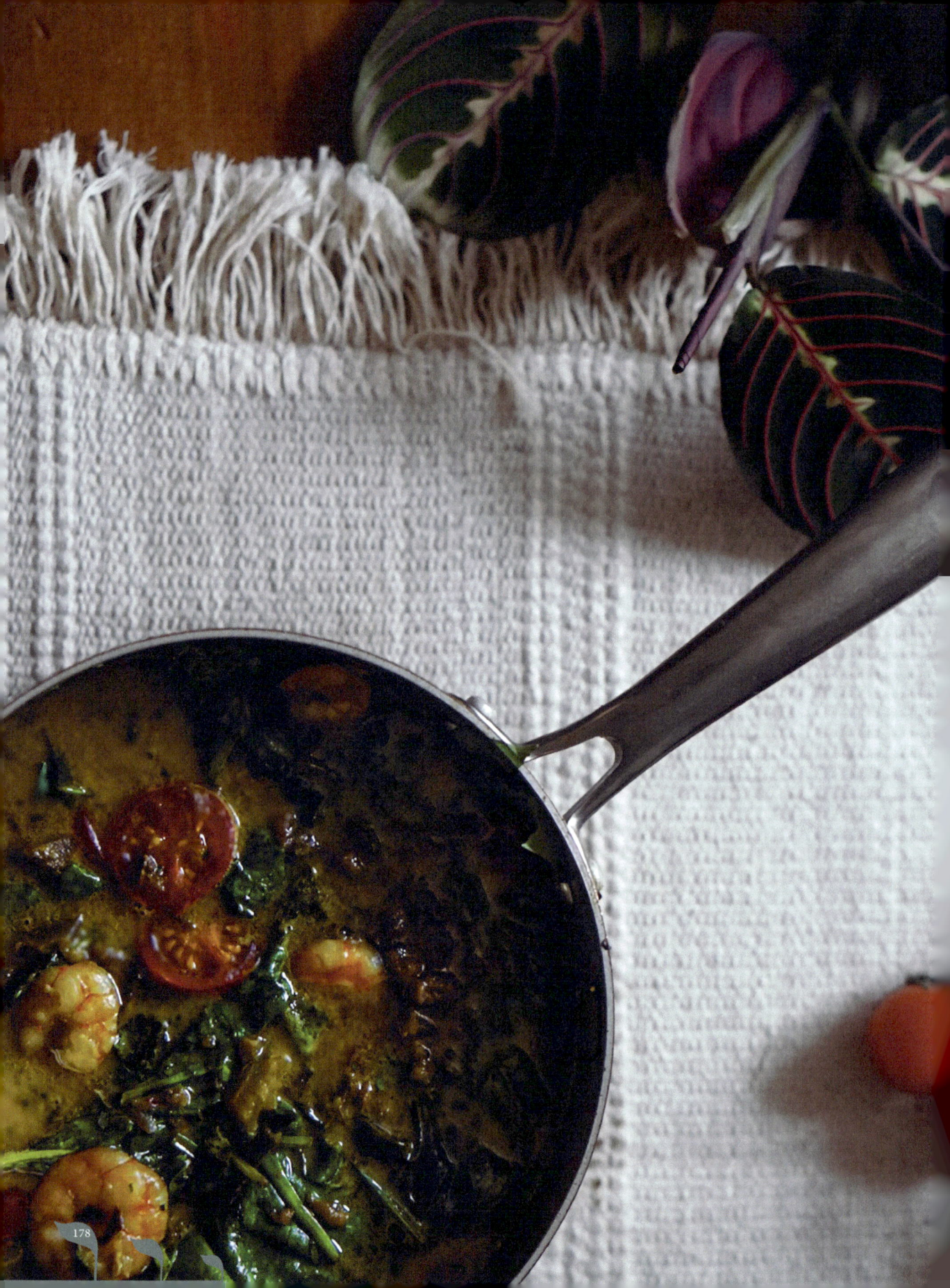

PRAWN CURRY

SERVES 4 | 🕐 40 MINS | GF NF

"A deliciously vibrant dish full of wondrous nutrients to fill your seafood soul. So quick and simple, it's a perfect midweek number to spice up your life."

With an array of spices and herbs, homemade curries generally make a fabulously filling and healthy meal and this is no exception.

It includes aubergine, spinach and tomatoes providing a good amount of fibre and packed with antioxidants.

Coconut milk and oil are an excellent source of energy. packed with antioxidants, coconut oil and milk for a good source of energy.

INGREDIENTS

2 tbsp	Coconut oil
½	Red onion
3	Garlic cloves
1	Red chilli
	(use ¼ of the seeds)
1cm²	Ginger
2 tsp	Cumin
1 tsp	Garam masala
1 tsp	Turmeric
½ tsp	Sea salt
½ tsp	Black pepper
2 tsp	Coriander
1	Celery stick
1	Aubergine
190ml	Vegetable stock
1 can	Coconut milk
1 thumbsize	Coconut cream chunk
150g	Cherry tomatoes
250g	Tiger prawns
250g	Spinach

METHOD

1. Heat the coconut oil until nicely melted in a large pan.

2. Finely chop the onion, garlic, chilli and ginger and add to the pan so that it lightly browns.

3. Add the additional herbs, spices, salt and pepper to cook so that all flavours unite while you cut the celery into thin slices to add into the pan.

4. Chop the aubergine into large-ish pieces and add it to the pan.

5. Add the stock and mix to ensure the flavours are spread evenly.

6. After 10 minutes, add in the coconut milk along with the coconut cream (which is used as a sauce thickener). Slice the tomatoes in half and just throw them in alongside the prawns. Wait until warm and the prawns are perfectly pink before adding the spinach to the top of the pan.

7. Put the lid on as the spinach steams, and open occasionally to mix it through.

8. The second the spinach has slightly wilted, it's ready to serve.

FISHIE PIE

SERVES 4 | 🕐 30 MINS | GF NF

"Serve with a lightly dressed and simple leafy salad, like rocket, spinach, watercress and tomatoes. This is one of my favourite bits that is twistable to however you are feeling. I love adding veg like leeks or peas to the filling, and changing the fish to whatever is tastily brought in by the local fishers."

A tasty, creamy fish pie can be the ultimate comfort food. Sweet potatoes are more nutrient dense than ordinary potatoes especially as they contain beta-carotene.

Most fish counters in supermarkets have off cuts of fish for fish pie so this dish can easily be kept within a budget. Frozen and well sourced fish is well worth it too.

Leek really lends itself well in flavour to fish and provides some good prebiotic fibre for feeding your microbiota. Mushrooms add additional protein and an array of therapeutic, immune boosting properties and is why they are one of our top ten anticancer foods.

INGREDIENTS

TOPPING
500g	Sweet potatoes
250g	Potatoes
Pinch of	Sea salt
30g	Butter
3 tbsp	Milk
Pinch of	Fresh nutmeg
Crack of	Black pepper

INSIDE THE PIE
20g	Butter
100ml	Milk
300g	White fish *(skinned & frozen)*
300g	Wild salmon *(skinned & frozen)*
200g	King prawns *(peeled & frozen)*
250g	Mushrooms
3	Garlic cloves
1	Leek
50g	Petit pois *(frozen)*
350ml	Double cream
100g	Cheddar cheese

METHOD

1. Preheat the oven to 180°C. First make the mash potato topping. Peel both varieties of potatoes, cut into even sized pieces and place in a pan. Cover with salted water, bring to the boil and simmer for 20 mins until soft. Drain well.

2. Return potatoes to the pan and stir on a low heat to rid excess moisture for a minute, then mash until smooth, adding the butter, milk, nutmeg and seasoning. Cover with a lid and place to one side.

3. Butter a roasting pan with another 10g butter, add the milk, white fish, salmon and prawns, cover with foil and cook for 10 mins. Remove from the oven and leave to cool.

4. In a pan melt the remaining 10g butter, slice the mushrooms finely, chop the garlic and add both to the pan. Cook on a medium heat until golden. Slice the leeks finely and add to the mushrooms and cook for a further 5 minutes. Add the petit pois and cream and bring to a gentle simmer for 2 minutes.

5. In a medium sized oven proof dish flake the cooked fish, discard the milk, add the prawns and top with the creamy mushroom and leek mix.

6. Carefully spoon on the mashed potato mix, and create a pattern with a fork, sprinkle the cheese onto and bake in the oven for 20 mins.

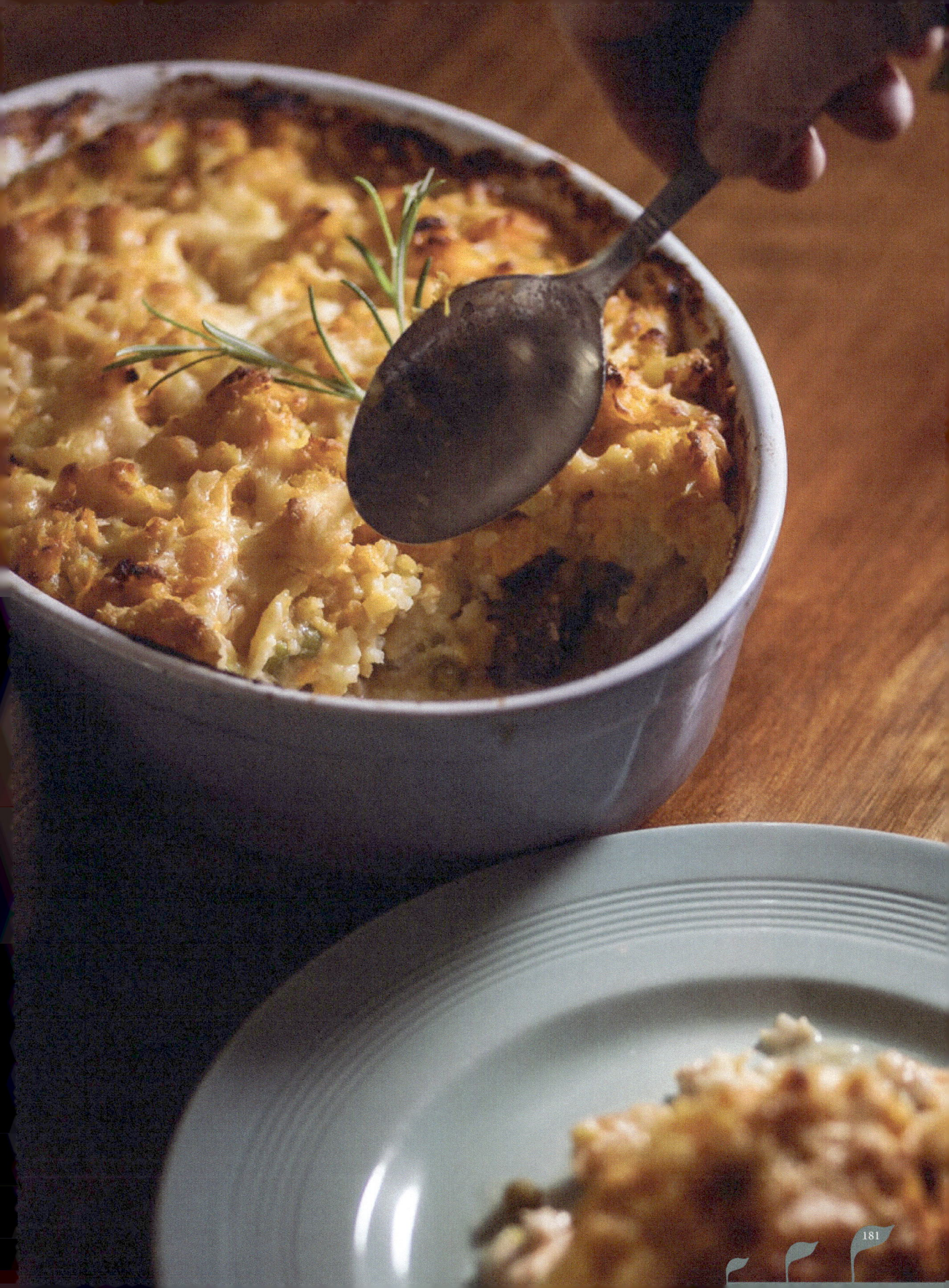

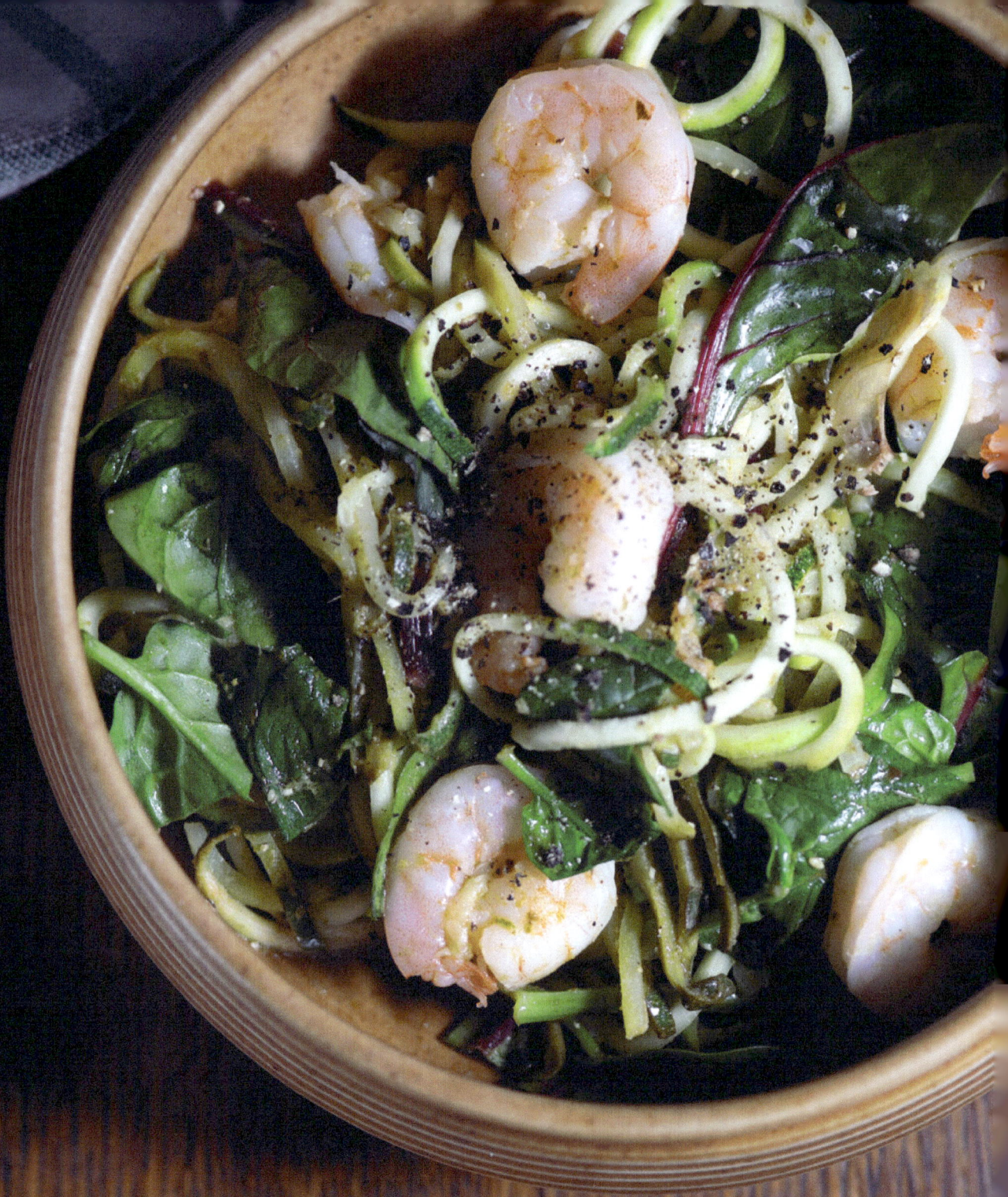

PRAWN COURGETTI SPAGHETTI

SERVES 4 | ⏱ 10 MINS | GF NF

"I pulled together some of the delicious leftover ingredients when spring was kicking in 'et voila'. I think that the courgetti is lighter than the classic pasta and gives you that mildly more crunchy and less weighted aftermath than spaghetti."

Courgetti spaghetti is a wonderful healthy low-carb alternative to wheat laden pasta. Along with the chard and spinach, you have 3 of your 8 a day in one dish. Topping with peas shoots adds in more nutrient value especially vitamin C. You can easily grow your own pea shoots on a window sill.

Prawns should be ethically sourced as prawn farming is a dirty industry! You can buy organically farmed which is the best choice.

Do not eat seafood if you are neutropenic (low white cell count) as you are more vulnerable to food poisoning.

INGREDIENTS

4	Courgettes
2 tsp	Coconut oil
400g	King prawns
8 tsp	Green pesto
2	Lemons
100g	Spinach
200g	Red chard
Pinch of	Sea salt
Twist of	Black pepper
4 tbsp	Crème fraîche
50g	Pea shoots

EQUIPMENT

Spiralizer

METHOD

1. Pull out your spiralizer and get to work on the courgettes. Quick and simple — very satisfying!

2. Heat the coconut oil in a large frying pan, add the prawns and just as they start to turn pink, add in your courgette and toss well, cooking for just 2 minutes. The easiest way to toss your courgette is using two large wooden spoons to keep turning the mixture over.

3. Spoon in the pesto and lemon juice along with the spinach, chard and seasoning. Toss well cook for a further minute.

4. As it cools, mix in the crème fraîche and garnish with pea shoots to enjoy.

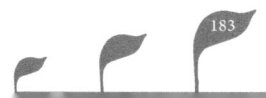

ALMOND COATED FISH & CHIPS

SERVES 4 | ⏱ 30 MINS | GF

"A great way of satisfying any cravings for fish and chips. Just a light twist with the type of oil and coating grains. A bit trickier than my other dishes, you need a trial or two get it right, or you can just grill the fish with lemon, salt and pepper!"

This recipe uses an ultra healthy batter to coat the fish, full of healthy fats from the almonds and no gluten. Frying the fish in coconut oil which is a saturated fat means that the oil is more stable and less damaged when heated to a high temperature. Cod/hake/halibut are classic fillets; go for de-boned deskinned.

Accompany with celeriac or sweet potato chips cooked in coconut oil (they are seriously delicious) and you don't have to feel guilty at all.

INGREDIENTS

100g	Almond flour
	(ground almonds)
25g	Coconut flour
1 tsp	Baking powder
Pinch of	Sea salt
Crack of	Black pepper
1	Egg
100ml	Double cream
600g (4x 125g)	Cod fillet
6 tbsp	Coconut oil
2	Limes

METHOD

1. In a bowl mix the almond and coconut flour, baking powder and seasoning. Whisk the egg and cream together. Make a well in the middle of the flour mix, add the liquid and whisk until smooth.*

2. Dip the fish pieces in a dusting of dry almond flour and then dunk in batter, coating all over.

3. Melt the coconut oil in a large nonstick pan.

4. Carefully place the battered fish in the oil and cook on each side until golden, approx. 2-3 minutes. If your pan is not big enough cook in batches and keep warm in the oven.

5. Remove and place onto kitchen paper to absorb excess oil, and serve with a segmented lime half.

Add a splash more milk to lighten your batter if needed.

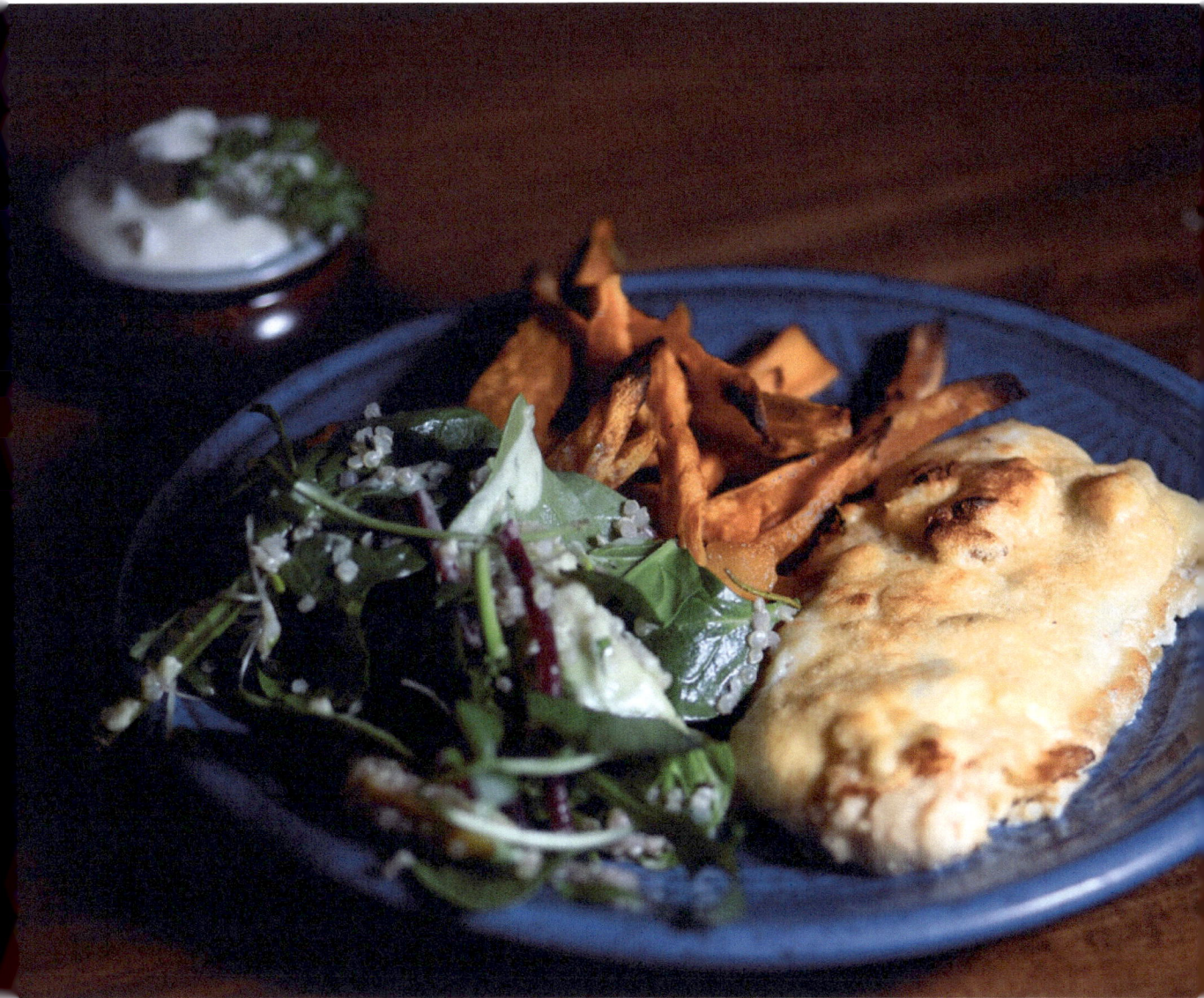

Lamb Kofta Salad & Spelt Flatbread Wrap

SERVES 4 | 🕐 1 HR | GF DF NF

SALAD | DF V VE NF

"This may seem lengthy, and have lots of different stages but believe me it makes a wonderful meal and is great for sharing. The flatbreads are made with baking powder so that they can immediately be made without having to prove."

The koftas can be made by spearing them, once shaped, onto 4 metal skewers, especially if using a low sided pan.

With plenty of herbs and spices, these koftas with this colourful salad provide a healthy low carb meal packed with protein, vitamins and minerals. If you are adding some carbs then these low gluten, homemade flat breads are a welcome addition.

-

Find the Spelt Wrap recipe on p208.

INGREDIENTS

KOFTA
Bunch of	Fresh mint
2	Garlic cloves
1 tsp	Coriander
400g	Minced lamb
1 tsp	Cumin
¼ tsp	Chilli powder
Pinch of	Sea salt
Crack of	Black pepper
Dribble of	Olive oil

SALAD
¼	Iceberg lettuce
½	Red onion
1	Tomato
1 bunch	Fresh mint
1 bunch	Fresh coriander
1	Carrot
1 tbsp	Olive oil
1	Lemon

METHOD

1. Start by chopping up the mint, peeling, crushing and chopping the garlic cloves, and mixing with the chopped coriander and all the other kofta ingredients. This is best done by hand to get a good even blend.

2. Divide the mixture into 4, shape and roll into sausages, and brush with olive oil.

3. Heat a griddle pan and when hot place the koftas on to cook for 4 minutes on each side. Do not move before or they will stick. Turn and repeat until cooked on all sides.

4. Slice up the lettuce, red onion, tomato and herbs. Grate the carrot and place with all other salad ingredients in a bowl and toss well, coating the salad with the oil and juice from the lemon.

5. Serve alongside the spelt flatbread (p208) and salad.

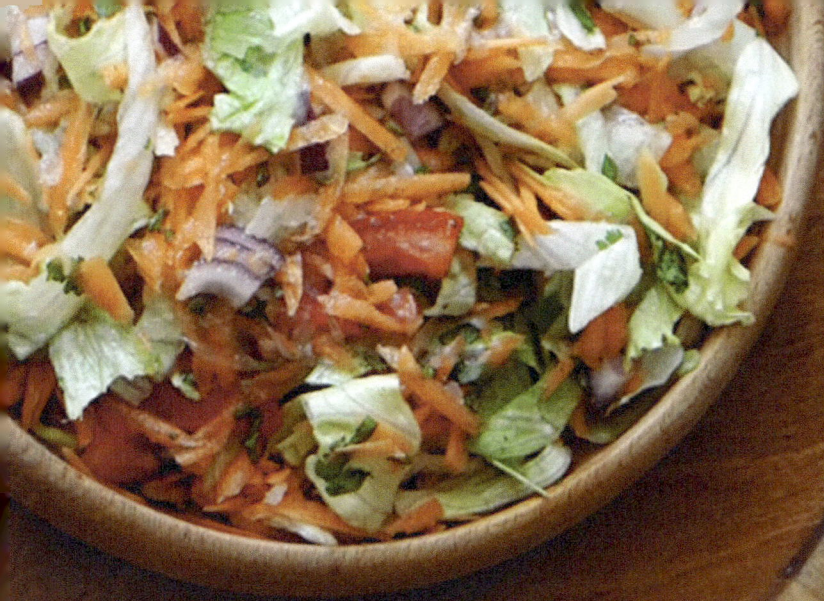
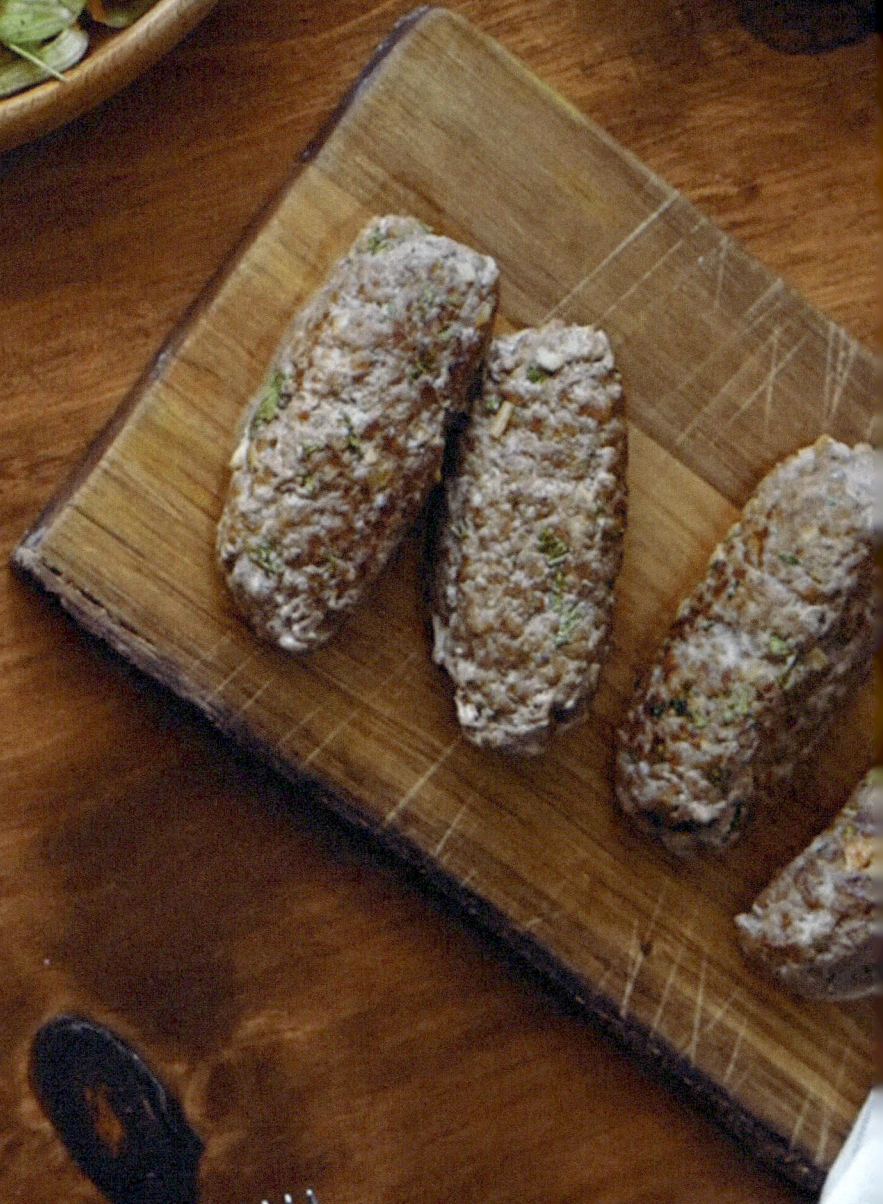
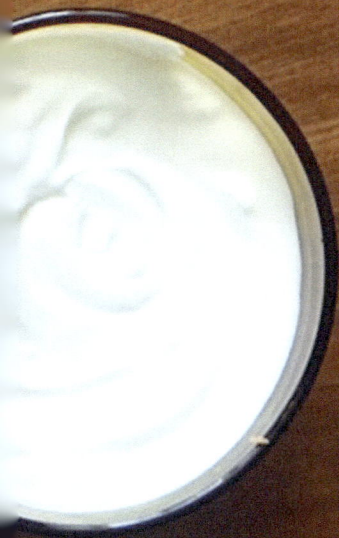
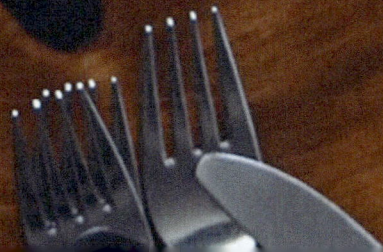

Lemon Chicken Freekeh

SERVES 4 | 🕐 45 MINS |

"This is a sort of take on risotto but without the cheese. It can be served with a spoonful of yoghurt and a scattering of pomegranate — (yes, I'm addicted pomegranate), if you wish to take it to a superior presentation level!"

Freekah is an ancient grain made from green durum wheat. It is high in fibre and protein and contains good levels of manganese, magnesium, niacin and phosphorus to support bone health.

The almonds provide healthy essential fatty acids and further protein. Onions are included in our top anticancer foods as they contain important sulphur compounds and flavonoids.

Lemons and their zest provide vitamin C and a plentiful supply of antioxidants. Chop in a good handful of parsley for its super detoxifying properties.

INGREDIENTS

25g	Butter
2 tbsp	Olive oil
2	Red onions
1	Garlic clove
4	Chicken breasts *(skinless)*
200g	Freekeh
½ tsp	All spice
400ml	Veg/Chicken stock
2	Unwaxed lemons
75g	Whole toasted almonds
Pinch of	Flat leaf parsley

METHOD

1. Melt the butter and oil in a large heavy based pan. Dice the onions and cook gently for 10 minutes until just coloured. Crush, peel and chop the garlic, then add to the pan to cook for a further 5 mins on a low heat.

2. Chop the chicken into even sized pieces, add to the pan and gently cook to seal the outside.

3. Add the freekeh, spice and mix well. Pour in the stock, stir and bring to the boil, then reduce the heat to a gentle simmer, place a lid on and cook on a low heat for 12 minutes.

4. Zest and juice the lemons, and set to the side.

5. Check and stir the liquid, which should have almost all gone. If not, increase the heat a little and stir to evaporate off.

6. Then remove from the heat and add the lemon juice, half of the almonds and half the parsley and stir through.

7. Sprinkle over the remaining almonds, parsley and lemon zest to serve.

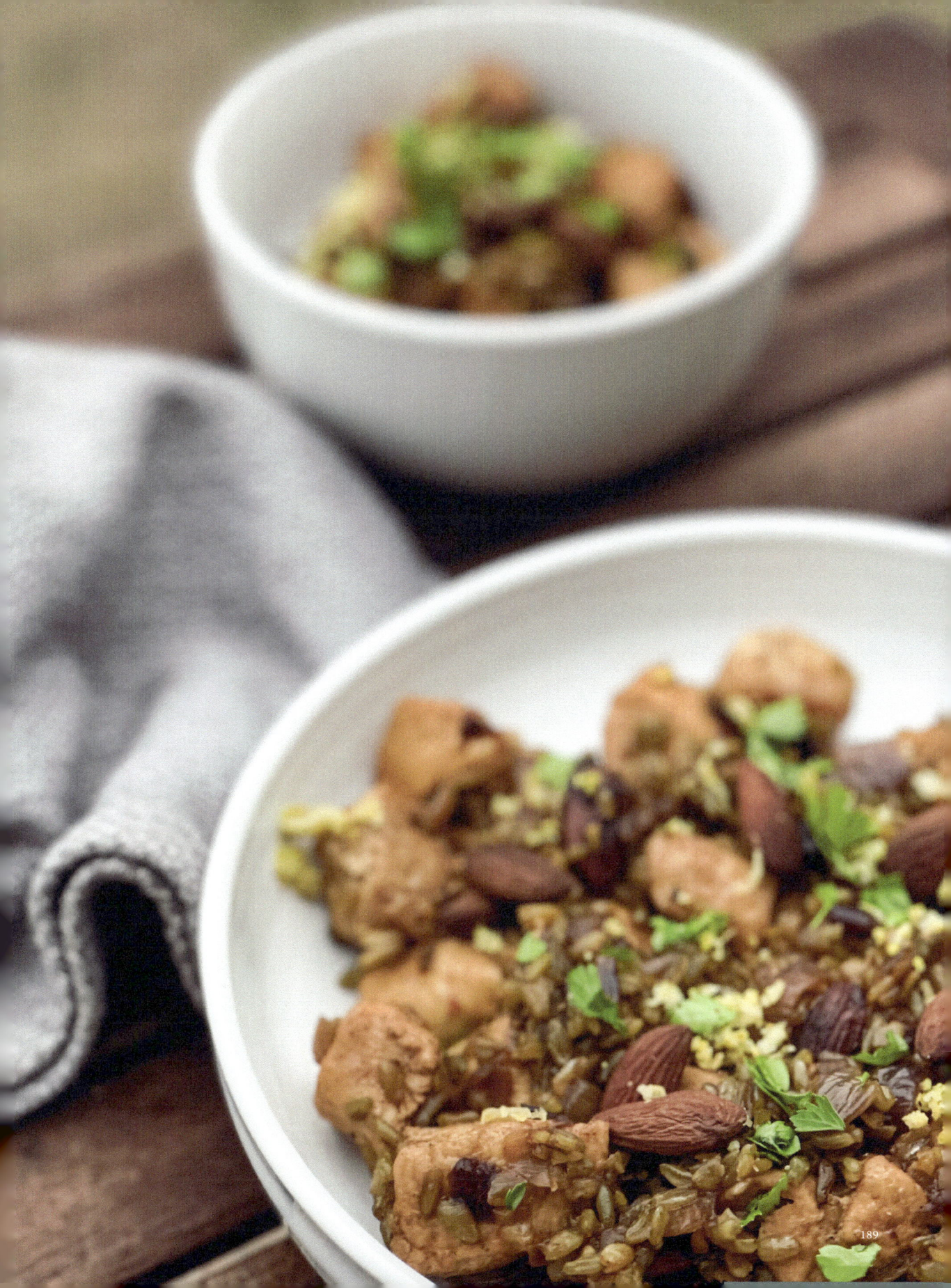

SPICES

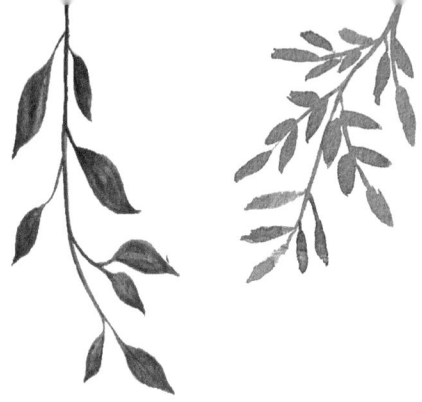

Cumin is one of my top delights, as it has a complex flavour which works well with so many foods. It can also be made into tea by boiling cumin seeds and then allowing to infuse for 10 minutes, and it's particularly known for its digestive properties as it stimulates the release of pancreatic enzymes (which benefits your digestion) and bicarbonate to neutralize stomach acid as it enters the small intestine.

Adding a variety of spices to your cooking literally does add to the spice of life! So many spices have been found to have very important anticancer and anti-inflammatory benefits.

Turmeric (Curcumin) has long been used in Ayurvedic medicine. Curcumin, the active ingredient in turmeric, is now hailed as one of the most important anti-inflammatory and anticancer compounds. There is a wealth of research to back this and I would recommend that you add raw turmeric (now easily available) as part of your daily diet. Three grams a day of fresh or dried turmeric is safe for most people to take.

Curcumin is not easily absorbed by the body but absorption can be aided by taking it alongside black pepper and fats.

Ginger is a similar spice to turmeric, and has also been shown to have many anticancer properties, one of the main ones being its anti-inflammatory effects. However some research on breast cancer stem cells demonstrated that a compound called 6-Shagaol found in ginger has powerful anticancer activity particularly in targeting stem cells which can be the cause of chemo resistance in some cancers. Ginger has also been shown to reduce fasting blood sugar levels and increase insulin sensitivity which is important for creating an environment in the body which is hostile to cancer cell growth.

Cinnamon has been shown to have the potential to stimulate circulation, aid digestion, act as an anti-convulsant and has antibiotic properties. It has also been shown that just a ¼ tsp a day can help to lower blood glucose levels over a period of time.

Chilli contains capsaicin which appears to have many anticancer properties. In a test tube it was found to induce cell death in prostate cancer cells.

Coriander has many health supporting and healing benefits. Use as a seed, ground or the leafy herb, where you can chop the stalks and the root into dishes for added health benefits. Research found that coriander seeds help to regulate blood glucose levels.

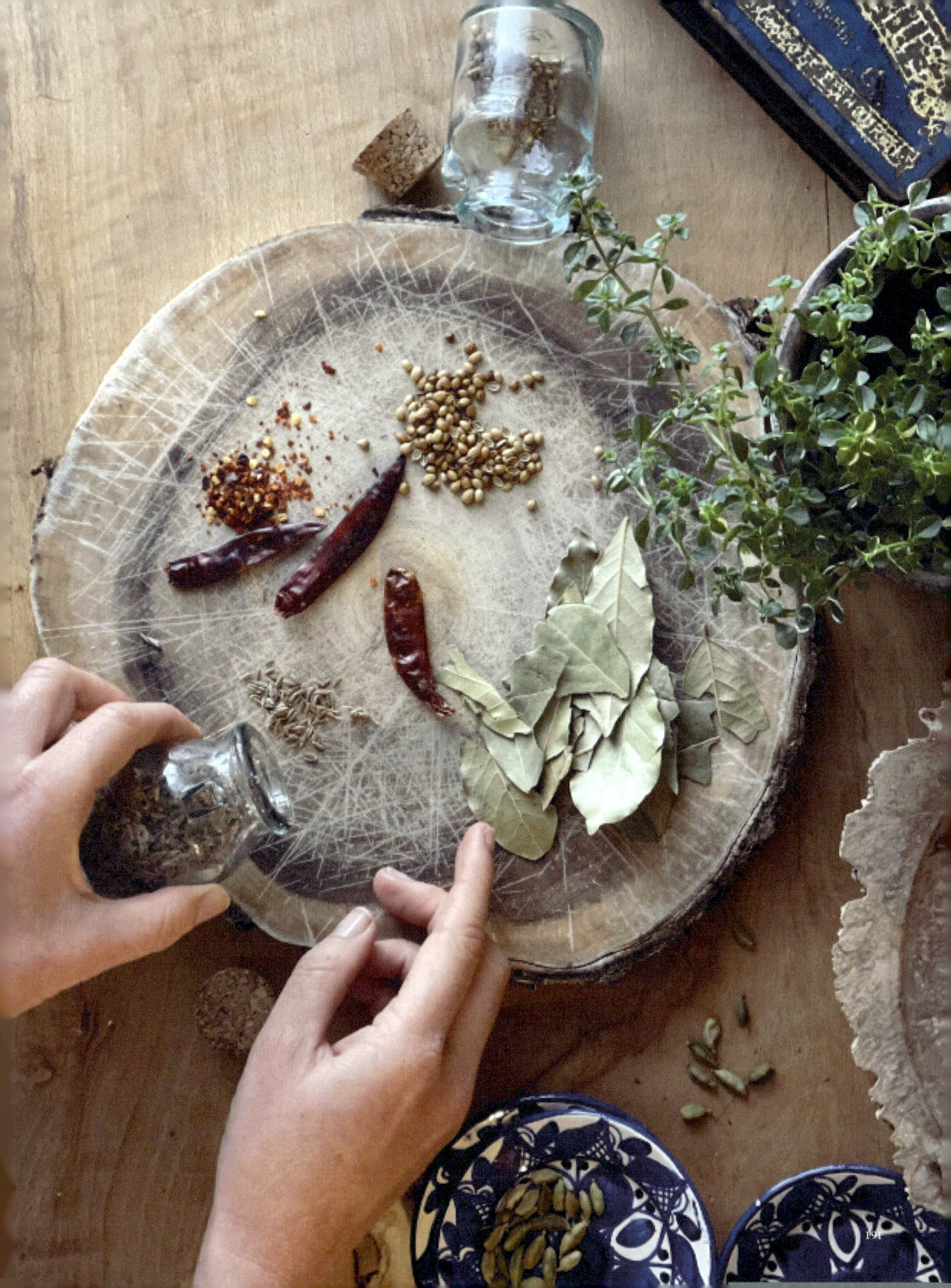

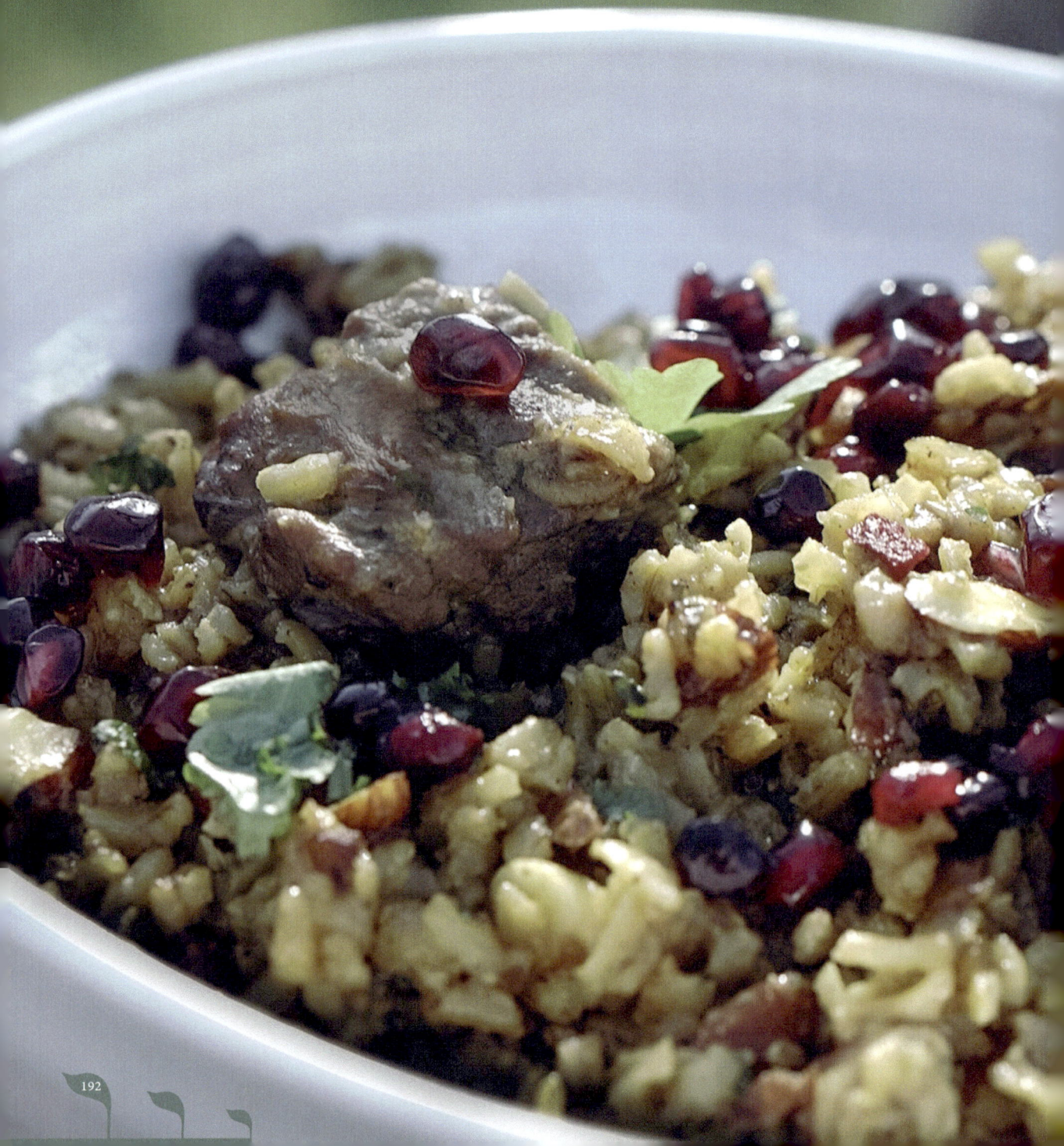

Iranian Lamb & Spiced Rice

SERVES 4 | 🕐 1 HR 30 MINS | GF DF

"A strongly satiating aromatic dish. It is smooth, but textured with nuts and freshened by the herbs and pomegranate."

The wonderful spices and herbs provide an anti-inflammatory profile to this dish.

Turmeric, which includes the important active compound curcumin, has had considerable research looking at its anti-inflammatory, anti-thrombotic and anticancer properties. Needless to say we should be adding turmeric to our food wherever we can. Best taken with black pepper as this aids the absorption of curcumin. Pomegranates are little gems of health benefits. They have been shown to protect against many cancers, particularly prostate cancer, and they are also protective of the heart and brain.

Lamb is a good choice of meat if you don't know the source as it is generally grass-fed. Adding the almonds and herbs to the rice raises the nutrient value with healthy fats and antioxidants.

INGREDIENTS

300g	Lamb *(neck fillet)*
2 tbsp	Olive oil
1	Onion
1	Garlic
3 tsp	Ground turmeric
1 tsp	Cinnamon
1 tsp	Cumin
¼ tsp	Nutmeg
1	Cinnamon stick
Pinch of	Sea salt
Crack of	Black pepper
1 litre	Chicken stock
150g	Brown rice
75g	Almonds
1 bunch	Mint
1 bunch	Flat leaf parsley
4 tbsp	Pomegranate jewels
	- seeds -

METHOD

1. Cut the lamb into 5cm discs, heat the oil in a shallow pan and brown off the lamb on a medium heat.

2. Chop the the onion, crush and dice the garlic, add to the pan, and cook for a further 5 minutes until soft. Sprinkle in the spices; turmeric, cinnamon, cumin, nutmeg, a cinnamon stick, and seasoning. Mix well.

3. Pour in the chicken stock and simmer with a lid on for 30 minutes.

4. Add the rice, mix well, place a tight fitting lid on and cook on a low heat for 40 minutes, stirring occasionally.

5. After this the liquid should have absorbed and the rice will be tender — if it needs further cooking add more liquid.

6. Roughly chop the almonds, mint and parsley, and add to the pan as well . Cook for 2 minutes whilst stirring, before topping with the pomegranate.

Ribbon Steak, Tender Stem & Asian Salad

SERVES 4 | 🕐 40 MINS | GF DF

"Really good with flat rice noodles if you need a hint more of a filler. This is a dish packed with healthy vegetables and flavouring. 'Studies show that grass-fed beef has less total fat than regular beef and contains more Omega-3 fatty acids, both of which are beneficial to your heart' [1]*"*

Lime juice and zest provides a good amount of vitamin C which will help to absorb the haem-iron from the meat.

The chilli contains capsaicin which gives it the pungent taste plus other antioxidant carotenoids which all provide numerous health benefits including anticancer benefits. Red chillis are richer in antioxidants than immature green ones.

The addition of beansprouts enhances the nutritional punch as sprouting greatly increases the nutritional value, protein, and digestibilty of the dish. Tenderstem broccoli is one of our top anticancer foods. The peanut butter, sesame seeds and oil provide some healthy fats, but make sure you heat them very gently so the fragile fats do not get damaged.

INGREDIENTS

1 tbsp	Olive oil
300g	Rump steak
-	
2	Unwaxed limes
1 tbsp	Peanut butter
2 tbsp	Soy sauce
4 tbsp	Sesame oil
1	Red chilli *(diced)*
1 clove	Garlic
400g	Tender stem brocolli
1	Carrot *(large)*
100g	Beansprouts
Bunch of	Coriander
1 tbsp	Toasted sesame seeds
Crack of	Black pepper

METHOD

1. Heat the oil in a pan and cook your steak for three minutes on each side for rare. Remove from the pan and place to one side allowing it to rest.

2. Prep the limes by getting them zested and juiced. In a small pan add the lime juice (save the zest for final stage), peanut butter, soy sauce, sesame oil and very gently heat, stirring frequently until smooth. Add a couple of tbsp of warm water if the sauce is too thick.

3. Dice the chilli and garlic, add them to the pan, and remove from heat and place to one side.

4. Trim the broccoli and cook for 2 minutes, then drain. Grate the carrot and mix together with the tender stem and bean sprouts. Chop the coriander and add alongside the dressing and toss well coating the vegetables. Arrange onto plates or one big platter.

5. Thinly slice the rested steak (across the muscle grain is best), it should be pink and juicy inside. Arrange on top of the salad, sprinkle with the toasted sesame seeds, a twist of pepper and lime zest.

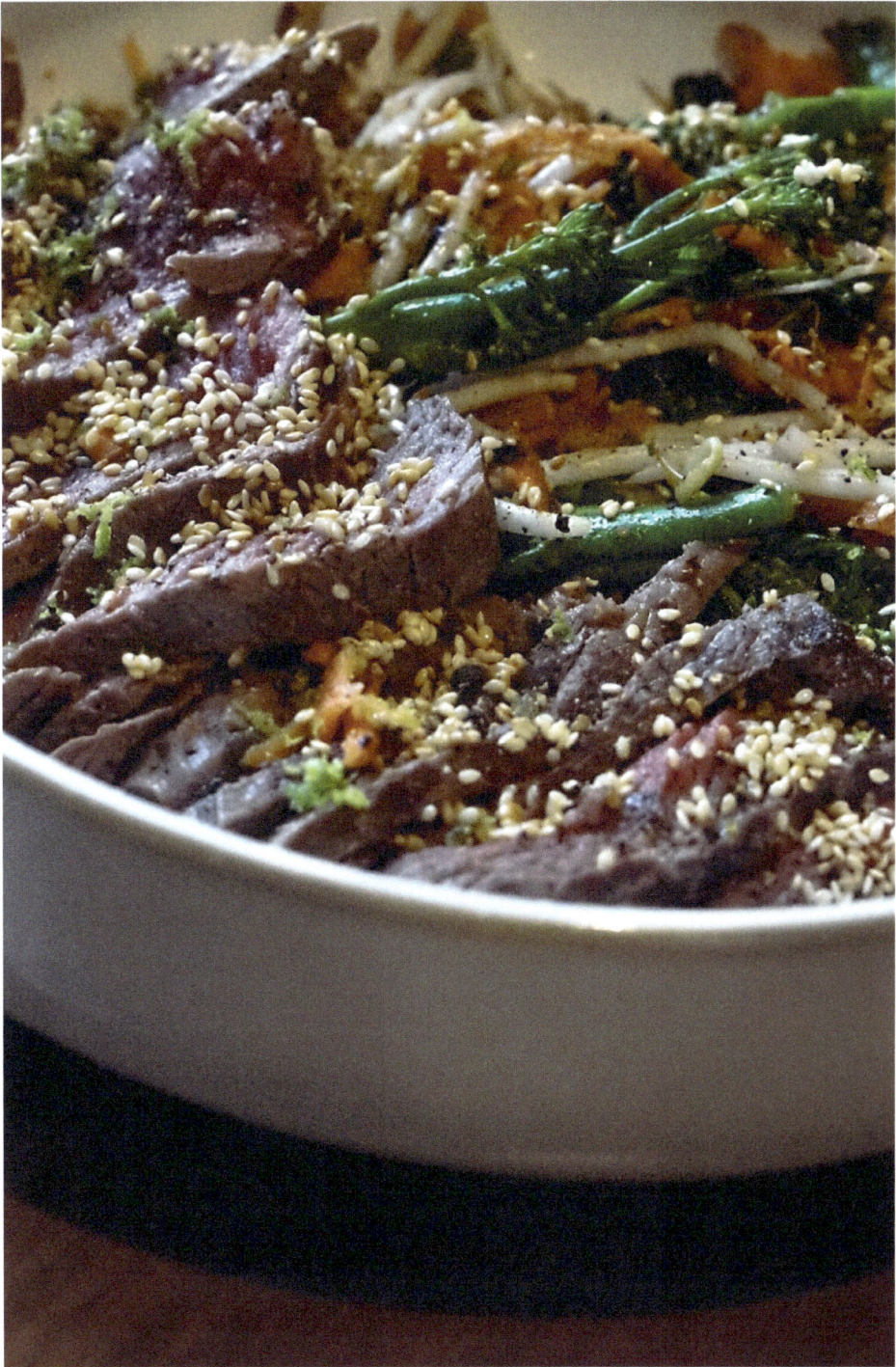

Zeba Saag Gosht

SERVES 4 | 🕐 45 MINS | GF DF NF

"A wedding present from my lovely Zeba & Soph. Deliciously nutritious, and I swear it's perfect for a low effort dish. Get it in the routine, and it swings down in time every time."

A curry is a great way to use a wonderful array of anti-inflammatory spices and herbs.

Turmeric is revered for its therapeutic properties and has a significant body of research to back its many effects that reduce the proliferation of cancer cells.

Chillis and ginger also have some good research on their many health and anticancer benefits. Capasaicin is the active component of chilli and one study found that it promoted apoptosis (cell death) in prostate cancer cells but not healthy cells. Ginger is one of our top ten anticancer foods.

Lamb is a good choice of meat if you are concerned about quality as it is in general naturally grass fed. Frozen spinach is a good standby as a convenient source of veg. It can be used easily in dishes without defrosting. Frozen veg is in general almost as good as fresh.

Really good to serve with mint yoghurt (p218) and wholegrain flatbread wrap (p210).

INGREDIENTS

1 tbsp	Coconut oil
1" cube	Ginger
2 cloves	Garlic
450g	Lamb, diced
1 tsp	Turmeric powder
1 tsp	Chilli powder
1 tsp	Coriander *(dried)*
500g	Frozen chopped spinach
Pinch of	Sea salt
Cracked	Black pepper
-	
Handful of	Coriander *(fresh)*
1 (20g)	Large green chilli *(garnish)*

METHOD

1. Heat up the pan with 1 tbsp coconut oil.

2. De-skin the ginger and garlic; then crush them, finely chop them and add them to the pan.

3. Add the chopped lamb, chunkily diced, to the pan, and stir until lightly bronzed.

4. Add the spices and cook for 45 mins on low heat, then add the spinach and cook for just 2-5 more mins to thaw and finish the dish. Taste and add salt and pepper.

5. Chunkily chop and garnish with fresh coriander and green chillies to taste.

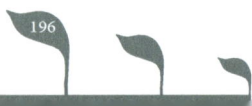

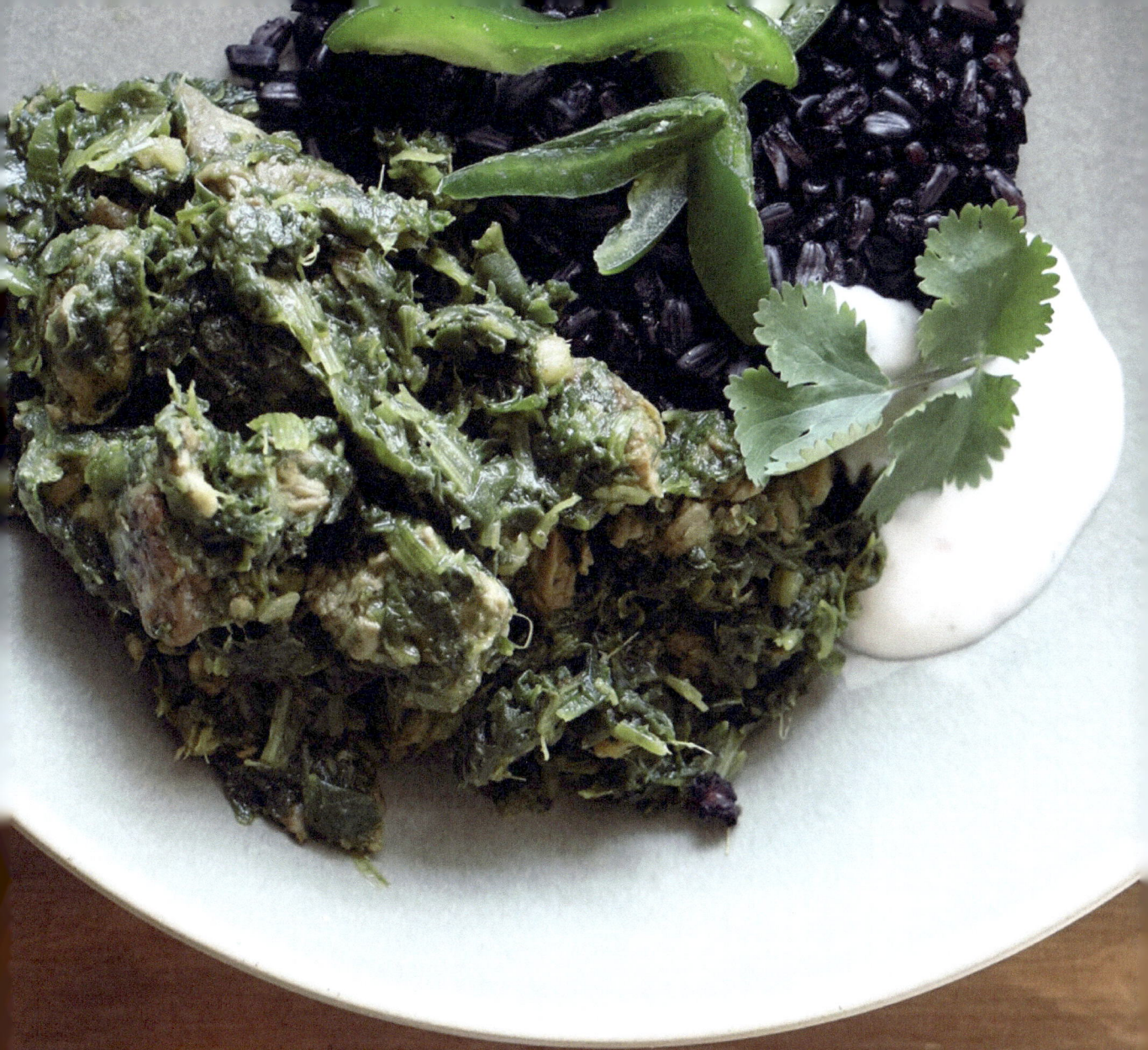

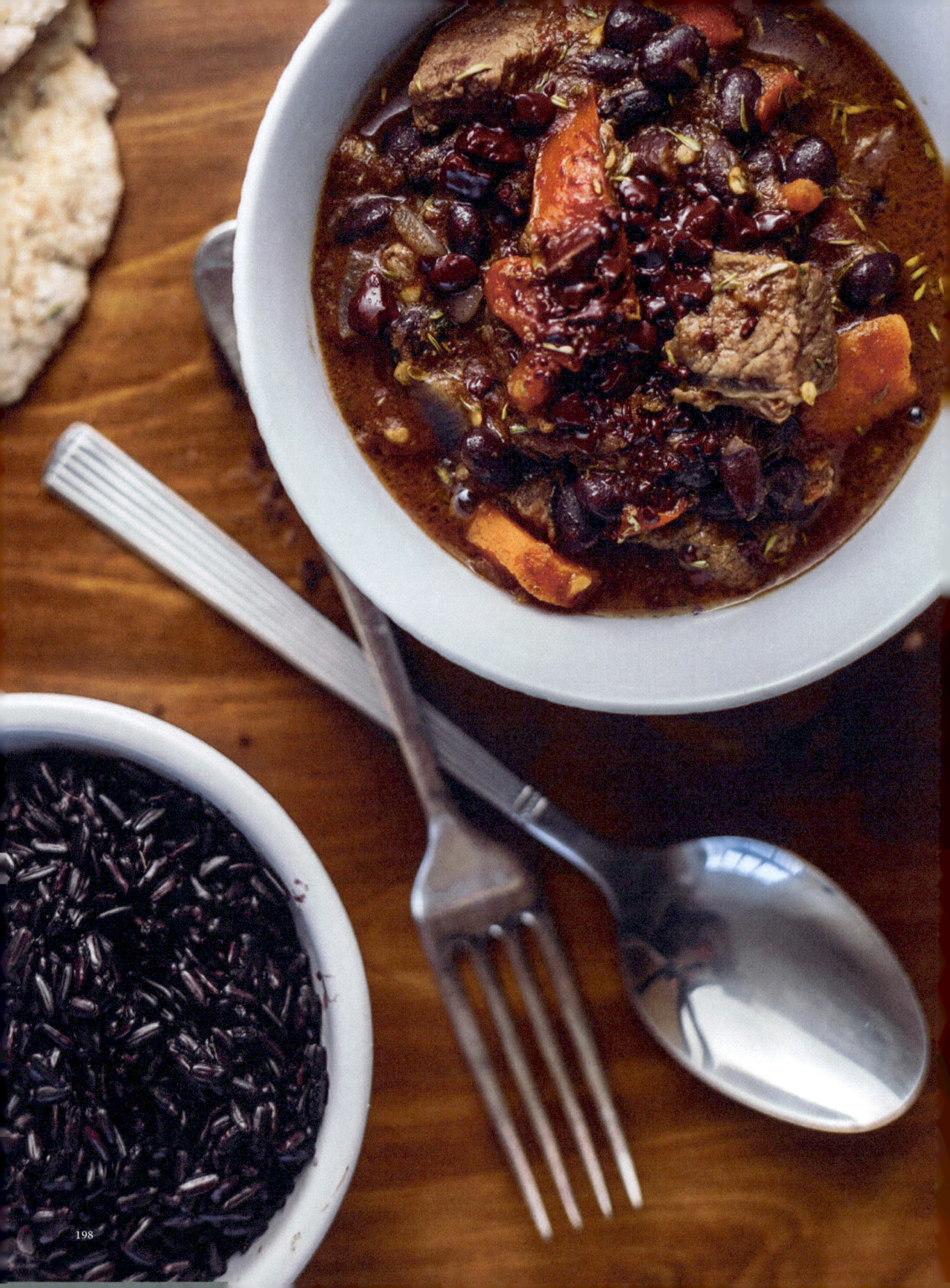

Beef Cacao Stew

SERVES 4 | 🕐 35 MINS | GF DF NF

"Chocolate and chilli, a wonderful combination! Make sure your chocolate is 85% cocoa solids for the health benefits. Cocoa solids are packed with antioxidants which means you can indulge in a little dark chocolate everyday."

Although red meat should be eaten infrequently (as much for the planet as health reasons), it can be a useful way of obtaining iron in your diet if you are prone to anaemia or just had surgery. The meat should be of good quality; organic, grass fed if possible. If cost is an issue then use less but better quality meat (quality over quantity) and pad out with extra beans.

Add fresh herbs if possible to gain all the wonderful therapeutic effects of rosemary, oregano and coriander.

It's great with black rice or wholemeal flatbread, and sour cream too!

INGREDIENTS

4 tbsp	Coconut oil
450g	Shin of organic beef *(cut into cubes)*
3	Garlic cloves
1	Red onion
3	Carrots
3	Large tomatoes
1	Red chilli
1	Red pepper
½ tsp	Dried oregano
½ tsp	Dried rosemary
150ml	Red wine
500ml	Beef stock
1 tbsp	Cacao nibs
Pinch of	Sea salt
Cracked	Black pepper
20g	85% Dark chocolate
400g (1 x tin)	Black beans

METHOD

1. Pre-heat the oven to 190°C.

2. Heat the coconut oil in a roasting pan or ovenproof dish. Once hot, add the beef and place in the oven for 20 mins until browned.

3. Finely chop the garlic and slice the onions.

4. Peel and chop the carrots and the tomato, keeping everything quite chunky. Add all to the browned beef, mix well then return to the oven for a further 10 mins.

5. Chop the chilli finely and red pepper into chunks. Then add the chilli, red pepper, oregano, rosemary, red wine, beef stock, cacao, seasoning and 10g dark chocolate, chopped. Mix well and cover well with a lid or foil.

6. Reduce the heat to 180°C and cook for 2.5 hours, checking every hour, stirring, and adding more liquid if needed. Add the pre cooked black beans, mix well, cover and return to the oven for a further 30 minutes.

7. Serve the beef topped with remaining grated chocolate.

SIDES & SAUCES

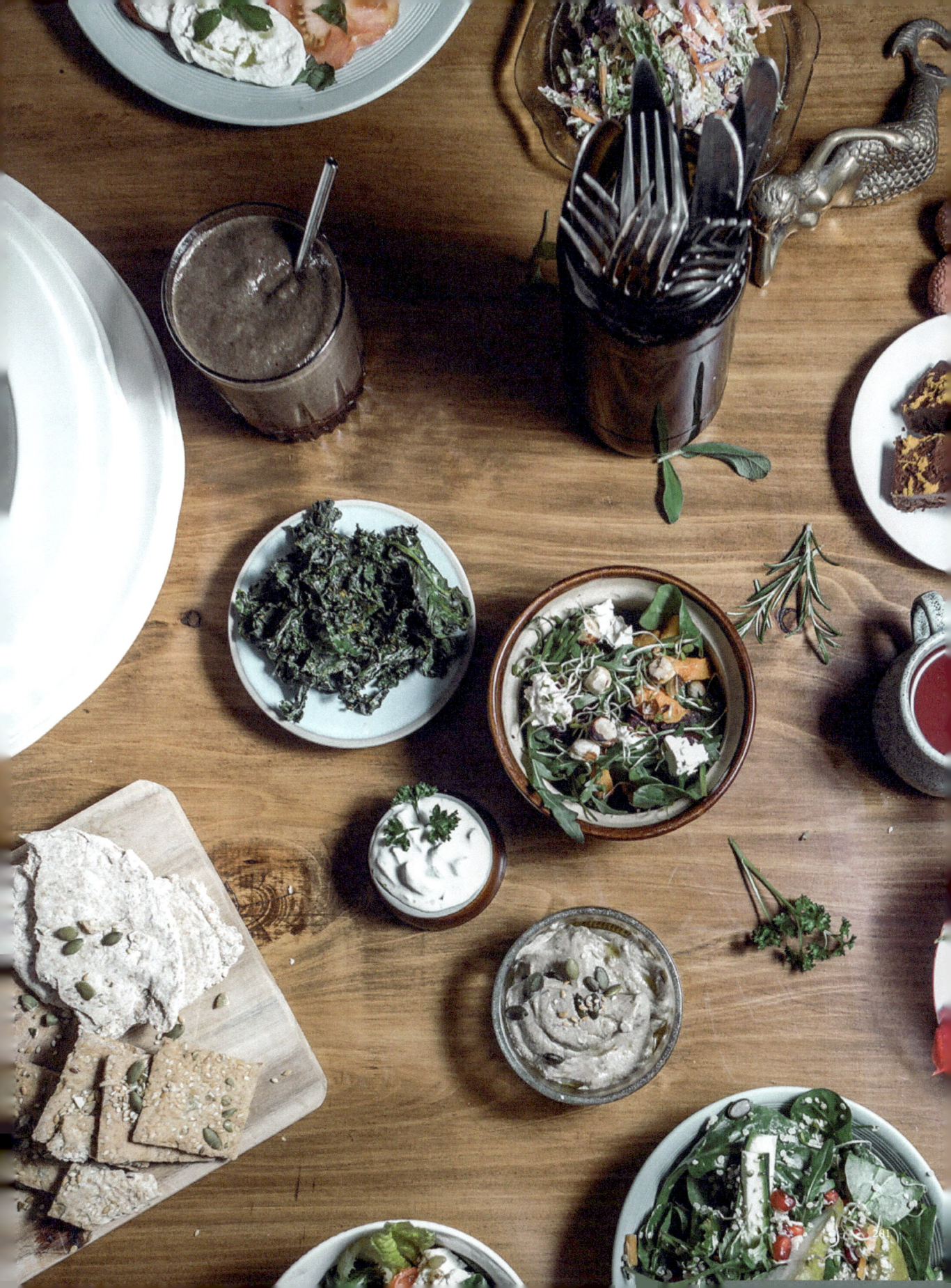

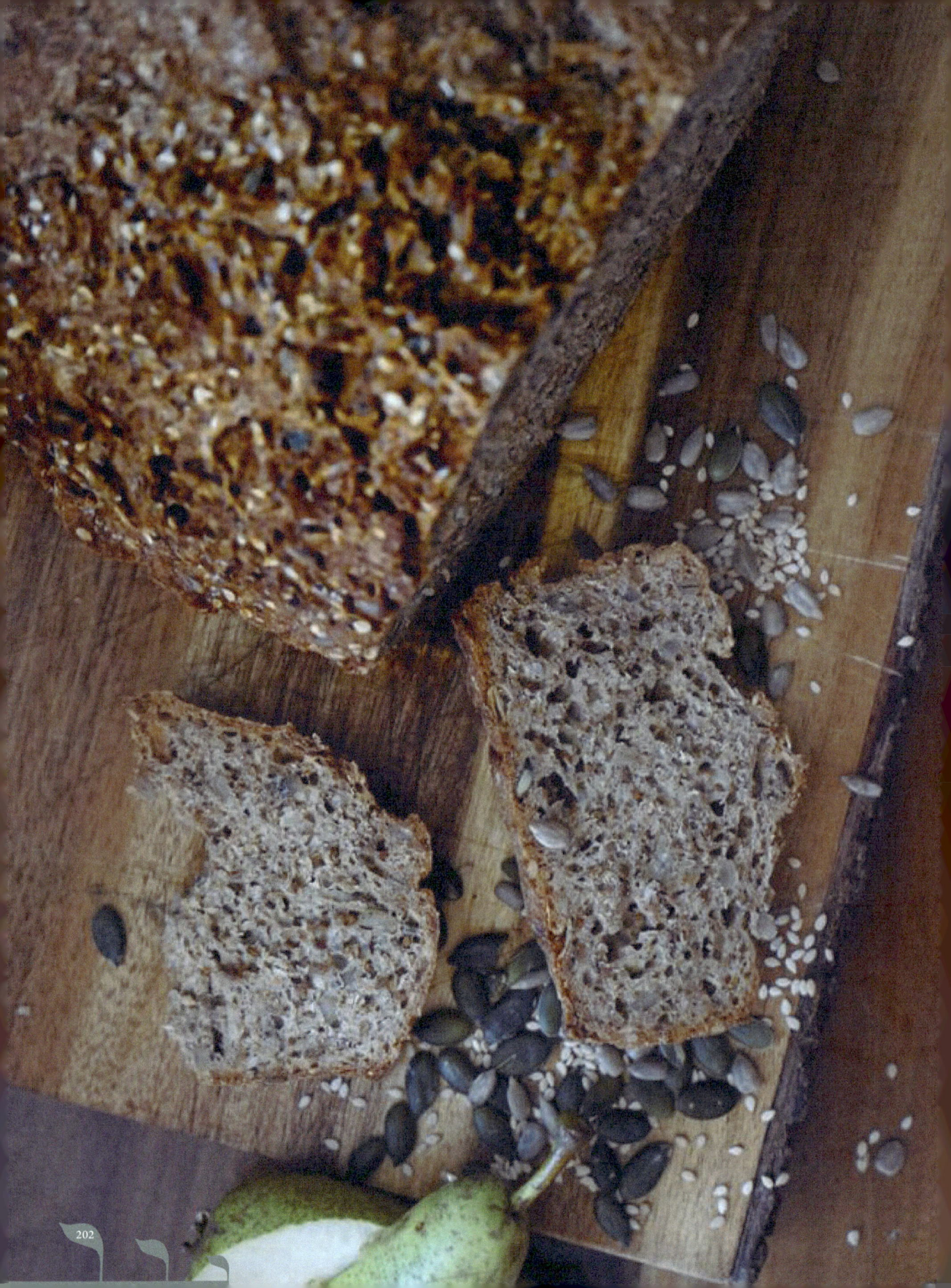

Seeded Spelt Pear Bread

6-8 SLICES | 🕐 1 HR 15 MINS | DF V VE

"Absolutely love finding out what you can create out of the standard vibe. I hurdled the filling from memory of an apple related bread, after ladening the fruit bowl and getting bored of them! So satisfying to waste not and want not, let alone twist the memories to nutritionally and mentally satisfy your day."

This 15 mins effort is so quick to make that there are really no excuses for not baking your own bread! So healthy, it really is worth persevering and giving up artificially fluffy bread full of additives and high in gluten. Spelt is a naturally low gluten grain which means the body can break it down so much more easily.

The seeds provide extra fibre and essential omega fats. The pear is an excellent source of soluble and insoluble fibre, plus folate, vitamin C and important antioxidants. This healthy loaf provides many benefits for gut health but to improve it further, try soaking the seeds for a few hours before using to aid digestion and improve the bioavailability of their nutrients.

INGREDIENTS

1	Pear
500g	Spelt flour
10g	Dried yeast
Pinch of	Sea salt
35g	Sunflower seeds
35g	Sesame seeds
35g	Pumpkin seeds
55g	Linseeds / Flaxseeds
-	
500ml	*Water*

METHOD

1. Heat the oven to 200°C.

2. Start by grating the pear into the mix bowl, then simply add all other dry ingredients and stir.

3. Add 500ml of water, warm, smooth the mix and add it to the tin. Use baking parchment to line if not silicone.

4. Bake for 1 hour, then remove to cool (if a non-silicone loaf tin, remove from the tin and turn off the oven, for an extra 5 mins to solidify the underside and then take out to cool).

Seeded Psyllium Bread

6 - 8 SLICES | 🕐 1 HR 30 MINS | GF DF V VE

This is a salubrious, gluten free loaf that just piles you full of goodness within your first bite. It's packed with seeds and so much healthier than the classic carbohydrate focused loaves."

The seeds plus the almonds will supply a good level of omega fats which are known for their anti-inflammatory effects. Psyllium husks are pure fibre but are perfect for binding ingredients together.

The oats add more prebiotic fibre to feed the little critters in our gut along with its numerous heart health benefits.

If you have the time, soak the chia and linseeds overnight in cold water, or just 10 mins before you start the recipe in warm water to ensure the nutrients are released from the 'shells' and more easily digested.

The bread lasts approximately a week if kept in an airtight container. It's good to keep any leftovers, sliced and frozen.

1 loaf serves approximately 8 small but filling slices. I recommend 2 per person.

INGREDIENTS

50g	Almonds
90g	Flax seeds
100g	Sunflower seeds
50g	Hemp seeds
	(or more sunflower seeeds!)
20g	Chia seeds
150g	Oats *(GF choice)*
55g	Psyllium husks
1 tsp	Sea salt
3 tbsp	Coconut oil

METHOD

1. Heat the oven to 180°C.

2. In a bowl place the almonds, flax, sunflower, hemp and chia seeds.

3. Remove 1 spoonful, and put to one side, place the rest of the nuts and seeds in a blender and blitz until roughly ground.

4. Place in a bowl and add the non-blitzed seeds, oats, psyllium and salt. Mix well.

5. Warm the coconut oil in a heatproof bowl for a couple of minutes in the oven to melt. Add the melted coconut oil and 350ml water to the nut mixture and mix well. A quick knead by hand is good to get an even mix.

6. Place and shape in the prepared, baking parchment lined bread tin, and cook in the oven for 40 mins.

7. Remove from the oven and carefully turn out of the loaf tin onto a sheet of baking parchment, and return to the oven to cook for a further 20 mins.

8. Remove when golden and leave to cool before enjoying.

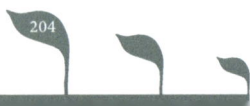

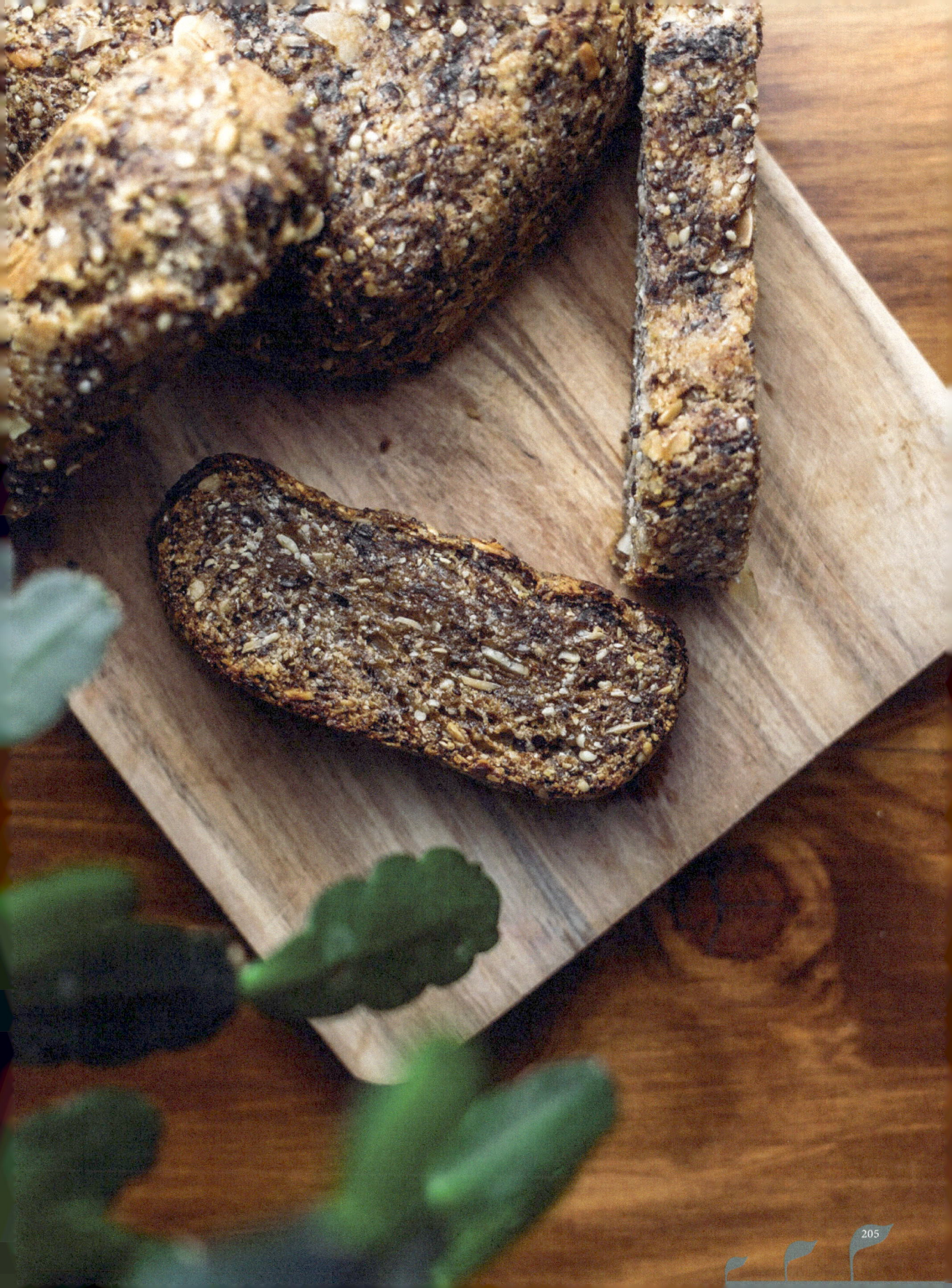

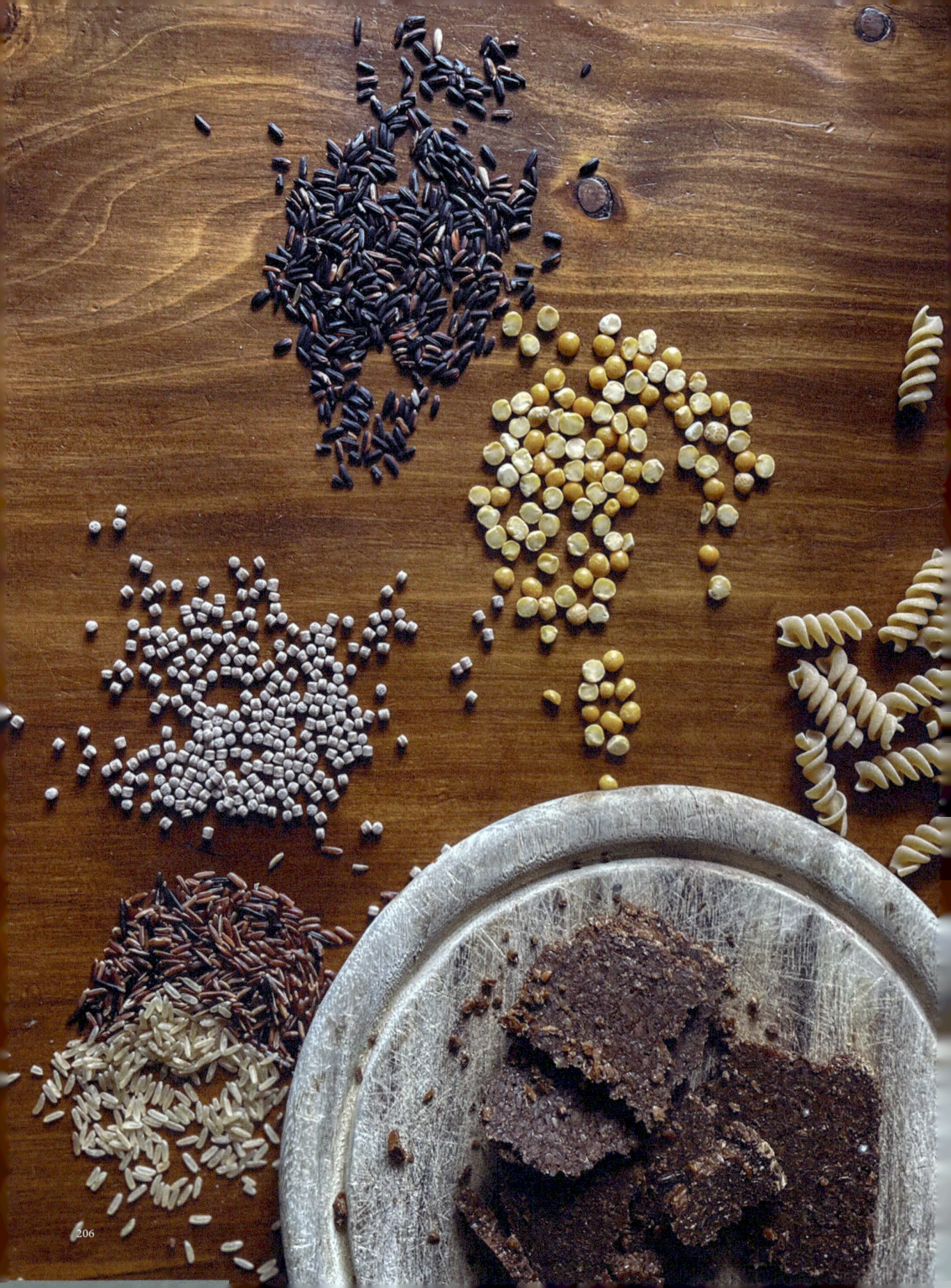

CARBOHYDRATES

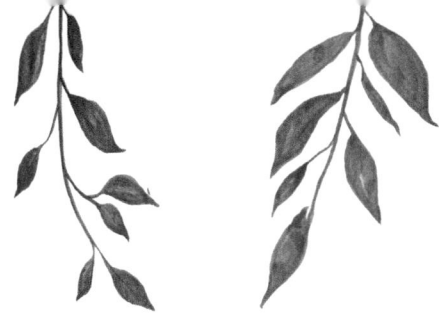

What are Carbohydrates?

Grains, vegetables and fruits which can be divided into sugars and starches. Both sugar and starch are broken down into glucose during digestion.

Unprocessed carbohydrates are known to contain an excellent profile of B vitamins, numerous minerals, and oodles of gut healthy fibre.

But when they are processed, essentially the fibre is taken away alongside many of the nutrients.

> "If it came from a plant, eat it; if it was made in a plant (i.e. factory), don't."
> - Michael Pollan

I think the above quote sums up what has changed in our era of carbs. Carbohydrate foods really are the most 'messed around with' foods on the planet.

Grains that are naturally low in gluten and unprocessed, such as spelt, rye, quinoa, millet, oats, amaranth, teff and so many more, retain their fibre, vitamins and minerals and feed our healthy gut bacteria.

As said before *(p16)*, maintaining a healthy microbiome is particularly beneficial to your brain and immune system, and is also involved in many other aspects of your health.

-

Even if we don't add 'sugar' to our food and drinks, we get natural sugars from the plant foods that we eat. Starchy carbs are grains, cereals and potatoes. Corn and legumes also contain high amounts of starch.

Glucose provides us with energy, but too much and it will be stored as fat. An imbalance in blood glucose levels or sudden high levels has a deleterious effect on many aspects of body functioning including the brain and the immune system.

In general, our diets are heavily biased towards starchy carbs from cereals, rice, white pasta, potatoes, white bread, biscuits, processed cereals and cakes.

For a healthy diet we should limit our intake of starchy carbs to once or twice daily and choose healthier wholegrain varieties rather than refined versions which are digested more quickly and so affect our blood sugar levels more radically.

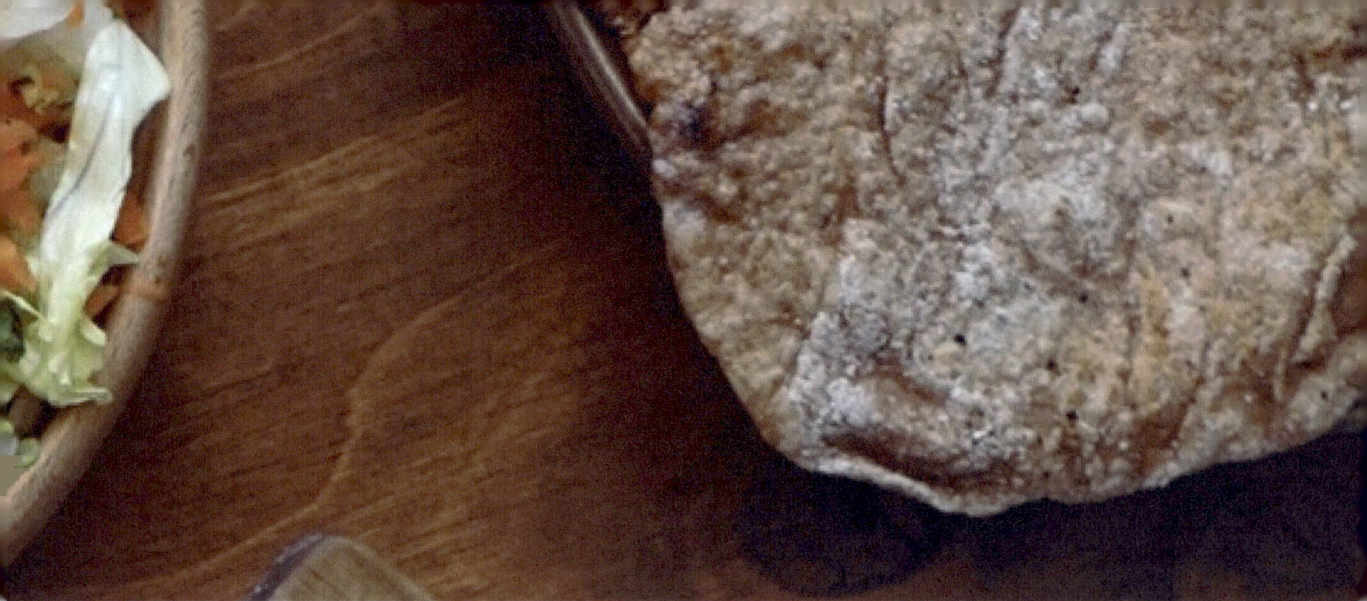

Spelt Wholegrain Flatbread

SERVES 4 | ⏱ 20 MINS | DF V Ve NF

"I love to treat myself to a side of whole grain flatbreads, with a classic curry or broth to soak up the sauciness. The perfect addition to many soups, curries, salads and mains."

Using spelt flour reduces the amount of gluten in these flatbreads compared with ordinary wheat flour ones which is always a good thing.

INGREDIENTS

200g	Spelt wholemeal flour
1 tsp	Baking powder
150 ml	Warm water
Pinch of	Sea salt
4 tsp +	Olive oil

METHOD

1. In a bowl mix together the spelt flour, baking powder, warm water, salt and oil, then combine until it all comes together in a scraggy dough.

2. Lightly dust a surface, quickly knead until it becomes soft and even, divide into 4 portions. Roll into balls and then flatten with the palm of you hand and roll out until the size of a side plate.

3. Heat a thick based large skillet pan, add a little oil and cook on a medium heat for 3 minutes until bubbled and brown, carefully turning with a palette knife. Cook for a further 2-3 minutes on the remaining side, repeat until all done.

4. Then reduce the heat to low, return the flat breads to the pan, place a tight fitting lid on and leave them to gently cook for a further 5-7 minutes, turning half way through.

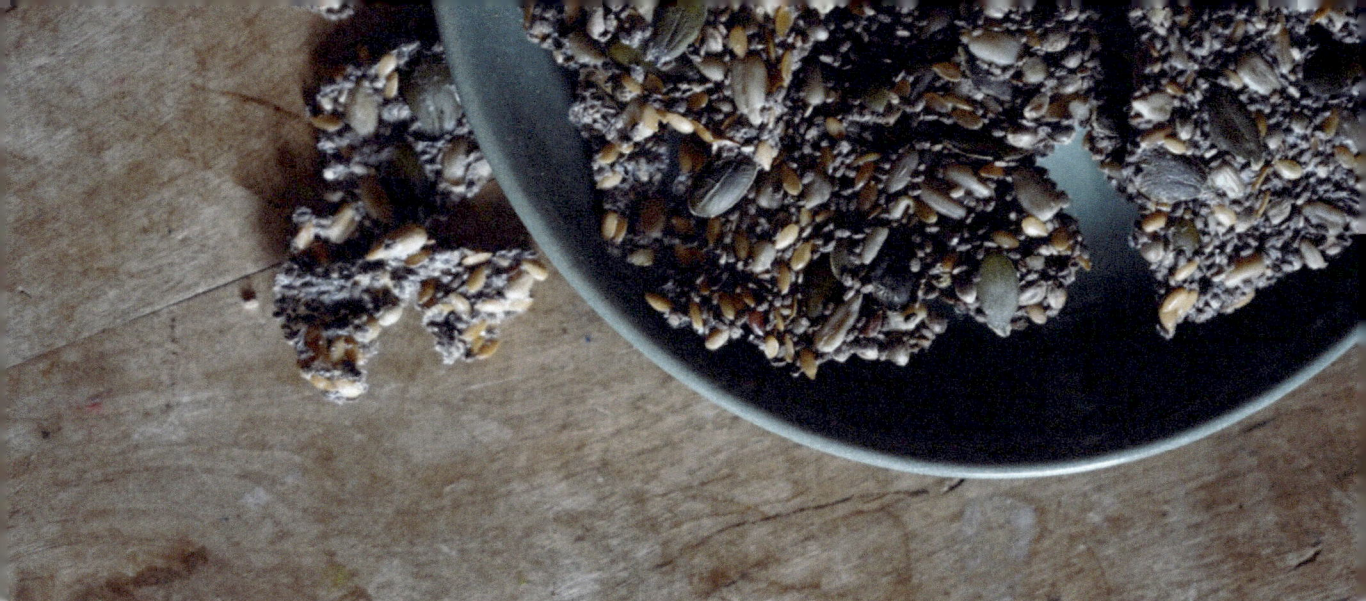

Thin Seeded Crispbread

SERVES 10 | ⏱ 90 MINS | GF DF V Ve NF

"These seedy biscuits are great for nibbling on, especially with cheese or dips, to benefit from a whole host of nutrients."

Seeds are best soaked for at least 8 hours to help us digest them so if you have time you may like to do this and drain them, then use as per recipe. You could even add some turmeric to these for added nutrient value as long as you are happy with yellow biscuits.

The great thing about these crispbreads, as opposed to bought ones, is that they contain no grains and therefore don't form acrylamides (carcinogenic chemicals) when baked. They are also packed with anti-inflammatory omega fats.

INGREDIENTS

50g	Pumpkin seeds
40g	Linseeds (Flax seeds)
70g	Chia seeds
50g	Sunflower seeds
Pinch of	Sea salt
Crack of	Black pepper
1 tsp	Oregano

METHOD

1. Turn oven on to 150°C.

2. Mix all ingredients, add 250ml water, mix.

3. Leave to become a firmer mix for 10 mins.

4. Spread thinly onto a baking tray lined with baking parchment.

5. Leave in the oven for 30-40 mins, then turn over using a new layer of baking parchment between 2 solid surfaces (e.g. chopping boards), when it de-humidifies (when it is no longer sticking to the baking parchment) and has stopped sweating, put back in the oven and bake for another 30 mins. Worth checking towards the end of the cooking time; you want it to have a good light brown crispiness, and for solidity if you turn off the oven, and leave crackers inside to cool and dehydrate.

6. Break them into chunks and store airtight, so they will easily last a week.

DILL TROUT GRAVLAX

SERVES 4 | 🕐 1 HR 15 MINS | GF DF NF

"Gravlax is cured, not smoked. It is done so by normally settling it with mixed herbs and aquavit in Scandinavia, Trout is a forest lover of low temperature water, because it holds more oxygen when cooler."

The trout is a treat, full of omega 3, giving it a very high anti-inflammtory profile.

Dill is a good source of manganese, which is an essential mineral for healthy functioning of the brain and nervous system. It also contains vitamins A and C and folate and iron, so do add a reasonable quantity.

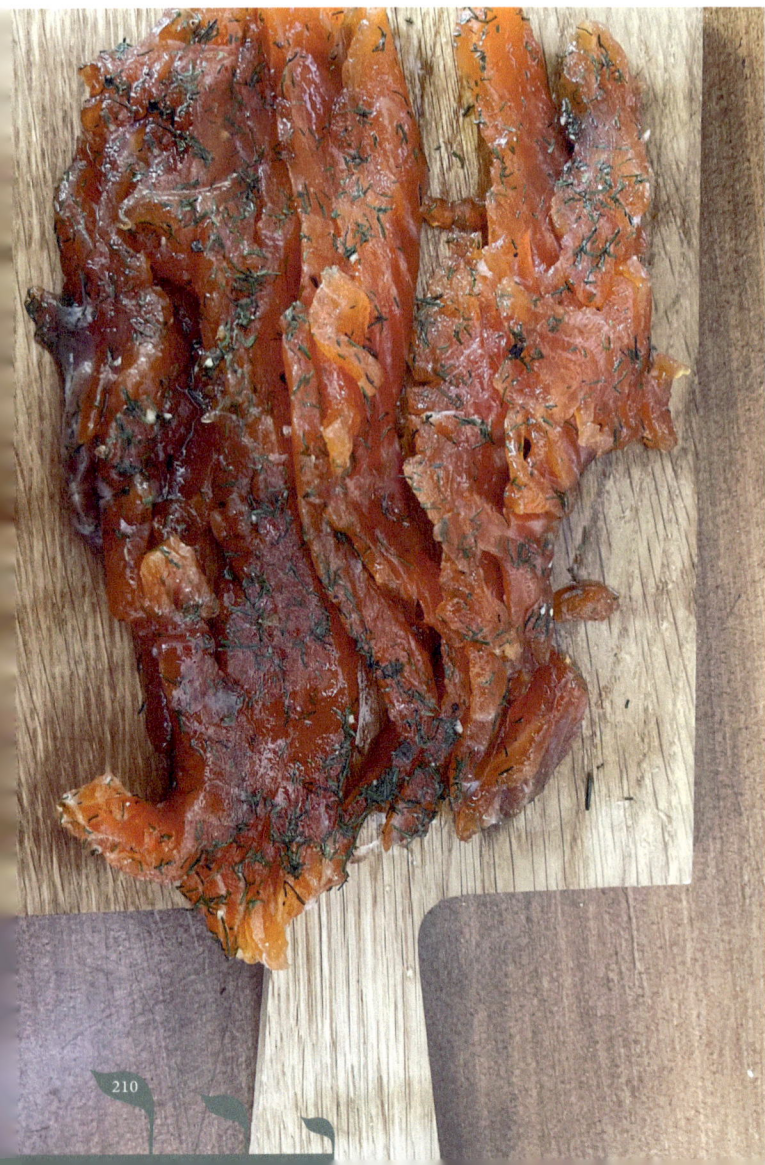

INGREDIENTS

250g	Trout Fillet *(skinned)*
2 tbsp	Salt *(flaked)*
1 tbsp	Runny honey
25 ml	Gin
1 bunch	Dill *(fresh)*
Crack of	Black pepper

METHOD

1. Add the trout to a baking dish and sprinkle the fillet with the salt. Cover with a layer of baking parchment, and weigh down with a pan to dehydrate. Transfer to the fridge and leave for 20 mins.

2. Remove from the fridge, carefully rinse off all the salt and pat dry.

3. Mix the honey and gin. Then once combined, de-stem and lightly chop the dill and add to the mix.

4. Slice the trout at an angle, to approx 2-3mm thick.

5. Spoon all the dressing on the trout, crack the black pepper. Re-cover the trout, weigh it down and pop back in the fridge for 30 mins (up to 24 hrs).

6. Pour out the fluid and serve.

TROUT GRAVLAX SPREAD

SERVES 4 | 🕐 5 MINS | GF NF SS

"Marscapone is the main add to this spread. It is the creamy, cheesy add on to the lone crackers. It is made by adding strong citric acid to classic cream. Protein and healthy fat infused galore. What other way is there to satiate yourself when you need something quick and easy than an hors d'oeuvre aka appetiser."

Mascarpone is an Italian creamy cheese. It's curdled cream with citric acid and has a strong and healthy fat content.

Lemon juice, surprisingly, aids an alkaline environment within the body.

A simple and delicious, nutrient dense dip to enjoy on a wholesome seeded cracker or crunchy vegetable stick, like celery.

INGREDIENTS

100g	Trout gravlax
200g	Marscapone
½	Lemon
1 dsp	Dill *(dried)*
Crack of	Black pepper
Pinch of	Sea salt

METHOD

1. Finely chop the trout into small pieces.

2. Add the mascarpone, squeeze in the lemon juice, the dried dill, and mix all together. Add the black pepper and sea salt to taste and complete.

3. Enjoy immediately or simply store in the fridge.

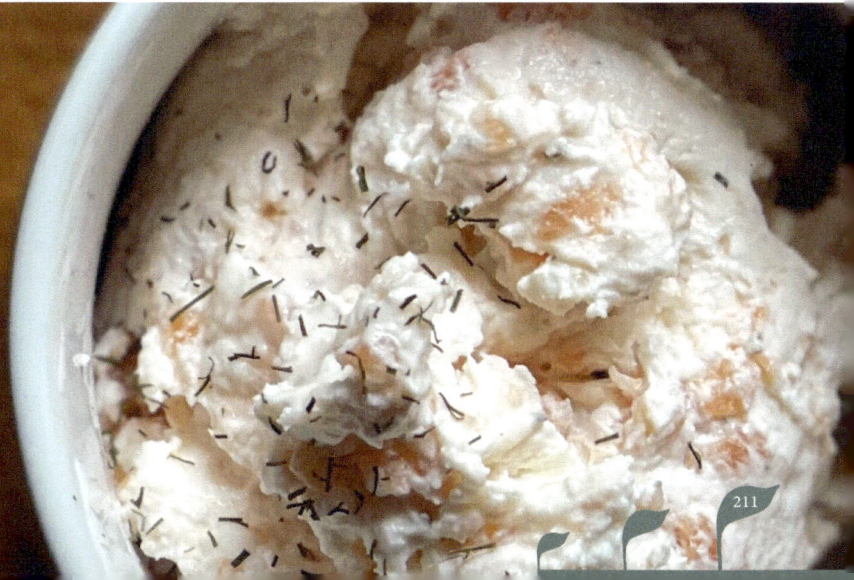

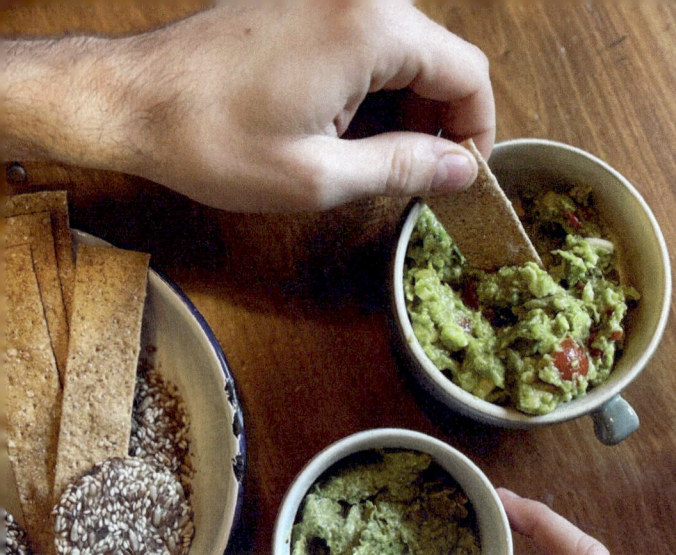

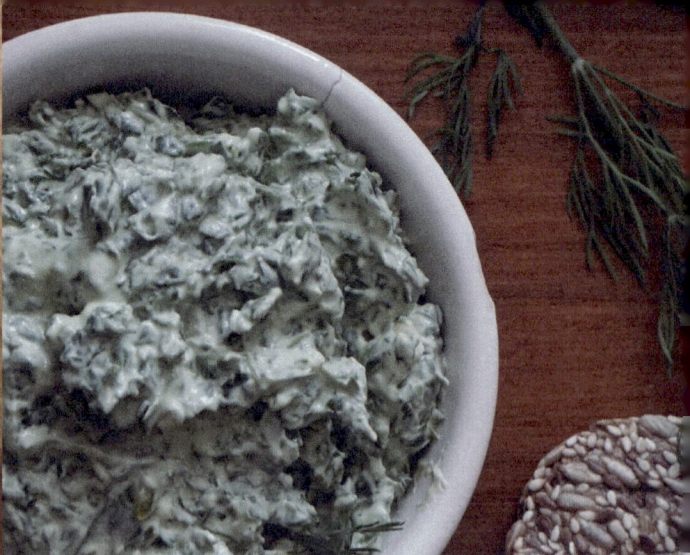

Guacamole

1 JAR | 🕐 30 MINS |

(GF) (DF) (V) (Ve) (NF)

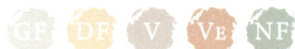

Avocados are rich in healthy monounsaturated fats and have been shown to have cholesterol and trigliceride lowering properties. It's classicly good with coriander if you switch out the parsley and a light mix finely chopped red onions.

INGREDIENTS

2	Avocados	Pinch of	Salt
2	Garlic cloves	Crack of	Pepper
Pinch of	Parsley		
½	Chilli		
½	Lime		
5	Cherry tomatoes		

METHOD

1. Chop the avocado into chunks and then semi mash with a fork.

2. Smash your garlic cloves after stripping them; you can use a garlic crusher or just crush with the knife sideways on them, then cut fairly finely. Add to the avocado.

3. Finely chop the parsley and the chilli. Add them along with the lime juice, which you chop in half and squeeze. Watch out for any seeds which will need removing. Give the mix a little stir.

4. Take your little tomatoes and chop into ½ cm chunks, then throw them in the guacamole, stir again and have a taste to add seasoning to suit.

Spinach & Feta Dill Dip

SERVES 4 | 🕐 10 MINS | (GF) (V) (NF) (SS)

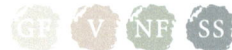

A deliciously creamy dip, made healthy with the raw garlic, which is super anti-inflammatory and antibacterial, and spinach for some green veg. Spinach contains high amounts of iron and vitamin C. Dill is calming on the gut and a potent detoxifier.

INGREDIENTS

50g	Feta	100g	Spinach
90g	Cream cheese	5 g (handful)	Fresh dill
2 tbsp	Sour cream	Crack of	Black pepper
1	Garlic clove		

METHOD

1. Mash the feta, add cream cheese and sour cream to a bowl, mash the feta and mix them together.

2. Finely chop the garlic and spinach, and stir them into the cheese mixture, followed by the de-stemmed and lightly chopped dill and add a crack of black pepper. Stir and serve with a garnish of fresh dill and seeded crackers.

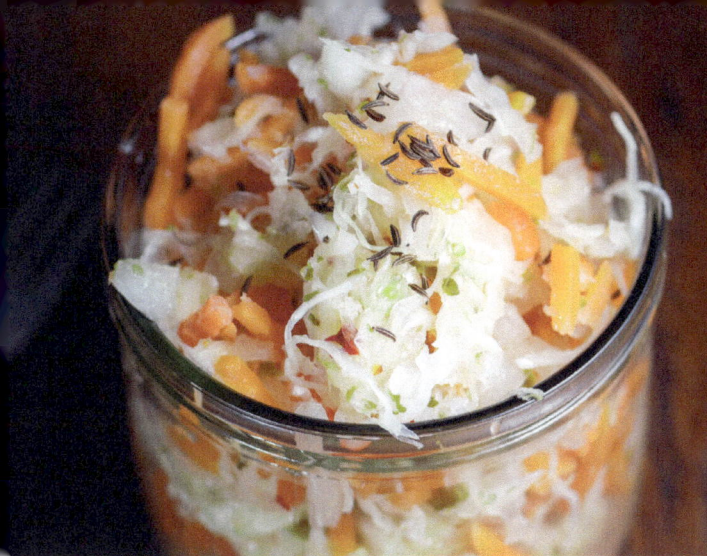

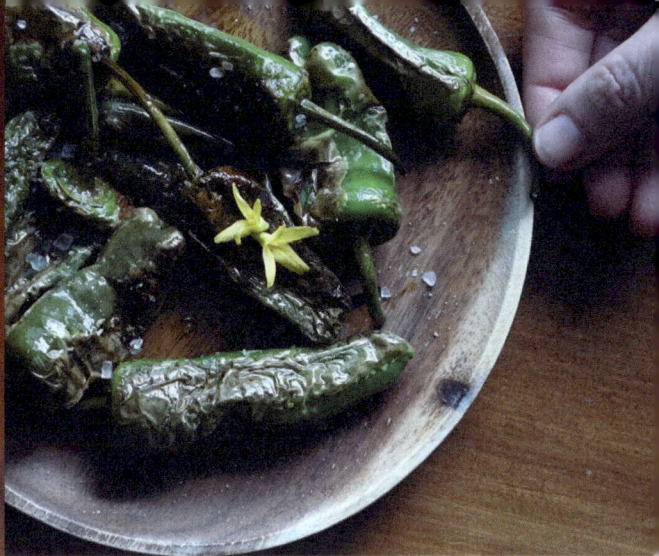

SAUERKRAUT

SERVES 40 | 🕐 30 MINS |

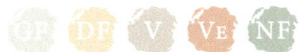

GF DF V Ve NF

This is the number one in fermented foods, which helps reinstate the gut flora after antibiotic and chemo treatments.

INGREDIENTS

600g	Cabbage	2	Jars
4	Carrots		approx.340g
5cm	Ginger		
2 tbsp	Sea salt		
½ tsp	Caraway seeds		
1 tsp	Black pepper		

METHOD

1. Sterilise your jars and allow them to cool.
2. Trim the cabbage, cut into quarters and finely slice into a bowl.
3. Peel and grate the carrots and ginger into the bowl.
4. Add the salt and massage by hand into the vegetables for 5-10 mins.
5. Add the caraway seeds and grind in the pepper. Give it one last massage.
6. Squeeze out the liquid as you add the mix to the jars. Pour off and save any liquid as you fill the jar with veg, then once full add enough of the saved liquid to exclude air and seal with the lid. Then store for 7-10 days. You will see fermentation bubbles after a few days. Once opened it should last 4-6 months if sealed when stored.

ROAST PADRON PEPPERS

SERVES 4 | 🕐 30 MINS |

GF DF V Ve NF

Padron Peppers are vitamin laden; A, B^1, B^2, C, & K. They are full of proteins, calcium and iron.

INGREDIENTS

300g	Padron peppers
1 tbsp	Olive oil
60g	Flaky sea salt

METHOD

1. Heat the oven to 180°C.
2. Line a baking tray and lay out the padron peppers. Mix in the oil and add to the oven for 20-30 mins.
3. Remove when they start browning, and sprinkle with the salt crystals.

CRISPY ROASTED KALE

SERVES 4 | ⏱ 30 MINS | GF DF V Ve NF

"The most nutrient filled simple side to watching TV, reading a book, or a general meal for me for sure! Simple and satisfying. If you're doing a large bowl, it's going to be easy to keep adding, as the kale crisps are great when left to cool while you make more to add to the serving."

Kale is the top of the pile when it comes to healthy greens. A handful of kale will provide you with vitamins A, K, C & B6. It is higher in vitamin C & K than most other vegetables. As a cruciferous vegetable it contains sulphoraphane and indole-3-carbinol which have been shown in numerous studies to be cancer protective. The vitamin A is converted from the high level of beta-carotene in kale. Vitamin A is vitally important for healthy vision and gut health. Kale is also a good source of magnesium and calcium, both necessary for strong bones.

Add turmeric and you increase the antioxidant and healing properties of this snack or side. Turmeric has exceptional anti-inflammatory properties. Be sure to use black pepper to aid the absorption of the therapeutic compound curcumin.

INGREDIENTS

1 dsp	Coconut oil
100g	Kale leaves
Sprinkle of	Sea salt
Crack of	Black pepper
-	
1 tsp	*Turmeric*

METHOD

1. Heat the oven to 150°C. While heating, add the coconut oil in a bowl to melt.

2. Take your kale, and de-stem it. Easiest if you hold the stem base and pull up, with the rest of the leaf held in your alternate hand.

3. With the de-stemmed leaves, simply rip them into reasonably sized pieces; 'half a playing card' is my standard.

4. Now wash the leaves and dry properly. You can spin dry, dab dry, or wait for them to dry — this will ensure they crisp in the oven.

5. Remove the melted coconut oil from the oven, and add the salt, pepper, *and the turmeric for a hit of health and flavour if wanted*, and add to the kale.

6. Cover your baking tray with baking parchment and lay out the kale thinly.

7. Bake for 10 mins, then turn-over the kale and put back in the oven for 10-15 mins.

8. Leave out for 5 minutes and they will have aired and crisped even further.

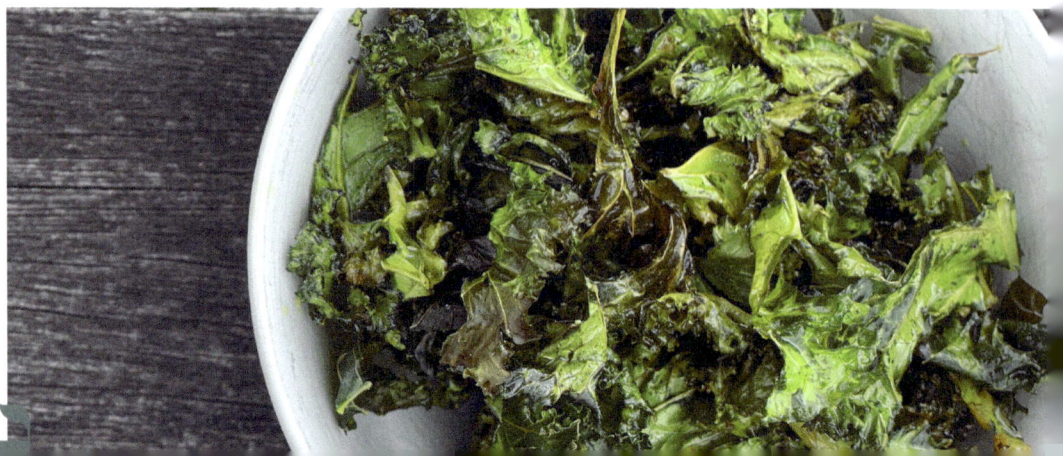

Sweet Potato Chips

SERVES 4 | 1HR 25 MINS | GF DF V Ve NF

Sweet potatoes contain less starch than ordinary potatoes and are rich in beneficial carotenes and vitamins. Leave the skins on for added fibre.

INGREDIENTS

3 tbsp	Coconut oil
800g	Sweet potatoes *(x3, large)*
Pinch of	Sea salt

METHOD

1. Set the oven to 220°C and add the baking tray to warm and the coconut oil in a jar to melt and scrub and rinse the sweet potatoes.

2. Cut the potatoes into ½ cm width chips. Throw them into a mixing bowl with the warm oil to coat and spread in the baking tin to a single layer.

3. After another 15 mins flip them over and add for another 15 to the oven. Ensure they crisp up and pull out to serve with a pinch of salt.

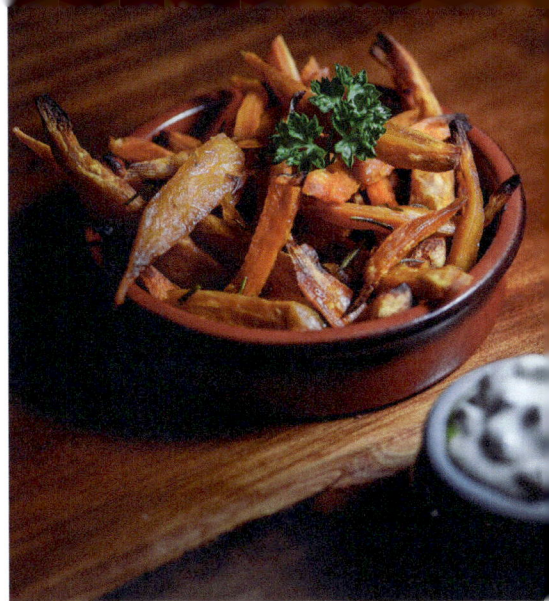

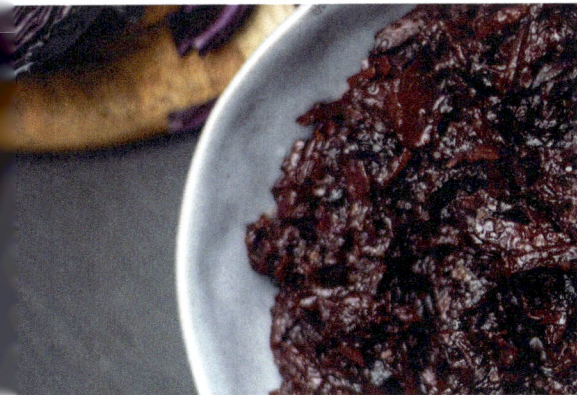

Red Cabbage, Pear & Beetroot

SERVES 4 | 1HR 25 MINS |

GF DF V Ve NF

Cabbage, classically delicious with plenty of spice, some gentle heat and some generous time. The beetroot adds to the earthiness and is packed with essential vitamins and minerals.

INGREDIENTS

¼	Red cabbage
1	Beetroot
1	Pear *(unripe)*
1 tbsp	Coconut oil
1	Red onion
1	Cinnamon stick
1	Star Anise
¼ tsp	Ground cloves
¼ tsp	Ground nutmeg
125ml	Red wine
1 tsp	Carob syrup

METHOD

1. Slice the cabbage as finely as you can. Peel the beetroot and cut it into fine matchsticks (or you can coarsely grate it to save time). Do the same with the pear – you needn't peel it though. Finely slice the onion.

2. Warm 1 tablespoon of oil in a large saucepan. Throw all ingredients in and pop a lid on and cook over a very gentle heat for 1 hour. Give it a stir every so often and make sure it isn't drying out; add a dash of water if it does.

3. Taste the cabbage and tweak the seasoning with salt to your liking. If you'd like it sweeter, add a bit of carob syrup at this stage, to your taste. Pop the lid back on and cook for a further 15-20 minutes, until completely soft and tender.

4. You can serve it straightaway, but it's arguably better reheated after a couple of days in the fridge.

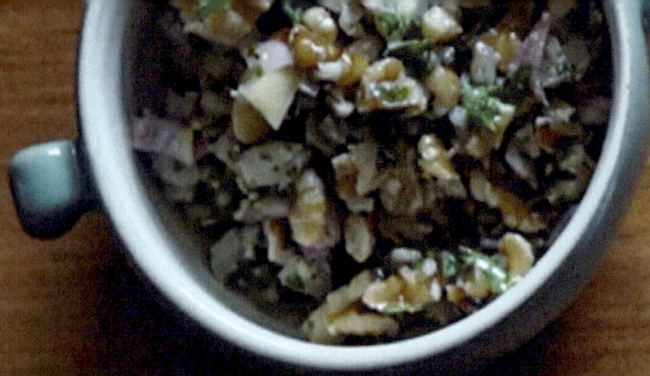

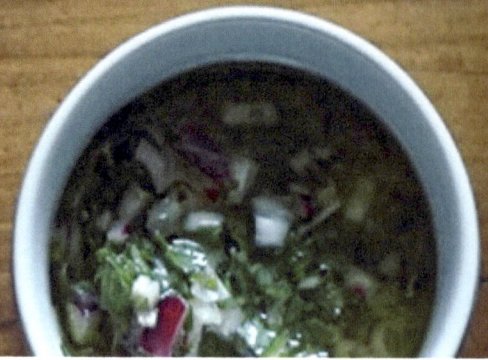

Walnut & Brazil Nut Salsa

SERVES 4 | 🕐 25 MINS

GF DF V Ve

This is a superb addition to a simply panfried piece of fish or cold meat or drizzled across some steamed or roasted vegetables, it is so good that it may become your 'always in the fridge' salsa.

INGREDIENTS

50g	Walnuts			
50g	Brazil nuts	1	Unwaxed	
1	Shallot		lemon	
Bunch of	Parsley	1 tbs	Red wine	
1	Garlic clove		vinegar	
Pinch of	Sea salt	5 tbsp	Olive oil	
Crack of	Black pepper			

METHOD

1. Chop the nuts into small even sized pieces and place in a bowl.

2. Finely dice the shallot and parsley, then add to the nuts.

3. Crush and very finely dice the garlic, add to the bowl along with the seasoning, lemon zest, juice, red wine vinegar and olive oil.

4. Whisk well until blended with a fork.

216

Herbalicious Dressing

SERVES 4 | 🕐 15 MINS

GF DF V Ve NF

Salad tossed in this herb rich dressing and mopped up with tasty bread is great. You can't have enough herbs so I'm always abundant with usage, you can always adjust the herbs to suit your kitchen or palate.

INGREDIENTS

1	Garlic		
½	Red onion		
2 tsp	Dijion mustard		
3 tbsp	White wine vinegar		
7 tbsp	Olive oil		
Pinch of	Sea salt	Bunch of	Basil
Crack of	Black	Bunch of	Chives
	pepper	Bunch of	Parsley
		Bunch of	Oregano
		Bunch of	Mint

METHOD

1. Crush, peel and finely chop the garlic, dice the onion, and mix together with the mustard and vinegar in a large jam jar or whisk in a bowl. Add the olive oil and seasoning again blend until emulsified.

2. Chop all the herbs and mix well making a bright green herb rich dressing, which will last 3-4 days in the fridge.

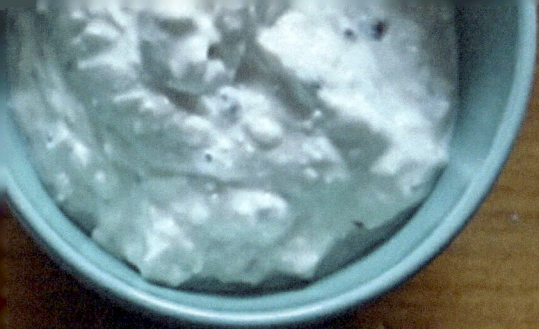

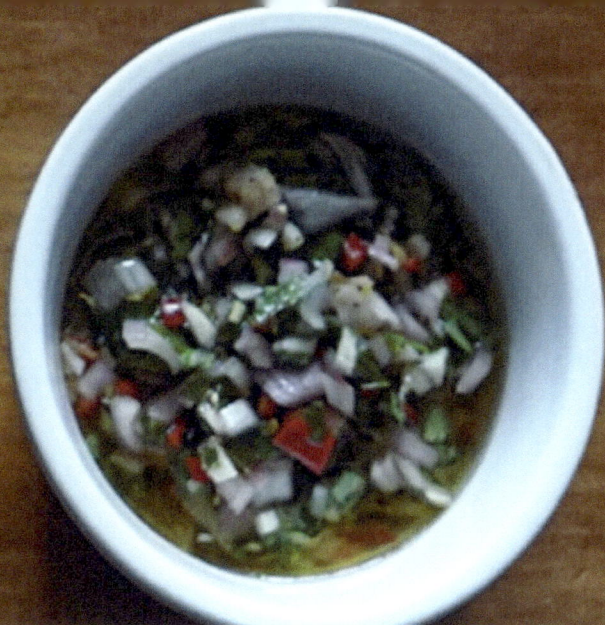

Cottage Cheese Spiced Sauciness

SERVES 4 | ⏲ 10 MINS

GF V NF SS

A great way of creating a rich creamy dressing that will add a little extra protein to your meal. Use as a salad dressing or serve with cold chicken or salmon. Try adding some of your favourite herbs as an additional variation, think basil, sorrel, parsley or chives.

INGREDIENTS

4 tbsp	Cottage cheese *(full fat)*
1	Unwaxed Lemon
1	Green chilli
1	Garlic clove
2 tbsp	Olive oil
Pinch of	Sea salt
Crack of	Black pepper

METHOD

1. Place the cottage cheese, lemon juice, zest, roughly chopped chilli, garlic, 2 tbsp of water, olive oil, and seasoning in a bowl.
2. Blend until smooth with a stick blender or place in a mini food processor and whizz until smooth. Taste and adjust if needed.

Chimichurri

SERVES 4 | ⏲ 15 MINS

GF DF V Ve NF

This classic Argentinian fresh herb sauce is frequently served with grilled meats but believe me it also goes extremely well with fish adding zest and freshness that lifts a simple grilled piece of meat or fish; a summer must.

INGREDIENTS

Bunch of	Parsley	4 tbsp	Olive oil
4 sprigs	Oregano	1 tbsp	Red wine
2	Garlic cloves		vinegar
1	Shallot	1	Unwaxed
1	Red chilli		lemon
		Pinch of	Sea salt
		Crack of	Black pepper

METHOD

1. Chop the parsley, and oregano leaves finely.

2. Finely chop the garlic and add to a mixing bowl with the prepared herbs.

3. Dice the shallot finely and also the red chilli, if you like it hot leave the seeds in, if not remove. Add to the herbs, mix well adding the olive oil, vinegar, lemon zest, juice, and seasoning, mix well and taste adjust if needed.

4. Leave to sit for 30 minutes before using.

Mint Yoghurt

SERVES 4 | 2 MINS | GF V NF SS

Yogurt is a source of protein and fat, laden with calcium for bone health. This delicious yoghurt provide vitamin A, B, zinc and potassium.

INGREDIENTS

10g	Mint
250g	Yoghurt
Pinch of	Salt
1	Chilli *(m)*

METHOD

1. Blend the fresh mint leaves with 2 tsps of yoghurt with a pinch of salt and the fresh chilli.
2. Mix in with the rest of the yoghurt, and serve.

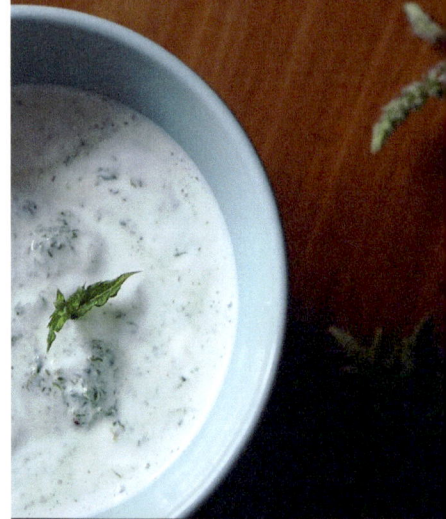

Tzatziki

SERVES 4 | 2 MINS | GF V NF SS

Leave the peel on the cucumber to retain the fibre, vitamins, minerals and antioxidants. Mint leaves act as a carminative on the digestive tract.

INGREDIENTS

Handful of	Peppermint
1	Garlic Clove
½	Cucumber
1	Unwaxed lemon
250ml	Yoghurt

METHOD

1. De-stem the mint and finely chop with the garlic.
2. Remove the cucumber's wet centre and grate it. Grate the lemon skin and then slice it in half and add the juice.
3. Mix all ingredients together with the yoghurt and enjoy.

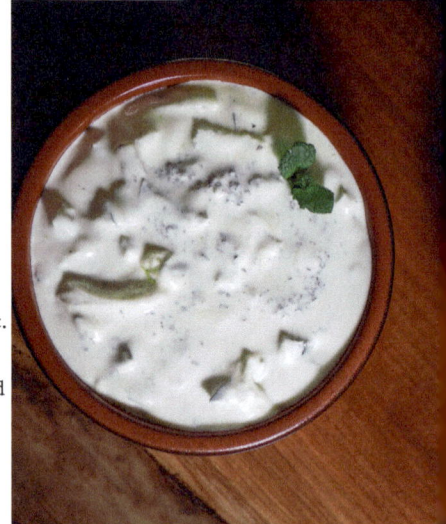

Baba Ganouch

SERVES 4 | 45 MINS | GF DF V Ve NF SS

Aubergines are purple and purple means an abundance of anticancer plant chemicals including the potent compound, solasodine rhamnosyl glycoside. They are also very rich in fibre and so beneficial to gut bacteria.

INGREDIENTS

3	Aubergines
3	Garlic cloves
4 tbsp	Olive oil
1	Lemon
3 tbsp	Tahini
Handful	Fresh parsley
Sprinkle of	Sea salt
-	
1 tsp	Olive oil
Crack of	Black pepper
Sprig of	Parsley

METHOD

1. Heat the oven to 180°C. Then lightly cover the garlic and whole aubergines with olive oil and heat them in the oven for 30 mins.
2. Remove the oven tray and lightly poke the aubergines with a knife to ensure softness, then slightly cool.
3. Remove the skin on both the aubergines and garlic. Now blend.
4. Once smooth, juice the lemon, to add to the blender followed by all other ingredients: olive oil, tahini, parsley leaves, light sea salt and black pepper (add more if needed, after you blend and taste).
5. Finish with a drizzle of olive oil, crack of black pepper and a garnish of parsley.

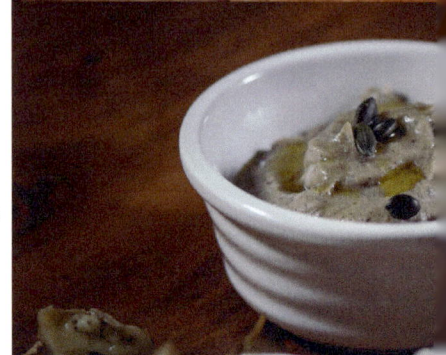

(Turmeric) Hummus

SERVES 6 | 🕐 2 MINS | GF DF V Ve NF SS

You're making approximately double the supermarket size of hummus.
Use non-salted, so you can use the liquid from the tin, so you lose less nutrients.

*Curcumin from turmeric and the piperine in black pepper have been shown to aid health
due to their anti-inflammatory, antioxidant and disease fighting qualities.*

INGREDIENTS

400g	Chickpeas *(1 can)*
25g	Tahini
½	Lemon
1	Garlic clove
1 tsp	Sea salt
Crack of	Black pepper
¼ tsp	*Turmeric*
25ml	Olive oil

METHOD

1. Drain the chickpeas, save the liquid, and tahini to the blender.

2. Squeeze in the lemon juice, crush the garlic to add, then season with the salt, pepper, *turmeric (if wanted)* and 100ml of the drained liquid or water.

3. For up to a minute, blend.

4. Add 30ml of olive oil to smooth the texture, and blend for a moment more.

5. Add more olive oil lightly to taste.

Beetroot Dip

SERVES 6 | 🕐 2 MINS | GF DF V Ve NF SS

Beetroots are easy to find all year round. Fresh are more laden with nutrients, vitamins, nutrients and antioxidants, but cooked are easy to use too.

INGREDIENTS

500g	Beetroot *(raw)*
1	Unwaxed lemon
3	Garlic cloves
2 tsp	Tahini
Pinch of	Sea salt
Crack of	Black pepper
2 tbsp	Olive oil
Pinch of	Cumin seeds

METHOD

1. Wash the beetroot bulbs and trim off the leaves.

2. Place in a large pan of simmering water and bring to the boil for 45 mins. Until it is soft for inserting a knife. When cooked, drain and set aside to cool approx 10 mins.

3. De-skin, roughly chop and add to a blender.

4. Finely zest and juice the lemon. Peel the garlic, and add to the blender, alongside the remaining ingredients. Blitz until smooth and you're finished.

COLESLAW

SERVES 4 | ⏲ 25 MINS | GF V NF

Coleslaw adds to your daily portion of raw food which increases the amount of nutrients, enzymes and fibre you consume. A big, colourful salad with coleslaw daily is a good approach to achieving a healthy diet.

INGREDIENTS

300g	Red cabbage
300g	Savoy cabbage
4	Radishes
2	Carrot
2	Garlic cloves
2 tsp	Parsley
40g	Sunflower seeds
100g	Yoghurt
1	Lemon
Pinch of	Sea salt
Crack of	Black pepper
Handful of	Micro herbs (sprouts)

METHOD

1. Thinly slice the cabbages and radishes using a mandoline or knife.

2. Coarsely grate the carrot, crush and finely chop the garlic, then roughly chop the parsley.

3. Add everything into a mixing bowl and add the sunflower seeds, yoghurt and squeeze in the lemon juice — make sure you remove the seeds.

4. Stir all together and add salt and pepper to taste.

5. Garnish with the micro herbs and serve.

TOMATO SALSA

SERVES 4 | ⏲ 25 MINS | GF DF V VE NF

Tomatoes are a good source of vitamins C & K, along with potassium and folate. They are laden with anti-inflammatory plant compounds. Raw onion and garlic aid detoxification pathways in the liver, are antimicrobial and contain quercetin, which has been shown to have anticancer properties. Added herbs and spices increase the anti-inflammatory credentials of this ultra healthy dip.

INGREDIENTS

150g	Cherry tomatoes
300g	Large tomatoes
½	Red onion
1	Garlic clove
Pinch of	Basil leaves
Pinch of	Parsley
1	Red chilli (mild)
8 tbsp	Olive oil
Pinch of	Sea salt
Crack of	Black pepper

METHOD

1. Halve the cherry tomatoes and chop up the large tomatoes, into 8ths.

2. Finely dice the onion, and garlic.

3. Thinly slice the basil and parsley, and finely chop the chillies.

4. Add all the ingredients, except the salt and pepper to taste.

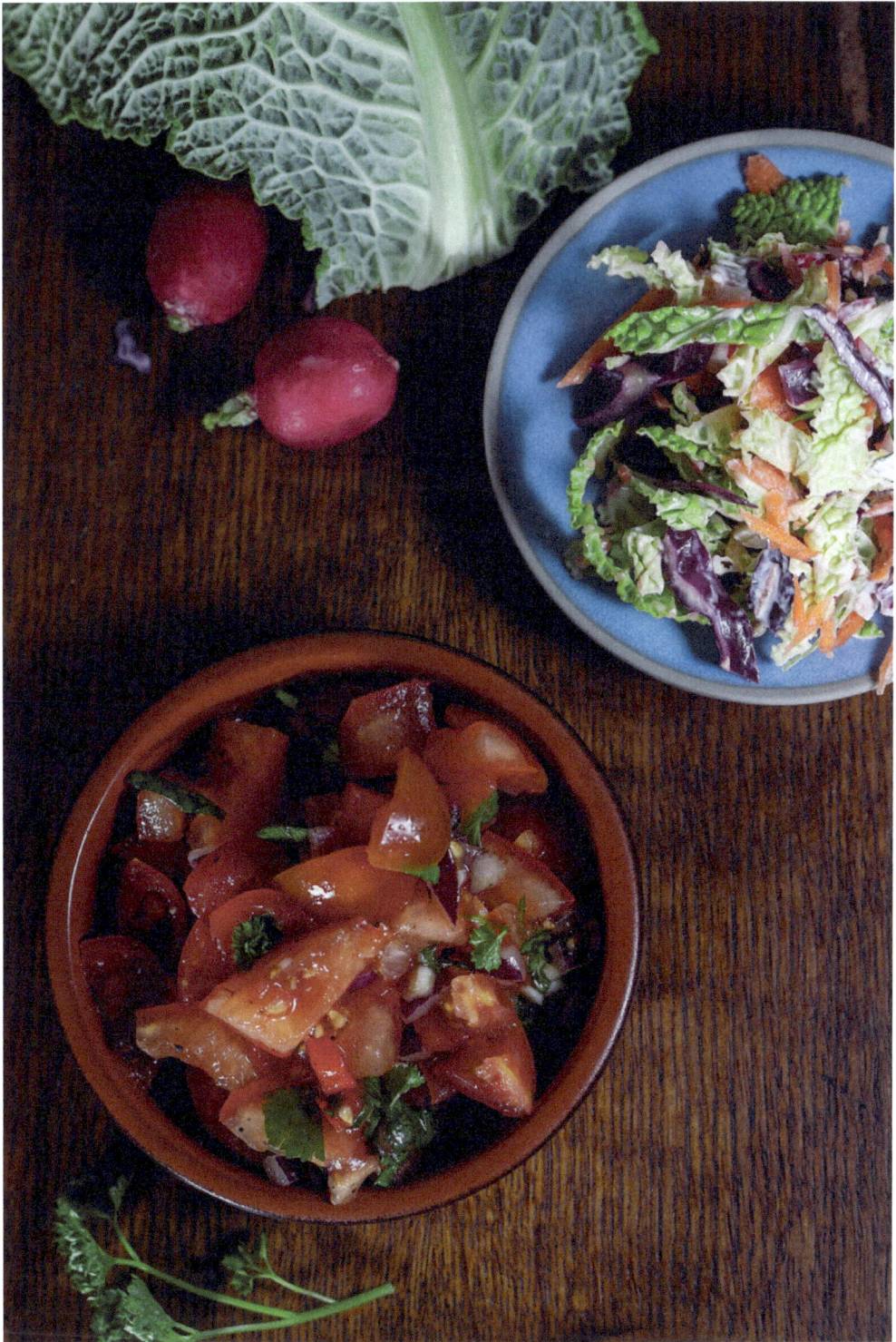

Vegetable Stock

1.5 LITRE | 🕐 1 HR | GF DF V VE NF

Below is a starter stock recipe which can be adjusted with the addition of fennel, tomatoes and any of your favourite herbs eg. rosemary, oregano, marjoram, sage etc. and if an extra richness is wanted replace 300ml of the water with white wine.

INGREDIENTS

2.5kg	Mixed vegetables
	onion
	garlic
	carrots
	celery
	leeks
	mushrooms
Handful of	Parsley stalks
Handful of	Thyme
3	Bay leaves
6	Black peppercorns

METHOD

1. Roughly chop the onions (skin on), into wedges, crush the garlic, roughly chop the carrots, celery, leeks, mushrooms and add to a stock pot and cover with cold water (approx 2 litres).

2. Add the herbs and peppercorns, place on the heat and bring to the boil, then reduce the heat and simmer for 1 hour removing, any scum that may rise to the top of the pot.

3. Strain the stock through a fine sieve and taste, if more flavour is needed return to the heat and simmer to reduce and intensify the flavour.

Fish Stock

1.5 LITRE | 🕐 1 HR | GF DF NF

Fish stocks should be light and blond in colour and do not need to be simmered for as long as other stocks.

INGREDIENTS

2.5kg	Fish bones
	heads/skin/crab lobster/prawn shell/head.
1	Onion
2	Garlic cloves
1	Leek
1	Carrot
1	Celery stick
Handful of	Parsley stalks
Handful of	Thyme
3	Bay leaves
6	Black peppercorns

METHOD

1. Place the fish bones etc in a stock pot.

2. Roughly chop the onions, (skin on) into wedges, crush the garlic, roughly chop the carrots, celery, leeks, mushrooms then add to a stock pot and cover with cold water (approx 2 litres).

3. Add the herbs and peppercorns, place on the heat and bring to the boil, then reduce the heat and simmer for 30 minutes, removing any scum that may rise to the top of the pot.

4. Strain the stock through a fine sieve and taste, if more flavour is needed return to the heat and simmer to reduce and intensify the flavour.

MEATY STOCK

1.5 LITRE | 🕐 4 HRS 30 MINS | GF DF NF

This makes a brown stock but if a blond stock is wanted do not roast the bones and vegetables or use red wine. If you are looking for other twists to the flavour, experiment with different herbs and spices like we do in the vegetable stock.

INGREDIENTS

2.5kg	Individual bones beef/lamb chicken/pork (do not mix)
1 tbsp	Olive oil
1	Onion
1	Leek
1	Carrot
1	Celery stick
Handful of	Parsley stalks
Handful of	Thyme
3	Bay leaves
6	Black peppercorns

METHOD

1. Heat the oven to 180°C gas mark 4 place the bones in a large oiled roasting pan and cook in the oven for 1 hour until dark and well coloured. Add all the roughly chopped vegetables, mix well and roast for a further 40 minutes. This caramelisation will add flavour depth and colour to your stock.

2. Into a stock pan add the roughly chopped vegetables, herbs and peppercorns, add the browned bones and cover with cold water (approx 2 litres), bring to a boil and then reduce the heat. Gently simmer for 3 hours — actually the longer you cook it the better the flavour so if you can cook it for 5 hours!

3. Skim off any scum that may rise to the top of the cooking stock and discard.

4. Once cooked strain the stock through a fine sieve and discard the bones, if a deeper flavour is desired return to a clean stock pot and gently simmer to reduce and intensify the flavour.

5. If the stock has a layer of fat onto carefully skim off with a metal spoon or cool and place in the fridge and the fat will harden and easily be lifted off.

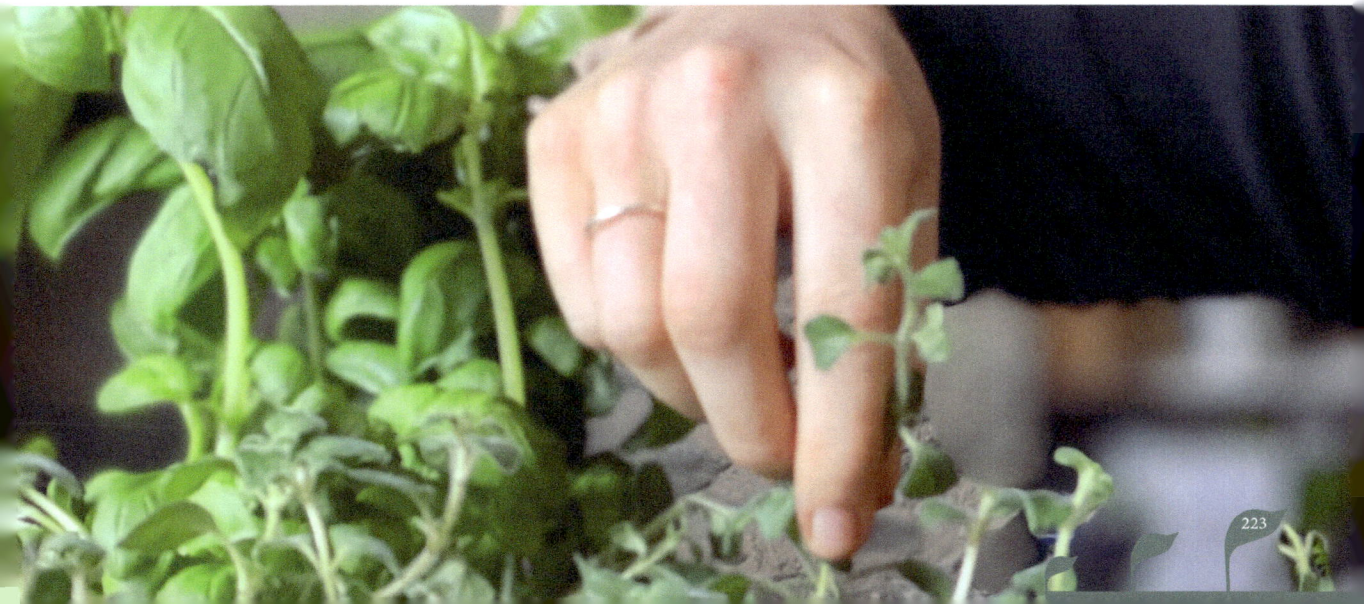

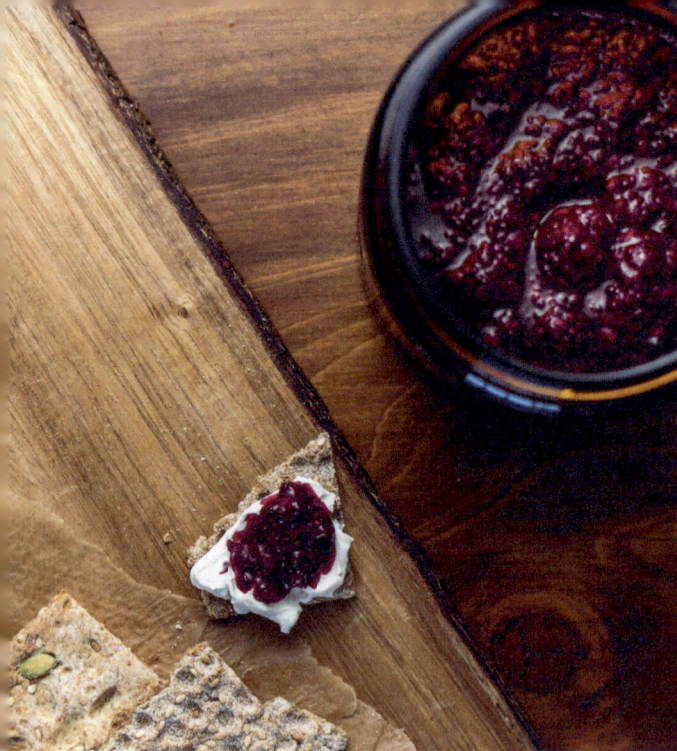

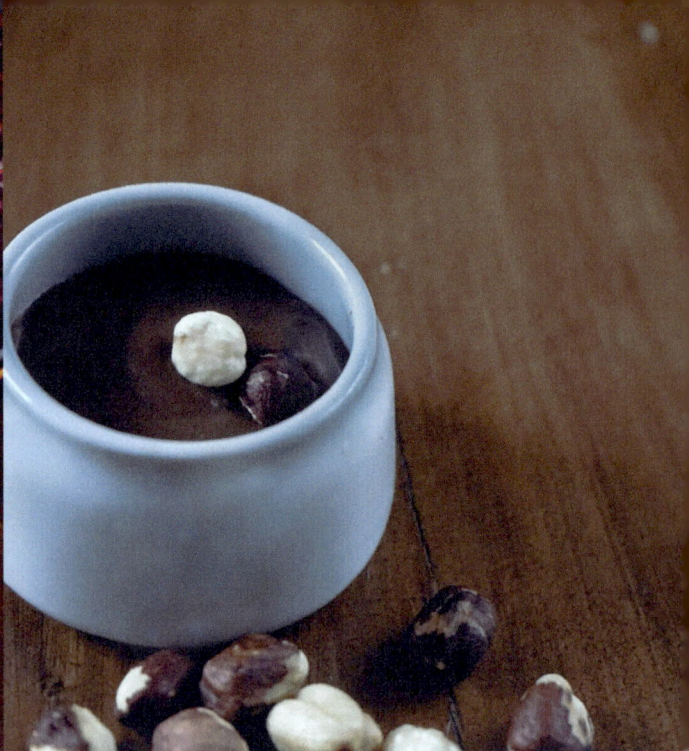

Blackberry Chia Jam

1 JAR | 🕐 1 HR 15 MINS |

GF DF V VE SS

Chia seeds will provide some protein and healthy fats to this easy to make jam.

INGREDIENTS

300g	Blackberries	60 ml	Apple juice
	(fresh or frozen)	1½ tbsp	Chia seeds
½	Lime	1 tbsp	Agave syrup

METHOD

1. Place the blackberries, juice and pulp of the lime and add apple juice in a medium saucepan.

2. Place on the heat, bring to the boil — then reduce and simmer for 2-3 minutes to break down the fruit.

3. Add the chia seeds and agave syrup, and stir through the mixture.

4. Cover and when cool, transfer to a jam jar, put a lid on, and place in the fridge to set.

*It will get thicker as the chia seeds swell, absorbing the liquid.

Cocoa Hazelnut Spread

1 JAR | 🕐 5 MINS | GF DF V VE SS

Pull away from the new age sugar by making your own sweet spread addiction.

The hazelnuts can be prepared from raw, simply oven heating until the skins can be rubbed off and the peeled hazelnuts can be added to the blender.

INGREDIENTS | EQUIPMENT

120g	Roast hazelnuts	Blender
50g	Cocoa powder	
80ml	Agave syrup	
150ml	Almond mylk	

METHOD

1. Grind the hazelnuts through the blender.

2. Simply add all ingredients to a blender for up to 3 minutes, until smooth and creamy.

3. Add to an airtight jar and it will taste to keep for 3 weeks.

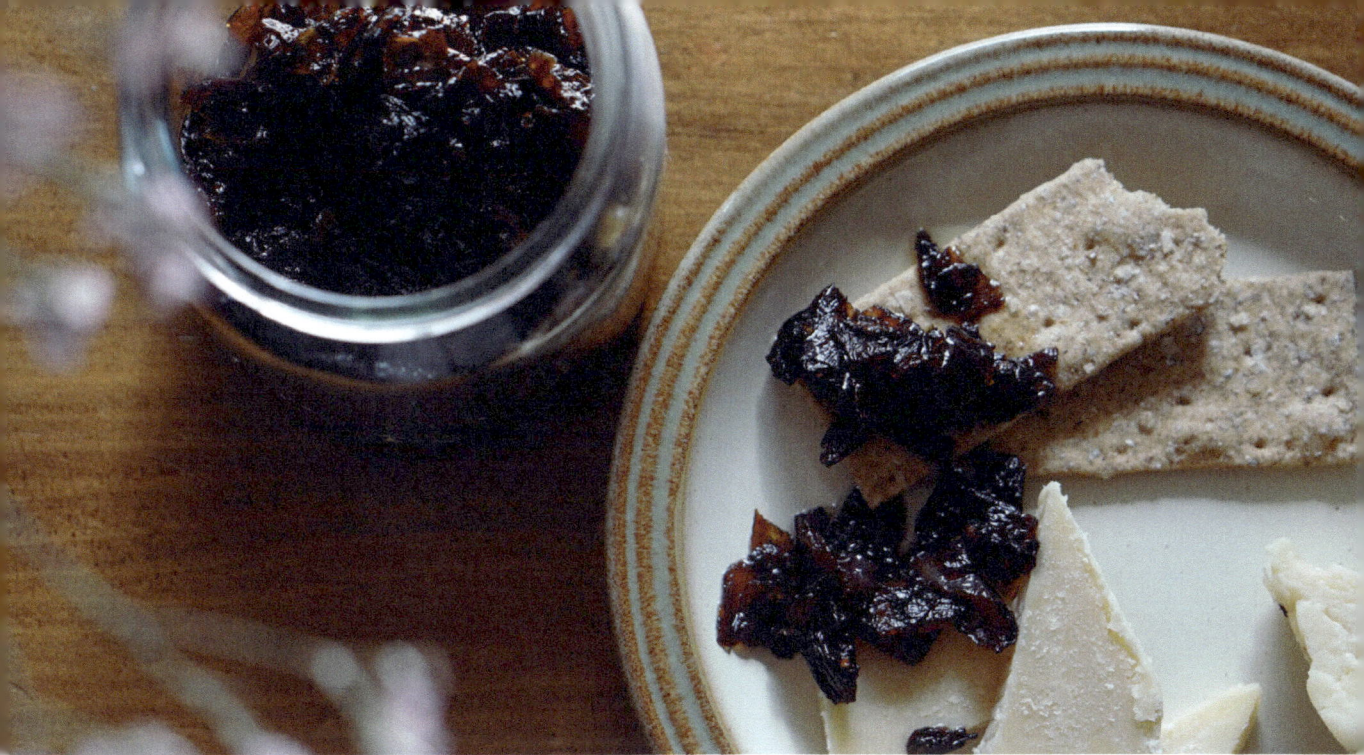

Red Onion Chutney

1 JAR | ⏱ 30 MINS | GF DF V Ve NF

"Delightful how I stumbled across this, at a hen party. When the men arrived to the same place with their stag session, they included an amazing chef. Absurdly while the surf was good in Cornwall, but an unforgttable weekend where a boat company manager introduced me to this sugar free chutney; just a little bit of honey, or carob syrup for the vegans. Delicious and delightfully healthy."

Red onions are slightly healthier nutritionally than white or brown onions due to the red colour providing increased levels of antioxidants. Onions and garlic are in our top recommended foods as they are full of therapeutic plant chemicals.

INGREDIENTS

4 tbsp	Rape seed oil
400g	Red onion
4	Garlic cloves
4 tbsp	Runny honey
60ml	Balsamic vinegar
1 tsp	Sea salt
1 tsp	Black pepper

METHOD

1. Turn the heat on to medium and add the oil to the pan while it warms.

2. Slice the red onions finely *(approx. 2x1 cm)* and add it to the pan for 10-15 minutes with a light but frequent stir so it doesn't burn.

3. While cooking, crush the garlic, and add the garlic, salt and honey and lightly stir for 5 minutes more.

4. Now add the balsamic vinegar and turn up the heat, so it will simmer away. Keep stirring for approx 2 mins until it has evaporated, turn off the heat and leave to cool for about 5 mins, before serving.

5. Add salt and pepper to taste.

DESSERTS

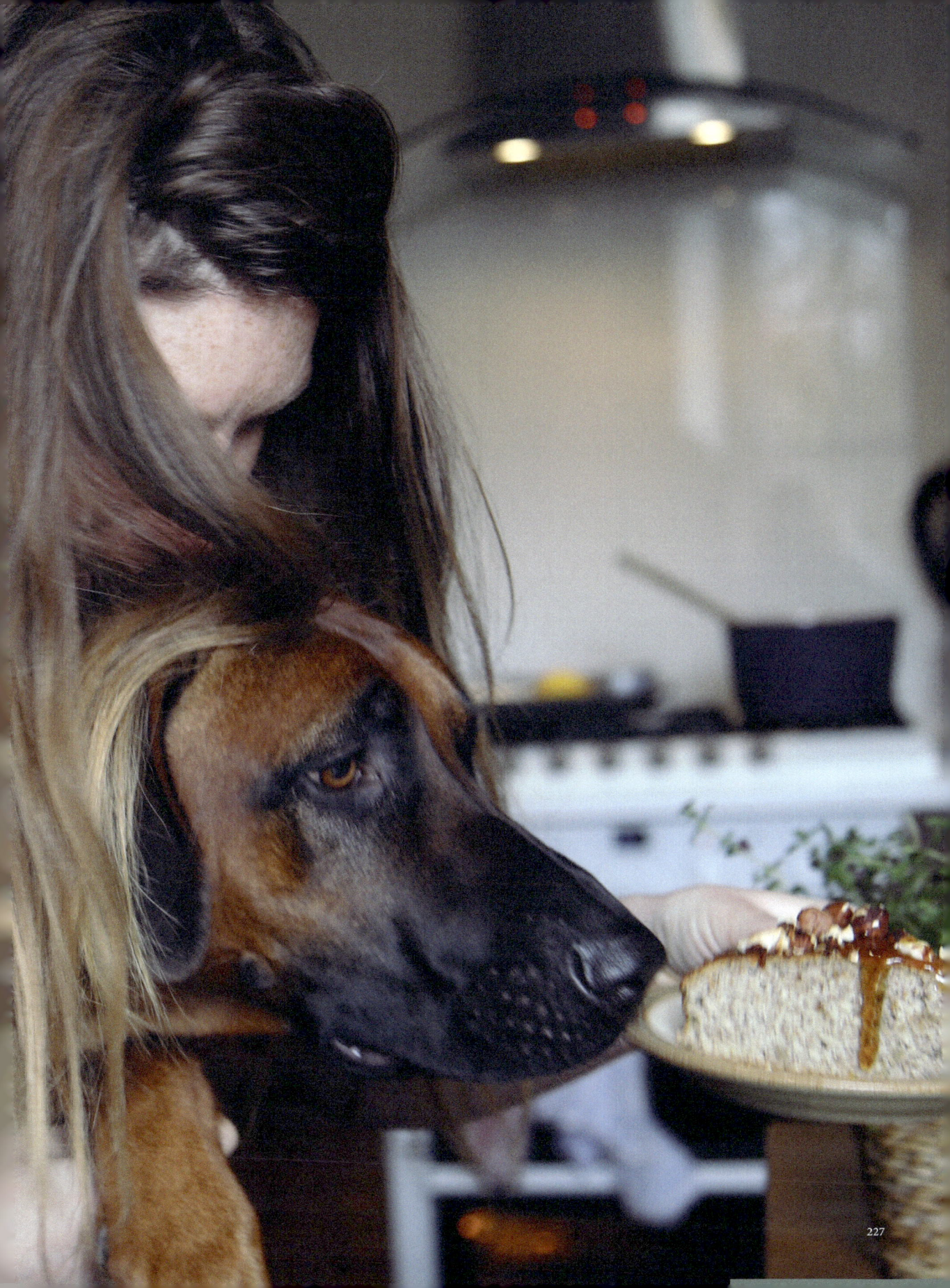

DARK CHOCOLATE FONDANT

SERVES 8 | 🕐 50 MINS | GF DF V

"Our aim is to make every mouthful of our recipe recommendations as nutrient dense as possible so using a combination of aubergine and chocolate makes a delicious dessert into an equally nutritious dessert."

Aubergines contain a particularly potent anticancer compound called solasodine rhamnosyl glycoside, plus they are rich in other antioxidants which are powerful free radical scavengers and also contain important vitamins and minerals.

Dark chocolate is an equally powerful source of antioxidants, polyphenols and flavenols and is rich in minerals such as zinc, iron and magnesium. Eggs and almonds provide you with protein and some healthy fats. If possible choose raw honey for a more nutrient dense sweetener. Serve with some dark coloured berries for added anticancer properties and top with creamy full fat yoghurt, or coconut milk yoghurt would be a perfect combination.

INGREDIENTS

1	Aubergine *(m)*
200g	Dark chocolate
80g	Runny honey
1 tsp	Salt
½ tsp	Vanilla extract
2	Eggs
70g	Ground almonds
1 tsp	Baking powder
10g	Cacao
1 tbsp	*Coconut oil spray*

EQUIPMENT

x8 Silicone cupcake vessels / ramekins
< 7cm >

METHOD

1. Heat the oven to 200°C.

2. Simply pierce the aubergine from head to toe on each side, I do x3 piercings per ¼, and set to roast for 30 mins.

3. Take 75g of the dark chocolate, break it up, and add to the oven in a heat proof vessel for 5-10 mins. This is perfect timing for when you get the aubergine out, as it needs that time to cool. Simply cut them in half, head to toe, to do so.

4. Scrape the aubergine centre into a blender, add the melted chocolate, honey and vanilla extract. Now blend together for 30 seconds, until smooth.

5. Lightly whisk your eggs and add the blended mix.

6. Mix together the dry ingredients; ground almonds, baking powder and cacao, before sieving and stirring them into the wet ingredients.

7. Grease the cases with coconut oil spray and divide the mixture equally between the 8 cup cake holders; cut the remaining chocolate and evenly press into the centre of each.

8. Cook for 15-20 mins and indulge in them whilst warm and runny.
   *You can prep them and store them in the fridge before the final cook if served after dinner. Pop them in as you serve the main course.

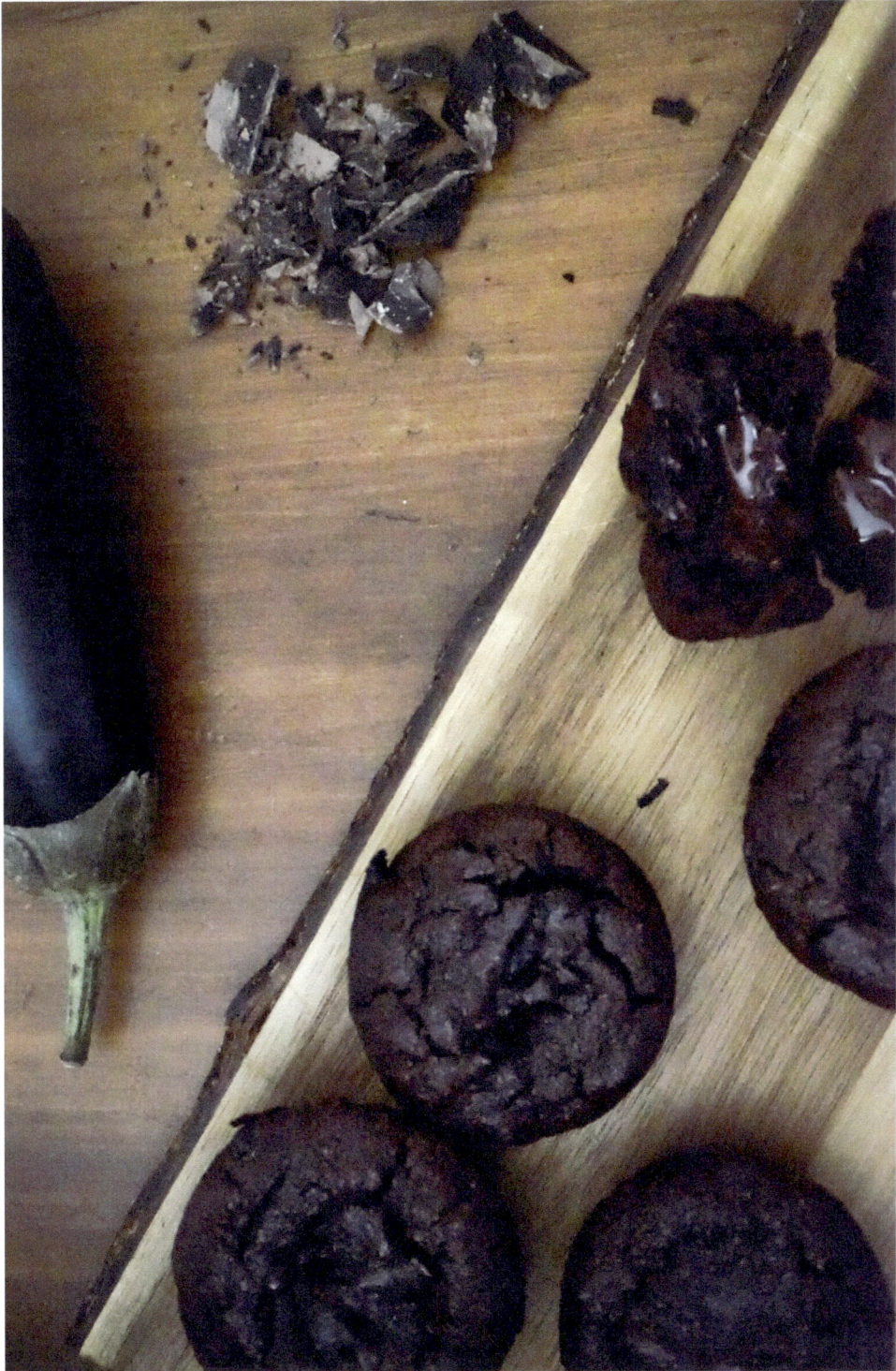

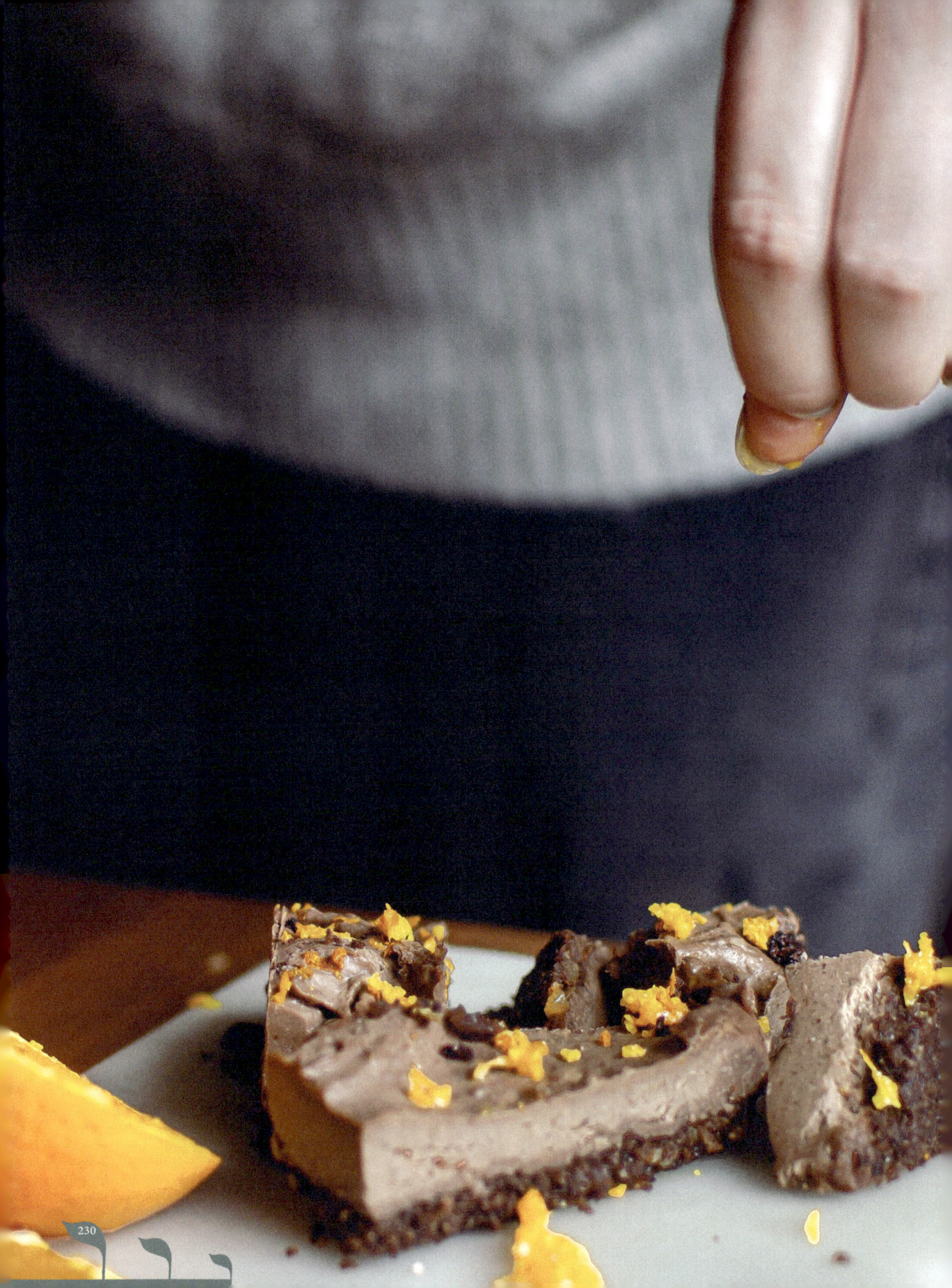

CHESTNUT TORTE

SERVES 8 | 🕐 1 HR 30 MINS | GF V

"As ever, my cupboards were full after crimble, and chestnuts are my favourite little Xmas element which helps lower your blood cholesterol, and contains fibre and vitamins to thrive you (even after eating dessert!) It's a fairly good and quick dish to make all year round though, as it's chilled perfectly for summer garden tea and cake in the garden — good times.
The torte uses raw (delicious) eggs, so it's important to have fresh organic eggs."

Make use of chestnuts all year round as a good source of vitamin C, B vitamins and folic acid.

The ground linseeds and pecan nuts will provide more of the healthy fatty acids especially omega 3. Remember it is always healthier to grind linseeds when needed to stop them oxidising.

INGREDIENTS

BASE
100g	Pecans
100g	Currants

TOPPING
300g	Roast chestnuts *(shells removed)*
2	Eggs
100g	Dark chocolate
270ml	Double cream
2	Unwaxed oranges

EQUIPMENT

9" Expandable cake tin

METHOD

1. Set the oven to 180°C.

2. Chop ¼ of your base pecans to small chunks and then blend the rest with the currants. Mix together and then squash into the base of the cake tin, pre-lined with baking parchment. Slip into the oven for 10 mins. Set to the side to cool once out.

3. Blend the chestnuts until smooth. Separate your eggs into yolks and whites, and add the yolks to the chestnuts for a quick final blend to combine.

4. Chop the chocolate into small chunks and melt it, in a vessel over a pan of boiling water, aka bain-marie.

5. Then, once warm and mostly melted, mix with ½ the cream (185ml).

6. Once fully mixed, pour into the bowl with the chestnuts and stir.

7. Whisk the remaining cream (185ml) and fold into the chestnuts.

8. Whisk the egg whites and add to the mix.

9. Finely grate the orange zest, squeeze out the juice and scrape out the pulp. Mix in half of the pulp with the juice to the chestnut mix, the other half will be scattered for texture and decoration. Simply add it to the base, once cooled and pop into the fridge to set. Best to wait approx 1 hr for it to set in the fridge, left in to the cake holder to maintain its structure.

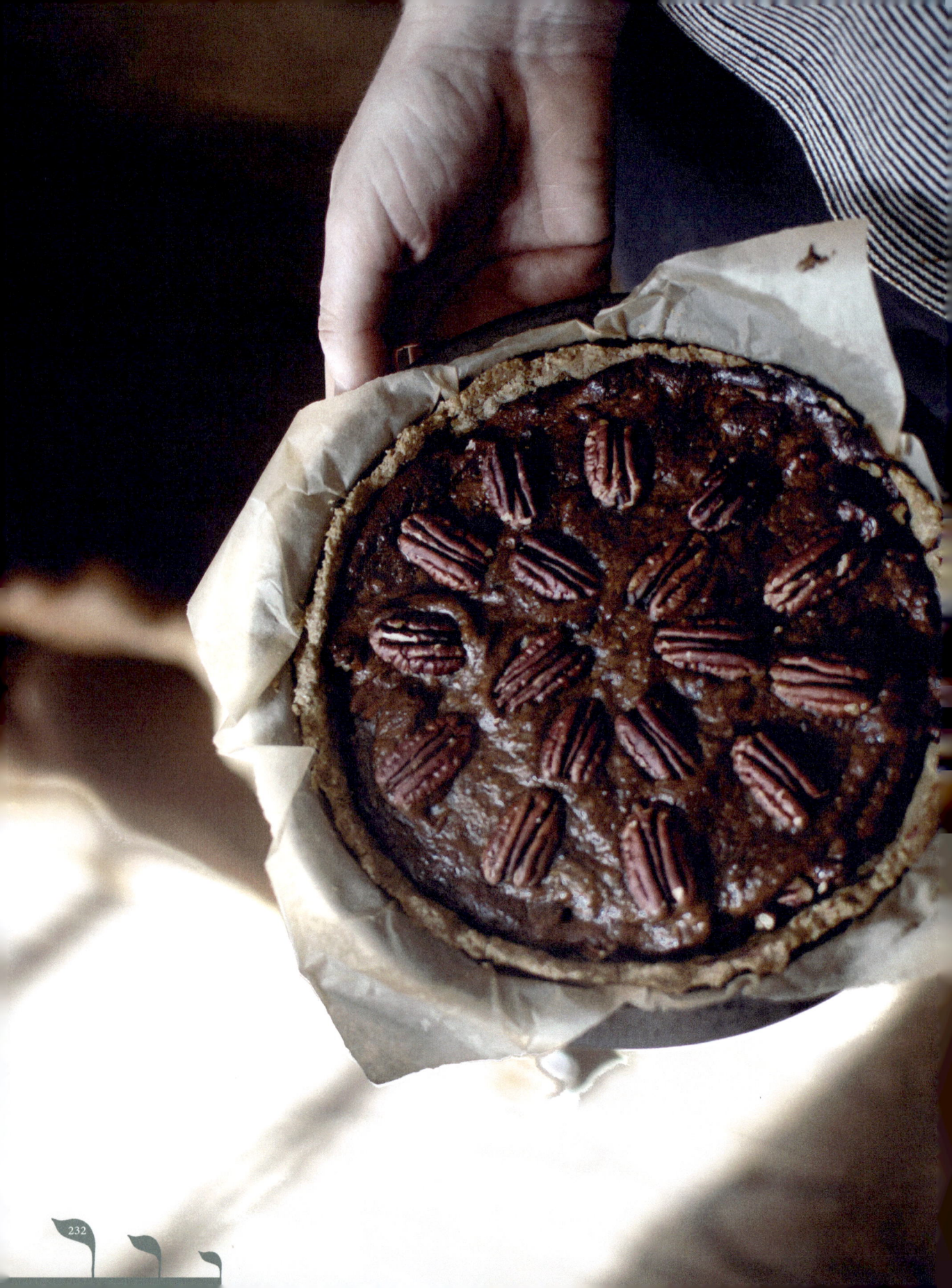

PECAN PIE

SERVES 8 | ⏱   10 MINS | DF   V

"Just one of those moments when you just throw together what is within arms length, to satisfy your want. This was created with and for my dreamboat of a mama and only needed 4 trials to be satisfied both through taste and health."

This provides plenty of fibre by way of the pecans, dates and linseeds which slow down the release of the sugars from the honey, dates and flour thus making this a lower glycaemic choice than regular pecan pie. Healthy fats are provided in the seeds, nuts and coconut oil.

INGREDIENTS

BASE

40ml	Coconut oil
25ml	Honey
50g	Linseed
100g	Rye flour

FILLING

79g (*1 can*)	Coconut milk
100g	De-stoned medjool dates
100g	Pecans
1	Egg
1 tsp	Cinnamon
1 tsp	Vanilla extract
Pinch of	Sea salt

EQUIPMENT

8" Cake tin, round
Baking weights (OR dried chick peas)

METHOD

1. Turn on the oven to 190°C.

2. Melt the coconut oil, with the honey in the oven.

3. In the meantime, blend the the linseed, and mix it in with the flour, coconut oil and honey when melted, followed by 25ml water — start with half, and add more if needed.

4. Knead the pastry together. Line the cake dish with baking parchment, and thinly add the base layer, no need to roll it out, just do it by hand.

5. Ensure it is covered with baking paper, which can be held down down with dried chickpeas or baking weights. Add to the oven for 20 mins to bake the pastry — blind.

6. Extract the solid coconut milk from the tin, and blend with the dates, egg, cinnamon, vanilla and a pinch of sea salt.

7. Remove the weight and cover. Pop back in the oven for 5 mins, and lower to 150°C.

8. Set aside about 12 pecans for decoration, chop the rest and spread them over the pie case, before filling with the delicious content. Decorate with your saved pecans and pop back in to the oven for 45 mins, when it must be left to cool.

- Keep an eye on the pie whilst cooking and cover with baking paper if you feel it's on the edge of a burn. Every oven is different!

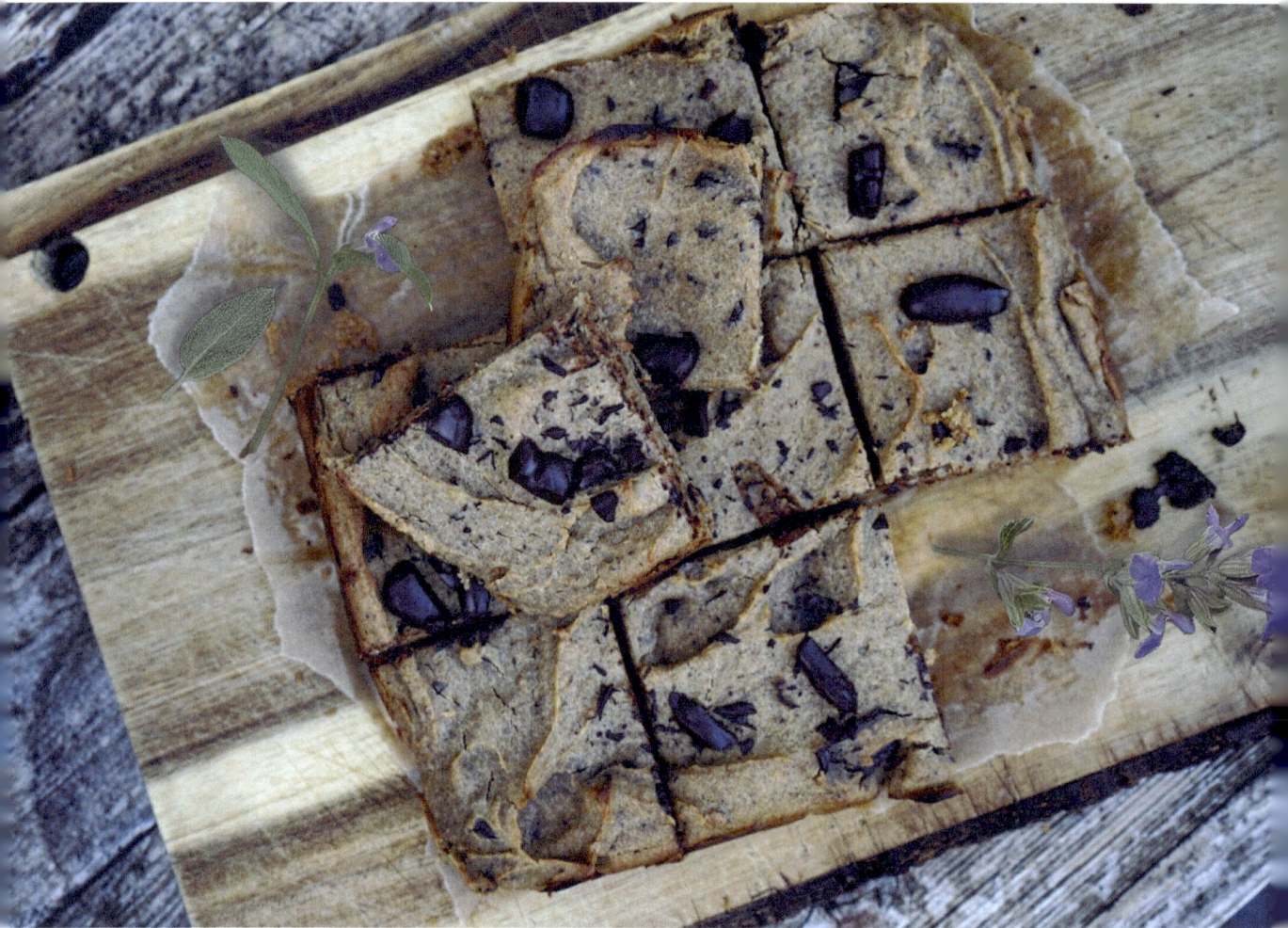

BEAUTIFUL BLONDIES

SERVES 8 | ⏱ 35 MINS | GF DF V Ve NF SS

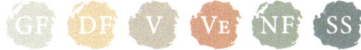

"Blondies. What more could one ask for? These fudgy blondies are grain, gluten, dairy and sugar-free. I'd say the quirkiest element of it is the arrowroot, It works as a thickening agent and keeps the dish held together. One of the good things is that it holds dark chocolate, which can be anywhere from 80%. It's well worth to have taste sessions so you can learn which brand fits you best. And yes I have added the VEGAN tab, so go for the vegan chocolate if wanted, I love the hazelnut mylk chocolate that I find in Hotel Chocolate."

These bars are packed with fibre from the butter beans, dates and arrowroot and are an ideal snack to have with you when you need a boost of energy. They have plenty of healthy carbohydrate, alongside protein, which together help to keep you fuller for longer.

Much of the carbohydrate content is resistant starch, which means it is resistant to digestion and therefore a perfect food source for the microbiome. Optimising our microbiome has so many health benefits, including bowel health, balancing hormones and stimulating the immune system. Arrowroot is a great choice as a thickening agent and is considered a health food. Being high in folate adds to its nutritional benefits. Other gluten free options are cornstarch, tapioca flour, potato starch and rice flour.

Medjool dates, despite their high sugar content, have many beneficial antioxidants and provide iron, potassium, B vitamins, calcium and magnesium. The tahini adds some healthy omega fats to the mix and the dark chocolate provides more healthy fats and antioxidants. Brownies, or rather Blondies, need no longer be a guilty pleasure!

INGREDIENTS

400g	Butter beans
110g	Tahini
110g	Medjool dates x8
50g	Arrowroot powder
75g	Dark chocolate - 80%
¼ tsp	Baking powder
¼ tsp	Baking soda
1 tsp	Vanilla extract
Pinch	Sea salt
-	

Add sage flowers for decoration and a dusky delicate taste

EQUIPMENT

8" Cake tin, square

METHOD

1. Preheat the oven to 180°C.

2. Line the cake tin with baking parchment, or oil it.

3. Add all of the ingredients, bar the chocolate, into the food processor and blitz till the mixture is smooth; it may take a few mins as the mixture is quite thick.

4. Chop the dark chocolate into chunks and stir into the mixture.

5. Scoop the mixture into the lined baking tin and bake for 20-25 mins.

6. Remove from the oven and leave to cool before slicing up; they will firm up.

7. The blondies will store in an airtight container in the fridge for up to 3 days.

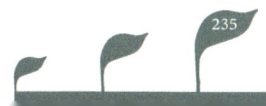

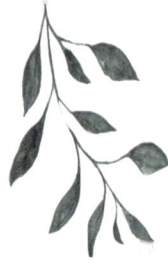
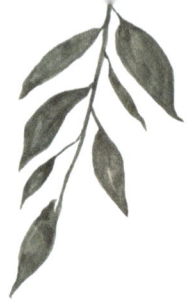

EDIBLE FLOWERS

Flowers are a beautiful part of our world: lovely to look at, enjoyable to grow and can even add a healthy twist to our diet.

Sowing seeds and watching them germinate, planting out the little seedlings in your garden or window box and eventually harvesting the leaves and flowers for decoration, flavour and wholesome nutrition is so satisfying!

I have borage flowers growing wild in my garden, and they are my absolute favourite (and no effort required!). They are usually a beautiful blue, but can also be white or pink. They taste peppery with a twist of cucumber, or coconut, so compliment many dishes. They bloom through the spring and summer here in England.

My next favourite are the nutty, spicy savoury nasturtium flower heads and leaves, which have strong flame coloured flowers. Nasturtiums grow and self seed in most soils and are such a cheerful sight! Add the flowers to salads for that spicy hint of peppery mustard.

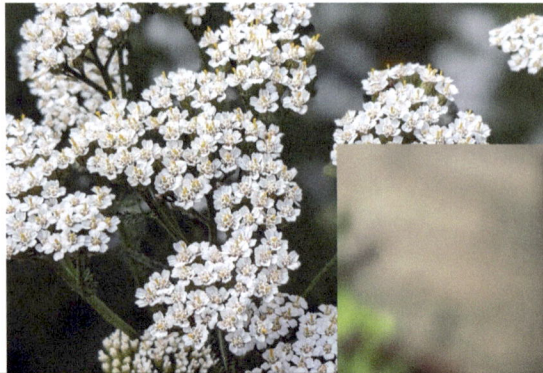

Yarrow >

< Borage Flowers | Nasturtium >

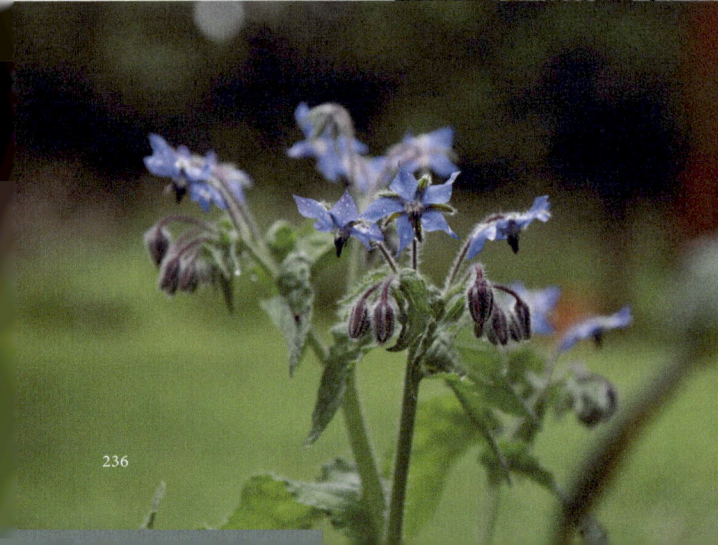

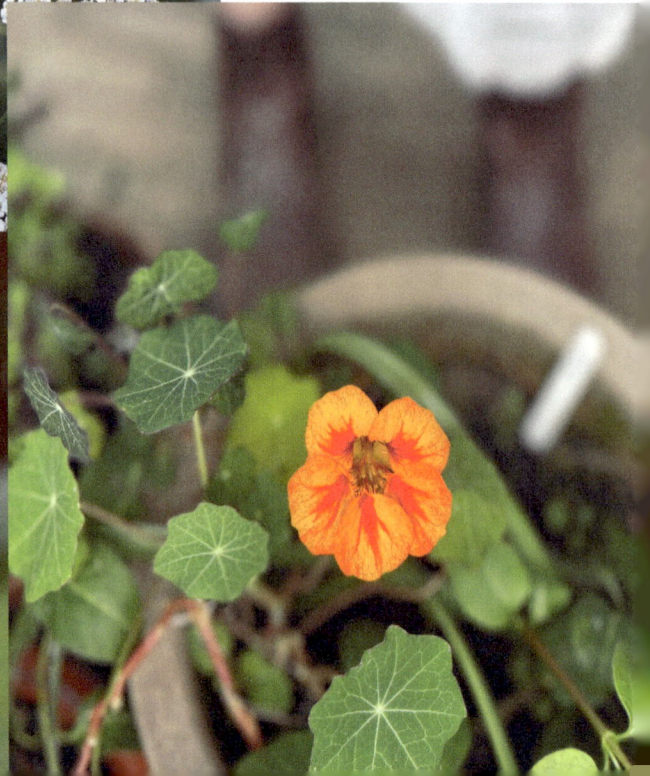

Other flowers you can enjoy — both sight and taste — sage flowers have a light dusky and delicate flavour (see p235) and grow well at home, for which the leaves are good in many other dishes. Calendula and tagetes which are both from the marigold family. Sunflowers, where you can even roast the buds like artichoke hearts and roses, which have a varied flavour set influenced by their perfumes, the flavours swinging widely from vanilla to sherbert...

If you have planted peas or beans you can eat the shoots and flowers (sadly not those beautiful sweet peas though - as they are toxic, but good to swipe for beauty) and herbs that have 'shot' ie flowered, like fennel, dill or basil have edible, flavoursome flowers. Your freshly picked herbs and flowers will have maximum vitamins. You can also dry some flowers such as rosemary or lavender for decorating out of season.

If you are a gardener you will know that some plants deter aphids and of course flowers attract bees and other pollinators. Planting hyssop, lavender, sage, garlic, onions and chives will deter certain pests such as aphids and carrot root flies. Earwigs will happily survive on aphids only attacking display plants and flowers if they get hungry or thirsty. Those useful, edible marigolds, particularly the strongly scented french variety are good to interlace with your herb and veg growings as they help deter whitefly and aphids and the nasturtium flowers do deter the classic black fly from your other growths. Fingers crossed they survive for you to munch!

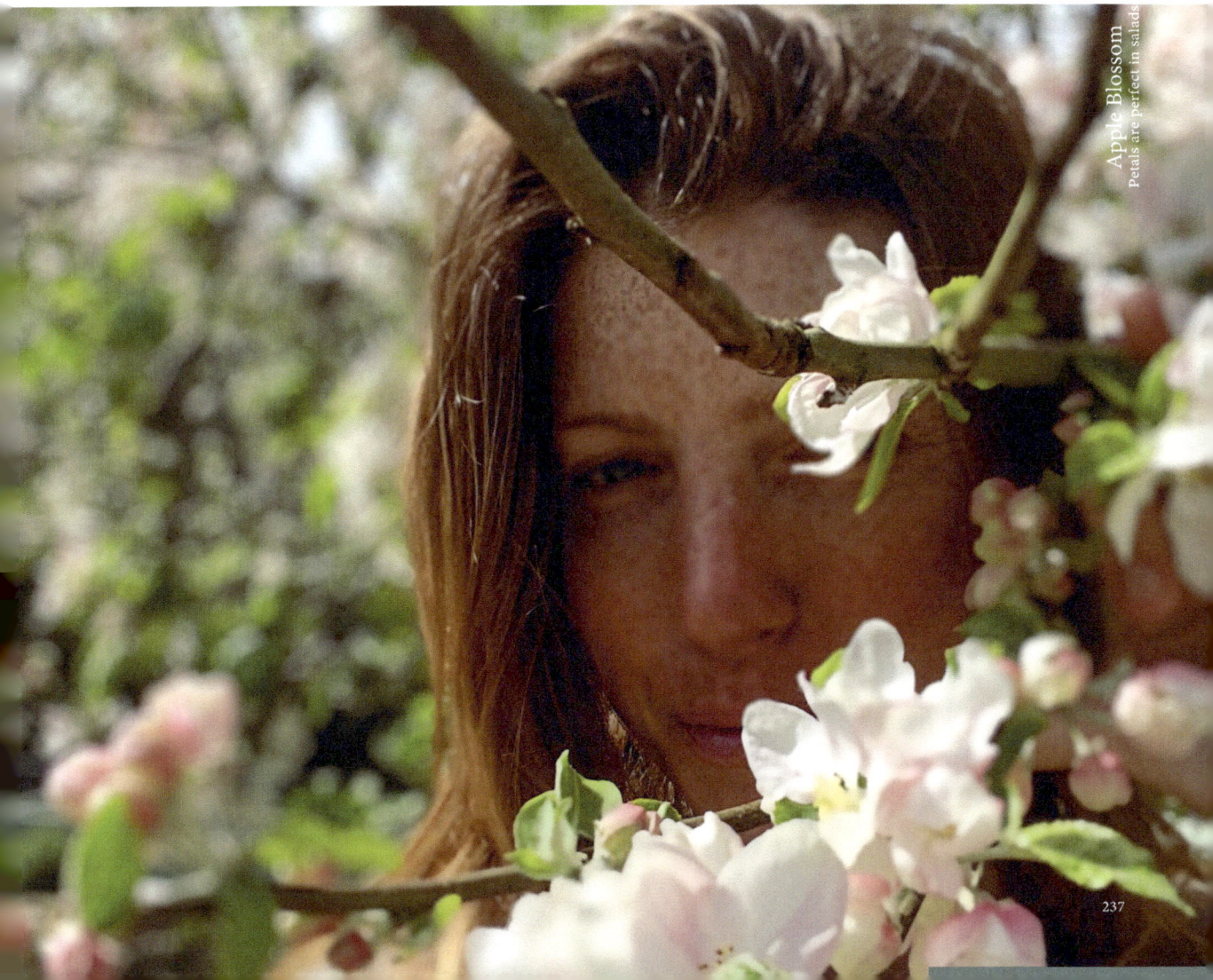

Apple Blossom
Petals are perfect in salads

Cookie Balls

SERVES 8 | 20 MINS | GF V VE

INGREDIENTS

100g	Dates
110g	Walnuts
2 tsp	Ground ginger
20g	Dark chocolate

METHOD

1. Pop the dates in a mug, cover with water, just let them sit for 5 mins.

2. While waiting, crush your dark chocolate which will be added last minute.

3. Blend the walnuts and ginger together, for 5 seconds, then add the dates when hydrated — simply throw them in the blender too for just up to 20 seconds.

4. Simply take the dough into a mixing bowl. Mix in the crushed dark chocolate, and roll into 8 balls. 25g each — aka a ping pong ball is best.

5. Pop them into the fridge, I like a 5 minute firm, but they are good at any time!

"I love simple recipes, life can be so full and hectic that I revoke as much complication from it as possible. When I make these little balls, I'll do so in batches to ensure at least a week's worth of guilt-free energy boosts. Filled with anticancer superfoods you can be safe in the knowledge that your mini-effort will be worth it. I particularly, like to serve the below balls after hosting friends or family too as an easy after-dinner treat."

Dark Chocolate Sesame Almond Balls

SERVES 6 | 30 MINS | GF DF V

INGREDIENTS

60g	Almonds
40g	Tahini
20g	Coconut oil
1 tsp	Cinnamon
1.5 tbsp	Agave oil
60g	Dark chocolate
1 tsp	Salt

METHOD

1. Roast the almonds for 5-10 mins at 180°C.

2. Take ½ of the almonds, crush them in the pestle and mortar and put to the side to mix in later.

3. The 2nd ½ of the almonds are to be blended — through pulses or a 2 blade bullet to create an oily butter.

4. Once created add in the tahini, coconut oil, cinnamon and agave.

5. Once blended, mix in the crushed almonds well and simply roll into 6 balls.

6. Pop in the freezer for 5 minutes, while you bain marie (melt) the dark chocolate.

7. Prong the balls with a skewer or toothpick and dip in the chocolate to cover. Let the excess melted chocolate drip off, sprinkle with the salt, then place on the baking paper to set in the fridge for approx 15 mins.

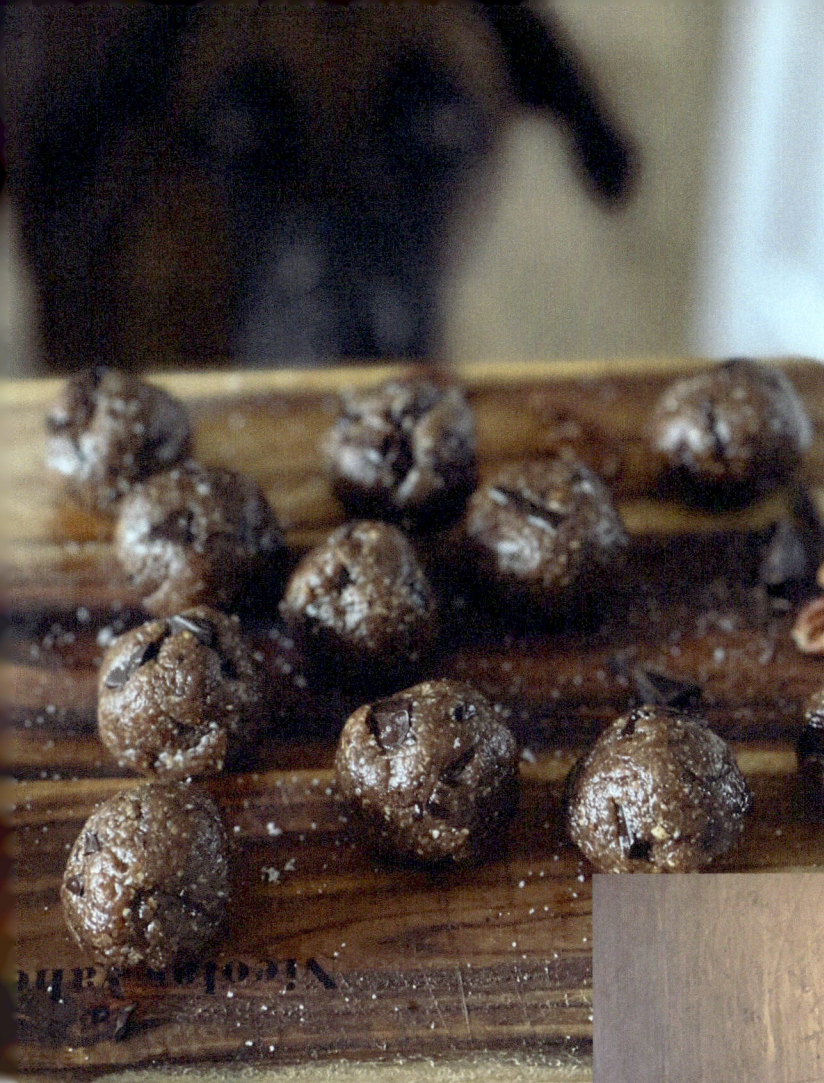

If you are wanting a little sweet treat these will hit the spot but provide you with some super anticancer foods.

Ginger is one of our top anticancer foods and dark chocolate is allowable in small quantities as it provides some exceptional antioxidants such as polyphenols, flavanols and catechins and some healthy fatty acids. Walnuts add to the healthy fatty acid profile with high amounts of anti-inflamatory omega 3. Dates are an excellent source of fibre.

"I personally have a strong memory of the soul the Cookie Balls were made for — Oscar the Grouch (the Cookie Monster from Sesame Street) — and I do believe they would be included in his obsession. Well worth the effort!

AND I say that the chocolate covered ball are perfect to be served as petit fours, that 'end of dinner' treat. The textures of a crunchable dark chocolate covered bite, work perfectly to balance the quality of the flavours."

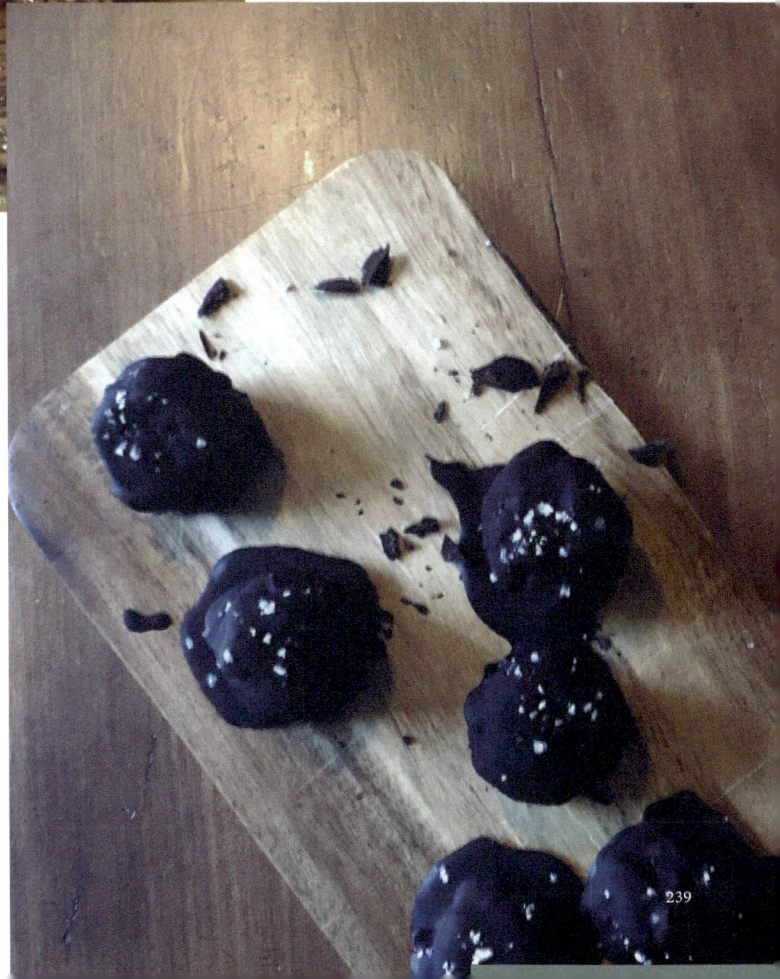

SEEDED APRICOT BALLS

SERVES 6 | 🕐 10 MINS | GF DF V Ve NF

"These are one of my addictions back in my London days. Everything you buy as a snack on the way to work, or at the hospital is seriously sweet. New age sugar or white processed carbs. I think that getting a softer sweetness with more nutrients, especially if it's on the edge of savoury and a 10th of the pre-made price is great. Done."

Apricots have been added to our top anticancer foods. The reason being that they are excellent sources of vitamin A and contain many antioxidants. They are also high in fibre, making a good choice for gut health. These seeded balls are in fact a perfect blend for a gut friendly food. The seeds provide the essential anti-inflammatory omega fats and are another good source of fibre.

INGREDIENTS

55g	Dried apricots
10g	Sunflower seeds
50g	Pumpkin seeds
10g	Desiccated coconut

METHOD

1. Blend all ingredients together bar the coconut.

2. Equally divide the mix into 6 segments, hand roll into balls and roll in the dessicated coconut to coat them and finish.

3. Simply keep in the fridge and enjoy your healthy snacks.

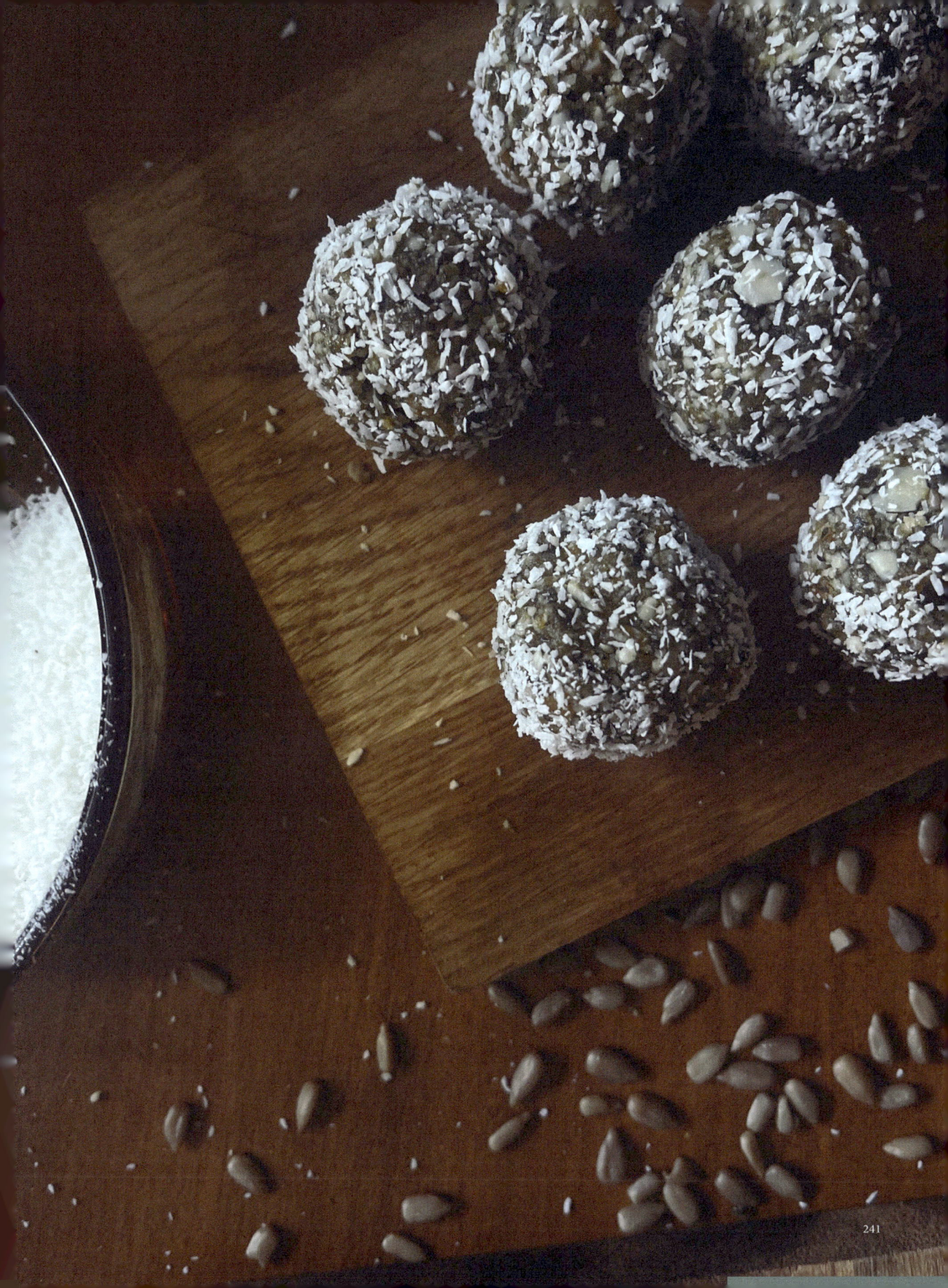

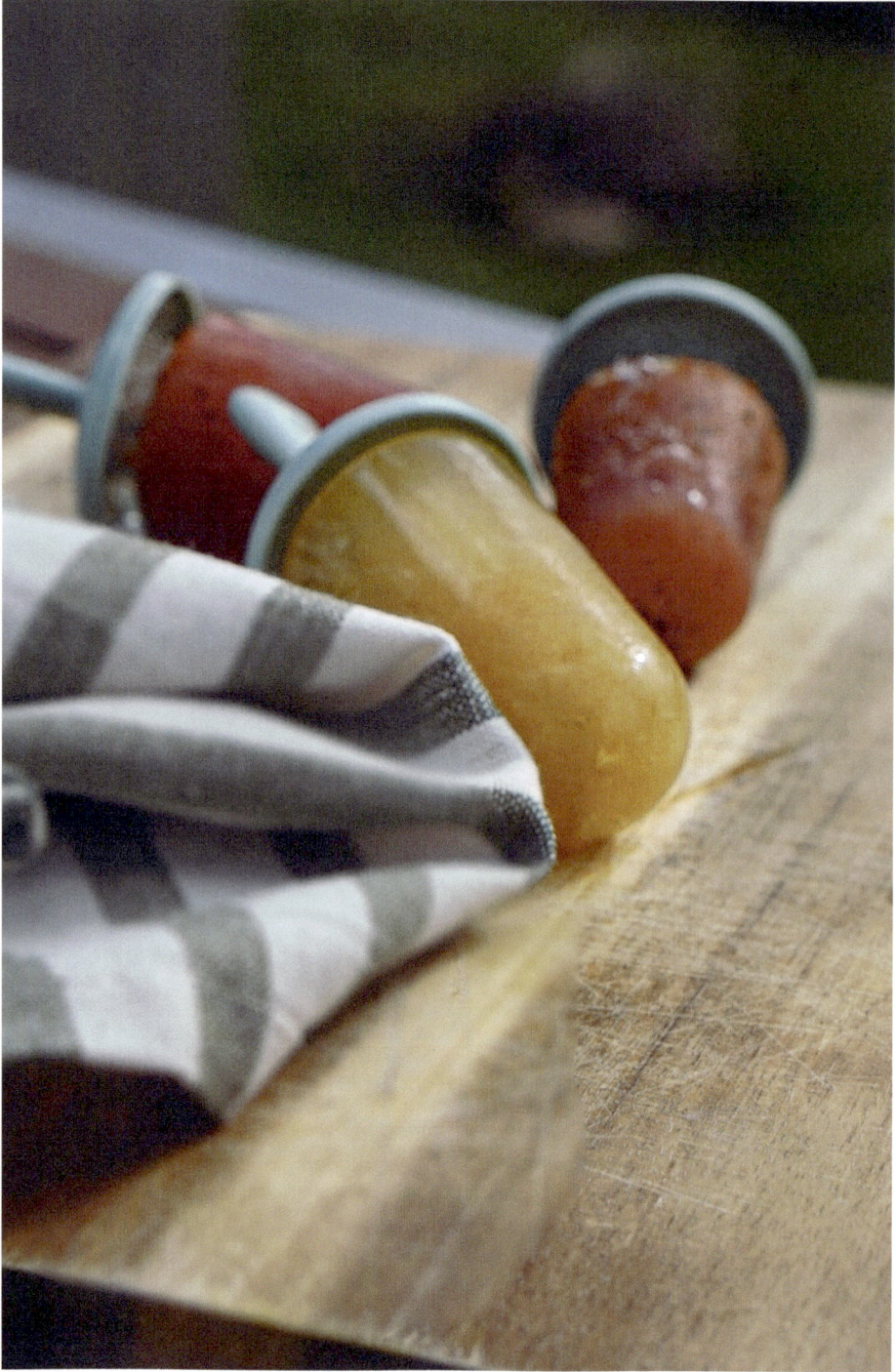

Lollipop Lollipop
Oh LOLLI LOLLI LOLLI (...pop)

SERVES 6 | 🕐 5 MINS (+ 5-6 HRS) |

"The song goes well and almost covers the time to make these genius little pops. I advise you to be open, as you will love finding your own niche of flavour; coconut, mango, raspberry, creamy coffee, lemonade... the list is never ending. Fresh and vitamin laden."

Minty Watermelon Pops GF DF V VE NF SS

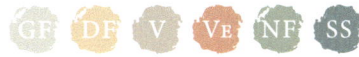

INGREDIENTS

800g	Watermelon
	approx. 600g deskinned
1	Lime
Handful	Fresh mint
mini pinch of	Sea salt

METHOD

1. Chunkily chop the watermelon, alongside juicing the lime and de-stemming the fresh mint leaves.

2. Blend all together and pour into the lolly moulds to pop into the freezer. They will require approx. 5-6 hrs to set.

Orangutang Pops GF DF V NF SS

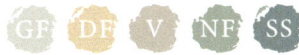

INGREDIENTS

800g / 6	Oranges
3cm	Fresh ginger knob
1 dsp	Honey

METHOD

1. Juice the oranges.

2. Scrape off the ginger skin, finely grate or chop it and then squash through a sieve into a bowl to mix with the oranges and stir in the honey.

3. Pour into the lolly moulds to pop into the freezer. They will require approx. 5-6 hrs to set.

"I think that if you see blood oranges, they are a perfect switcheroo for the classic."

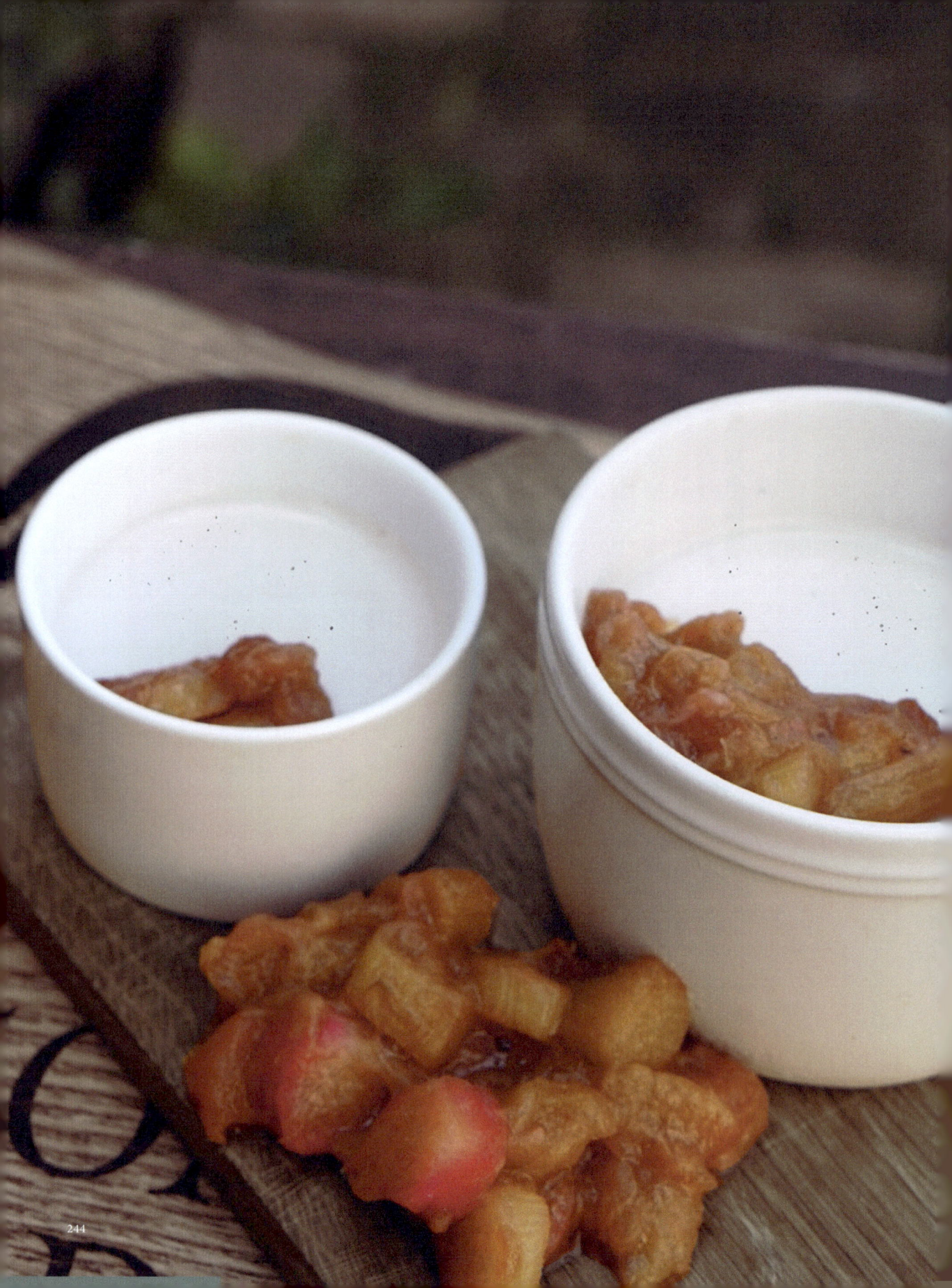

Rhubarb Panna Cotta

SERVES 4 | ⏱ 1 HR 30 MINS | GF DF NF SS

"Super simple, and works both hot and warm so can easily be made a little in advance and eaten later. Add other seasonal vegetables to cook if you have a favourite or an abundance of something. "

A delicious panna cotta made with coconut milk so great for those avoiding dairy. Rhubarb is a good source of fibre and the antioxidants called anthocyanins which have numerous health benefits.

INGREDIENTS

3 sheets	Gelatine leaf
1 tin	Coconut milk
	(full fat - 60%)
30g	Honey
1 tsp	Vanilla bean paste
-	
200g	Rhubarb
15g	Honey

METHOD

1. Put the gelatine sheets in a shallow bowl of cold tap water to soften. This will only take approx 5 mins.

2. Stir your can of coconut milk, add ½ to a pan to warm, not boil, on the stove. Stir in the honey and vanilla, and turn off the heat.

3. Add the gelatine to the pan, after squeezing out the excess water in your hand and stir in to dissolve.

4. To cool the mix, add the last of the coconut milk and stir in.

5. Pour into 4 holders (small glasses or ramekins are perfect) and add to the fridge.

6. Lightly chop the rhubarb and throw it into a pan to heat with 2 tbsp of water and 15g honey. Stir while heating and breaking down to a delicious compote, then just set aside to cool and simply dress the panna cotta when served.

Vanilla Sponge Cake

SERVES 10 | ⏲ 1 HR | GF V

"You can switch the honey for nutritional ingredients such as carob fruit, or agave syrup at equal measurements. To replace the eggs for vegans or those who prefer non dairy products... The 2 eggs can be switched for 3 tbsp of ground flax seeds, normally mix with 6 tbsps of water and rest for a minute or so to strengthen its hold."

Ground almonds hike up the nutritional content and provide a good level of anti-inflammatory omega 3.

The fruit provides a perfect contrast to the nuttiness of the cake and with lashings of double cream this is a delicious occasional treat on a day when you just must have cake!

INGREDIENTS

250g	Ground almonds
1 tsp	Baking powder
2	Eggs
65g (¼ jar)	Organic runny honey
Splash of	Vanilla extract
-	
500ml	Double cream
150g	Raspberries
100g	Pomegranate seeds

METHOD

1. Heat the oven to 180°C.

2. Mix the ground almonds and baking powder together, add the honey alongside the eggs and vanilla, and stir to create a paste.

3. Slowly stir in 250ml of water to the mix to create the perfect cake batter consistency.

4. Seperate into 2 cake tins and pop in the oven.

5. Cook for 20 mins, check by inserting a skewer; all done if it comes out clean.

6. Whip the cream while the cake cools and simply spread the cream on inbetween and top once cool and ready to serve.

7. Tumble on the raspberries and scatter the pomegranate seeds.

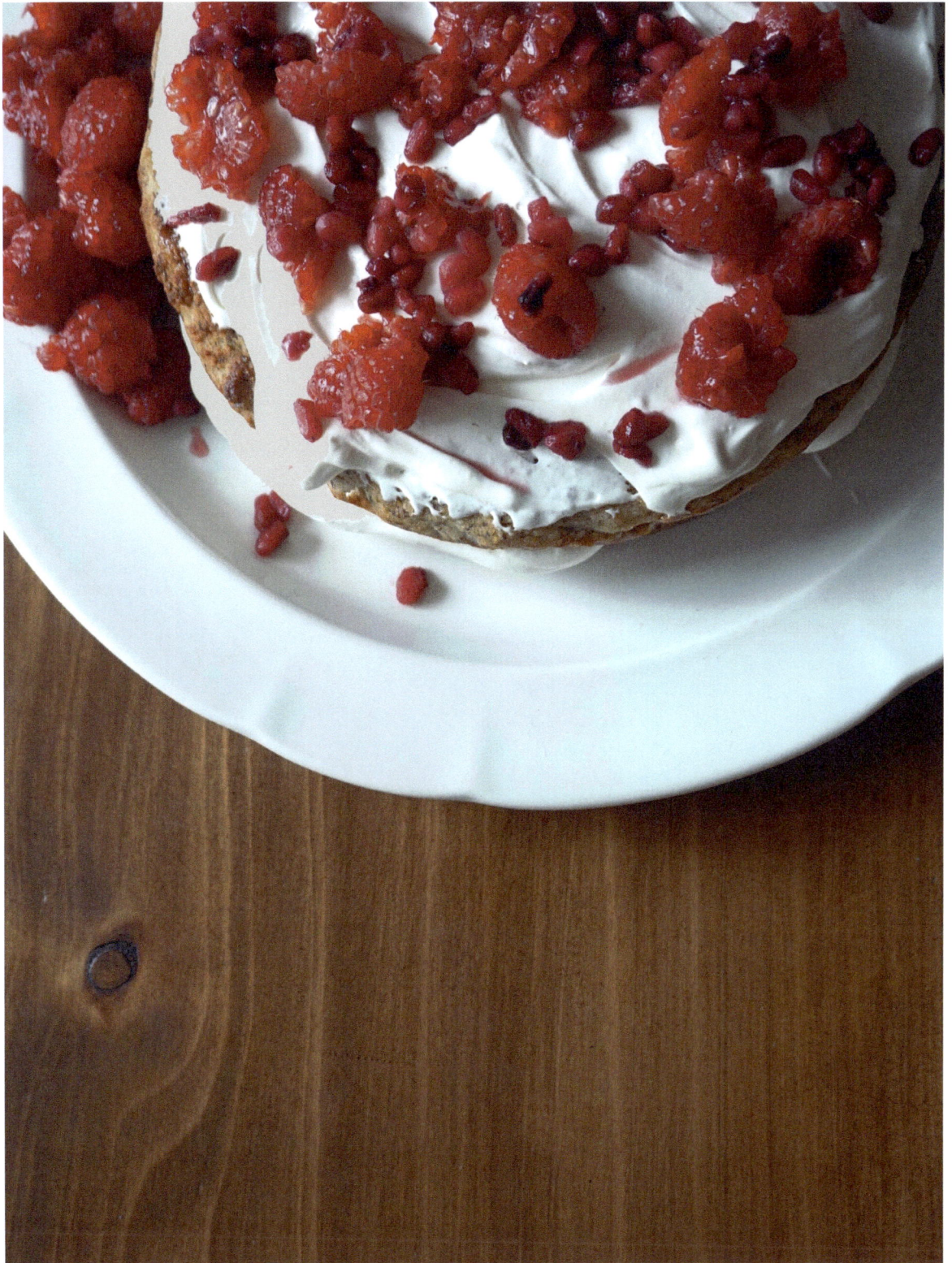

SUGAR LOVE

This is a big step, but once you get it, you add healthy to your happy bites. It is an understanding that makes you stop and appreciate every bite, knowing that it can be nourishing not just your taste, but your body's strength and health. There is both physical and mental satiation sultration.

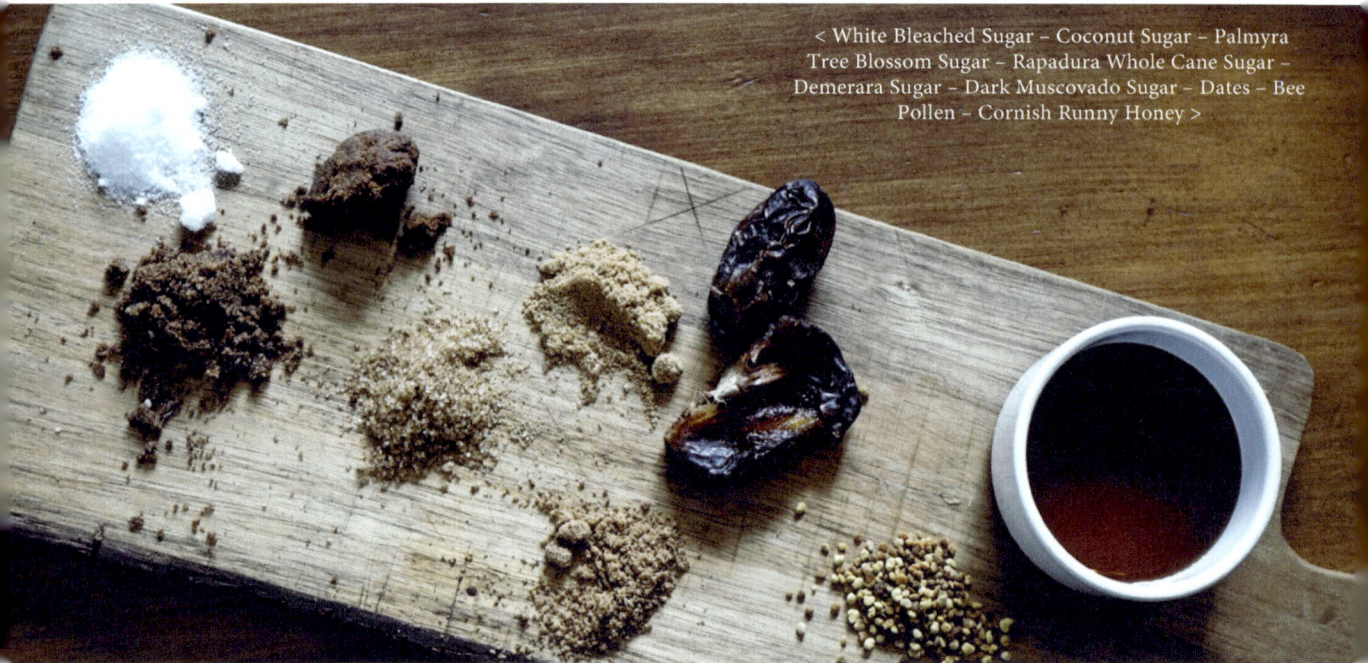

< White Bleached Sugar – Coconut Sugar – Palmyra Tree Blossom Sugar – Rapadura Whole Cane Sugar – Demerara Sugar – Dark Muscovado Sugar – Dates – Bee Pollen – Cornish Runny Honey >

Thankfully there has been much more emphasis in recent years about the evils of consuming too many sugars. Whilst many of us are probably aware now that added sugars in foods and drinks are not good for us, there are still mixed messages regarding the body needing sugar for energy.

We may require a small amount of sugar (glucose) in our blood stream but we certainly don't have to consume it to maintain this - glucose can be made and stored in the liver from the breakdown of fats or from the breakdown of amino acids within the body. This stored glucose is only released when necessary for energy.

Blood Sugar and Exercise

Insulin sensitivity is increased during exercise as your muscle cells increase glucose uptake during and after activity. It does depend on the intensity of the exercise, with short bursts of intensive exercise best at promoting the uptake of glucose. It therefore makes sense, if you are going to eat carbs to have them immediately before or after intense exercise.

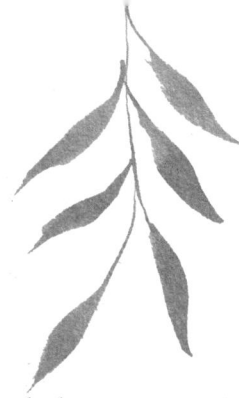

Sugar Bites

- Use natural sweeteners such as raw honey, maple syrup, blackstrap molasses which are more nutrient dense than ordinary sugar. Blackstrap molasses are very high in B vitamins, iron, calcium, magnesium, manganese and potassium.

- If you eat sugary foods, eat them after a protein and fat rich meal when the digestive process is longer. This slows the release of those sugars into the blood stream.

- Avoid foods with added sugar. If sugar is placed high up on the ingredient list of a food product, the product is best avoided.

- Artificial sweeteners are, in general, not a good choice as they are very sweet and stimulate our sweet taste buds and our brain's reward centre making us crave sweeter and sweeter food. It can create a vicious circle.

- Avoid all sugary drinks (diet and normal types) and concentrated fruit juices as this can add a considerable load to our sugar intake. Including artificial 'sugar free' drinks!

- The sweetener aspartame has been linked in some studies to an increased risk of cancer. It is also known to increase your appetite.

- Avoid **added** fructose which cannot be broken down easily in the body and gets stored as fat in the liver.

- Artificial sweeteners trick the body by sending a message to the gut to expect a release of glucose from a sweet food. When no glucose arrives, the body is already primed and has released some insulin in response. Insulin is known as the fat storage hormone, and this drives the body to store energy as fat. Thus, replacing sugar with sweeteners may actually drive weight gain.

- If we eat sugar in excess this will also be stored in our liver and fat cells, potentially increasing the risk of fatty liver associated with diabetes and other chronic disease.

- A high intake of refined sugar is linked to obesity, diabetes, cardiovascular disease, and cancer.

- Sugar increases inflammatory chemicals in our body which can damage our DNA and speed up the aging process.

- Although fruit is good for us in many respects, choosing less sweet fruits is preferable. Keep the very sweet tropical fruits as a treat and concentrate your fruit intake to berries, tart apples, rhubarb, green bananas etc.

- Ideally, we should be consuming more veg than fruit. Natural fruit sugars are still sugar. Choosing 80% veg to 20% fruit can help to reduce our sugar intake.

*Take a tip from the Wholesome Worlds delicious desserts and add vegetables such as beetroot and aubergine to slow down the release of the sugars.

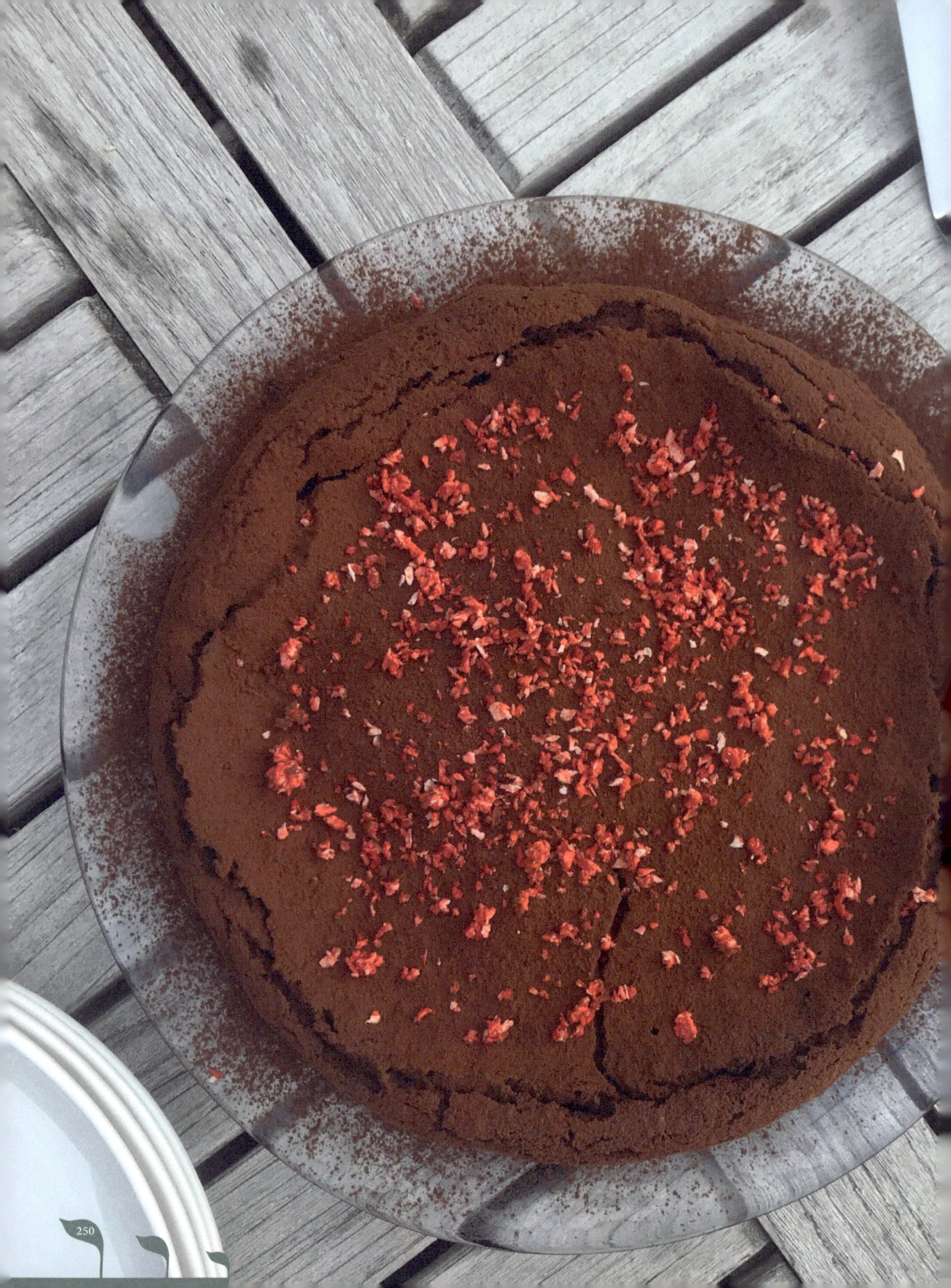

Choclatori Torte

SERVES 12 | ⏲ 10 MINS | GF V NF

"My go to dessert for a naughty treat or a show stopping sunday feast with friends. Inspired and taught by my lovely friend Tori, and so secretly hinted to in its title..."

If it lasts to the second day it tastes even better and is freezer friendly.

It may contain sugars (unrefined best) but this Torte is so rich and chocolatey you only need a sliver to satisfy any chocolate cravings. It's perfectly balanced with the addition of healthy fat and plenty of protein from the seven eggs. The combination of these macronutrients, and the high levels of flavenols shown to increase insulin sensitivity, help to reduce any potential glucose spike.

The dark chocolate also contributes to the nutrient density of this yummy treat. Dark chocolate is a powerful source of antioxidants, polyphenols and flavenols and is rich in minerals such as zinc, iron and magnesium.

It's gluten free, foolproof and satisfies your indulgent cravings.

Delicious on its own or paired with a sharp berry coulis or a whipped coconut cream.

INGREDIENTS

250g	Dark chocolate, 70%
50g	Coconut oil
200g	Butter
200g	Coconut sugar
120ml	Agave syrup
7	Eggs *(at room temp.)*
1 tsp	Vanilla extract
Pinch of	Cocoa powder

METHOD

1. Preheat the oven to 190°C. Grease and line a 9-inch springform pan with parchment paper.

2. Melt the chocolate, coconut oil and butter together in a bowl over a pan of simmering water, bain marie, until the chocolate is almost completely melted. Remove from heat and stir until smooth and totally melted. Stir in the sugar and agave, then let cool for a few minutes.

3. Add the eggs with a whisk, one at a time, fully combining between each addition. After all the eggs are added, continue to stir until the batter becomes thick, glossy, and utterly gorgeous. Add in the vanilla extract.

4. Pour the batter into the prepared tin. Bake 30-45 minutes, all ovens are different, until the torte jiggles slightly in the middle but is not completely set. Begin checking at the 30-minute mark to ensure the torte does not overbake. It might be cracked but don't worry this adds to its character.

5. Let cool in the pan for 10 minutes, and unmold. Dust with cocoa powder. Cut into wedges and serve alone or with whipped cream, berries, or anything else your heart desires.

MAPLE PEARS

SERVES 4 | ⏱ 30 MINS | GF DF V VE

"Quick, easy and ridiculously delicious! One of those healthy dishes that are perfect for a dinner party."

The skin of pears contains at least three to four times as many phenolic phytonutrients as the flesh.

These phytonutrients include antioxidant, anti-inflammatory flavonoids, and potentially anticancer phytonutrients like cinnamic acids.

INGREDIENTS

4	Pears
1	Vanilla pod
25g	Walnuts / Hazelnuts
2 tbsp	Maple syrup
1 tsps	Ground cinnamon
-	
400g	Coconut yoghurt

METHOD

1. Preheat your oven to 180°C and line a baking tray.

2. Cut your pears in half lengthways and use a teaspoon to remove the core and seeds.

3. Place on the baking tray inside the oven facing upwards.

4. Slit the vanilla pod lengthways and scrape the seeds out (keep the empty pod and use it to flavour jars of coconut sugar).

5. Chunkily chop and add the nuts to the oven.

6. In a ramekin, or small bowl, mix together the maple syrup, cinnamon and vanilla seeds. Pour almost all over the pears.

7. Pop into the oven, remove the nuts, and bake for 20-25 minutes until soft and golden. They may need slightly longer if they are not quite ripe enough.

8. Place 2 halves per plate with a little yoghurt and some of the syrup – don't forget the nuts!

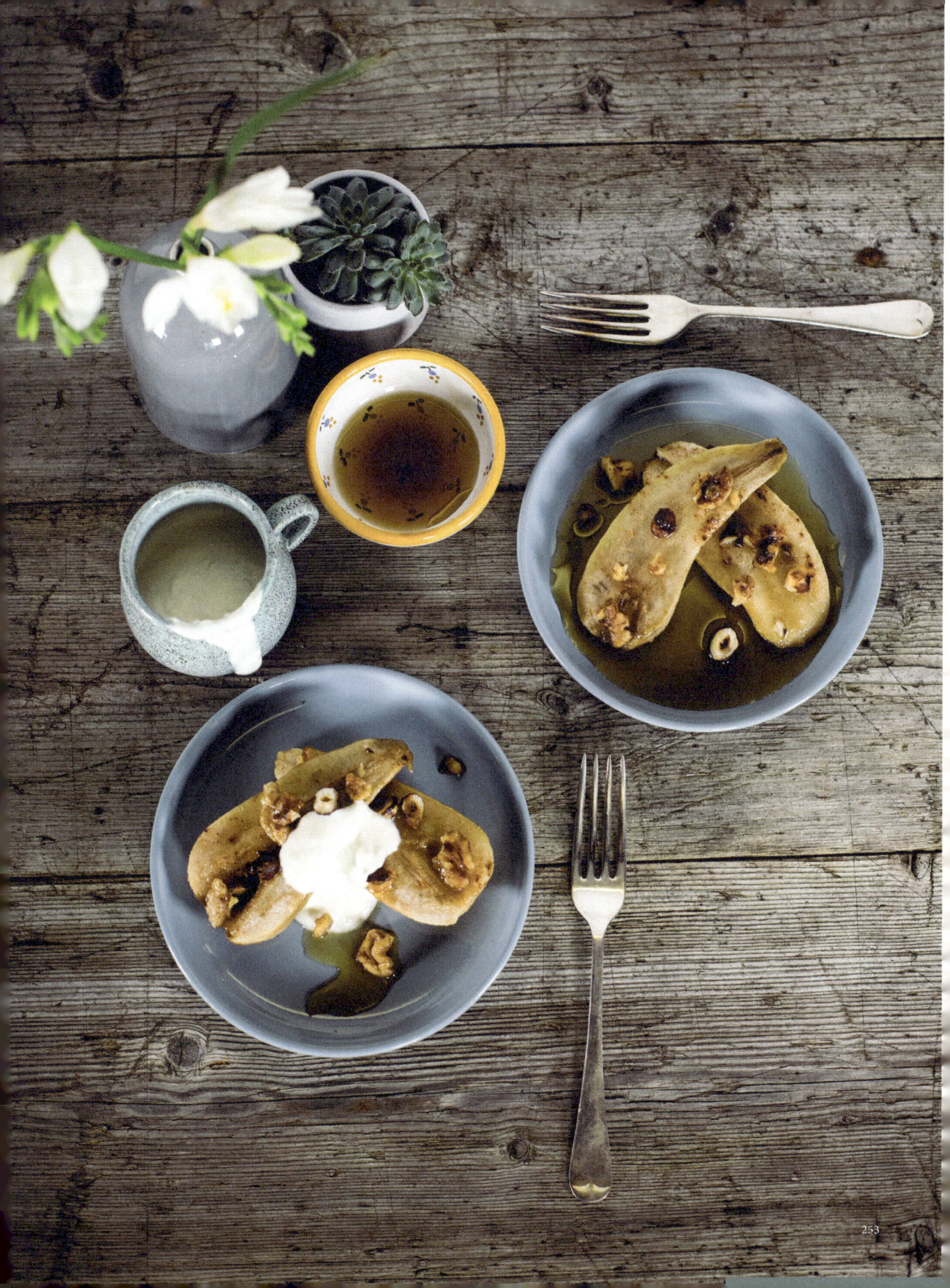

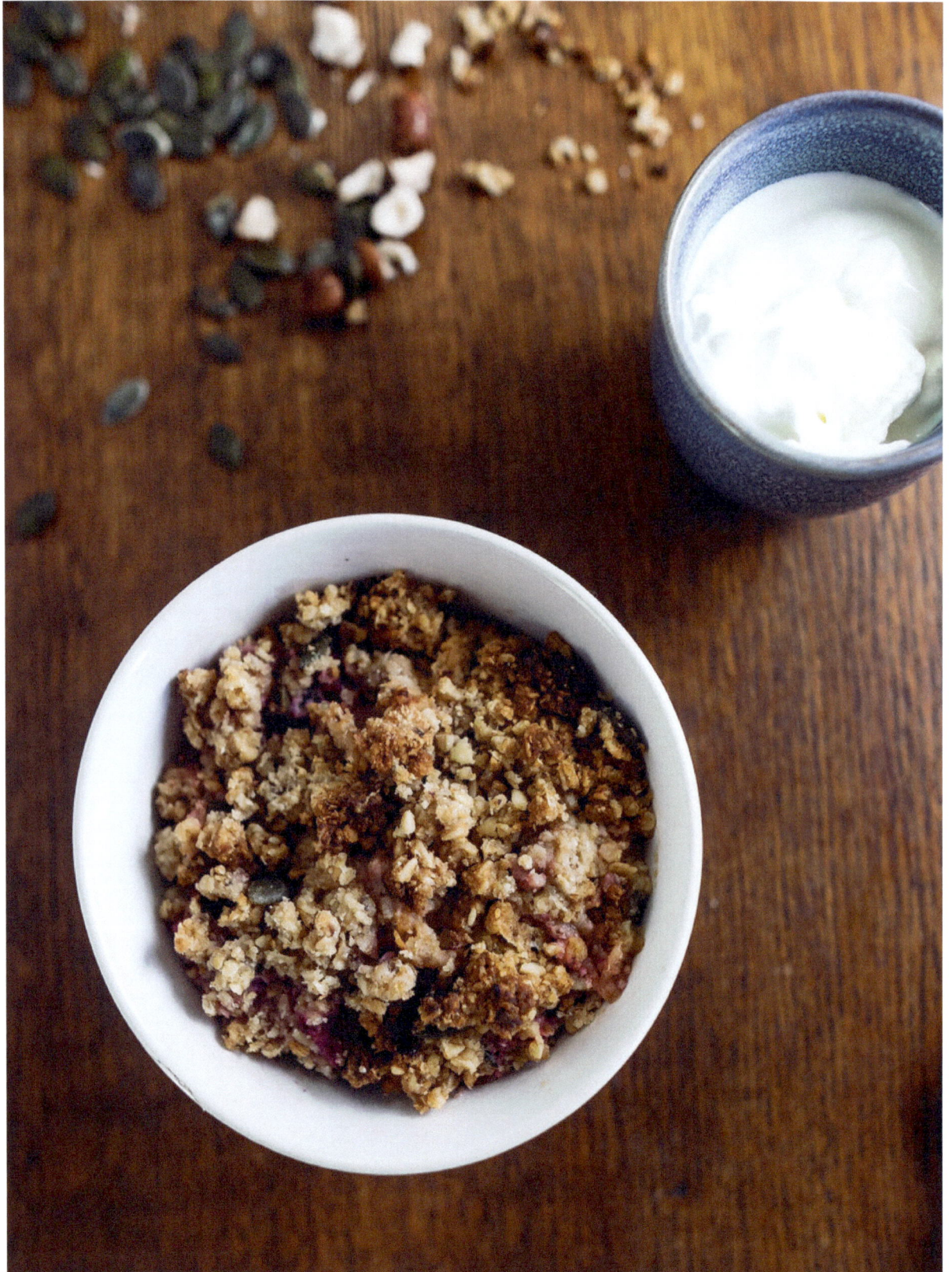

PLUM CRUMBLE

SERVES 6 | 🕐 1 HR 15 MINS | GF DF V

"My favourite flavours for crumble are apples and rhubarb from the garden, for which they are not always there, or in season! But plums are pretty good as well. I think a few hazelnuts, crushed and thrown in the topping is good too ."

Plums, although high in carbs tend to be more tart than other fruits and do not appear to have too much impact on blood glucose levels.

They contain ursolic acid which has anticancer properties and plenty of vitamins A, C & K, so good for bones and healing. Their fibre, antioxidant and potassium levels are also thought to be contributory to their heart protective benefits. Adding cardamom and cinnamon improves the anti-inflamatory profile of this dish, as do the almonds, hazelnuts, chia and pumpkin seeds.

Using oats as a base for the crumble makes this gluten free and provides some great prebiotic fibre.

INGREDIENTS

CRUMBLE DOWNSTAIRS
1kg	Plums
2 tsp	Ground cardamom
2 tsp	Ground cinnamon

CRUMBLE TOPPING
50g	Coconut oil
2 tbsp	Honey
150g	Rolled oats (GF)
150g	Ground almonds
50g	Flaked almonds
25g	Pumpkin seeds
20g	Chia seeds
Pinch of	Sea Salt

EQUIPMENT

20 x 20cm Baking dish

METHOD

1. Preheat the oven to 180°C.

2. Halve and destone the plums to add to the baking dish, sprinkle with the ground cardamom and cinnamon, cover with foil and place in the oven for 20 minutes.

3. In a small saucepan place the coconut oil and honey, put on a low heat, gently melt and mix together.

4. In a large mixing bowl mix the oats, ground almonds, flaked almonds, seeds and sea salt.

5. Pour the oil and honey into the dry ingredients. Mix with a spoon to create a crumb mixture.

6. Remove the foil from the cooked plums and add a little water if needed (50ml). Sprinkle the crumb in an evenly layered topping.

7. Return to the oven and bake for 20 minutes until golden.

FATS (good AND bad)

Fat is delicious and nutritious.

Over a number of years fats have been vilified as making you fat, increasing cholesterol and clogging your arteries.

Whilst this is true of manmade fats such as hydrogenated trans fats, other natural fats in the diet have many significant health benefits especially on brain health.

To break it down simply... there are good fats and bad fats.
We need it to be about 1/3 of our total diet intake.

Fats are easily damaged by heat and light, therefore many manufacturing processes can render fats into molecules that the body finds difficult to break down and utilise. This is certainly the case for hydrogenated fats often found in processed foods and is an important reason for choosing foods that have not been through a factory process. Equally fats found in animal products are healthiest if the animal has been fed a natural diet and has been allowed to graze or forage. Intensively reared cows and pigs and battery chickens do not have a healthy fat profile.

The Categories of Fats

- Saturated
- Monounsaturated
- Polyunsaturated

Saturated fats are derived from meat products, whole milk, butter, cream, cheese and lard. These should be eaten in moderation to avoid competing for absorbtion with the important essential fatty acids. Vegetarian sources are coconut and palm oil.

Monounsaturated fats are healthy and are found in a variety of oils, particularly olive oil. They are thought to be an important part of the highly regarded Mediterranean diet rich in healthy oils, nuts and seeds.

Polyunsaturated fats (PUFA's) include the very important omega fats which are known as Essential Fatty Acids (EFA's). PUFA's can also include some rather unhealthy refined oils which should be avoided such as sunflower, corn, canola and other cheap vegetable derived oils.

EFA's however should be eaten in abundance as they cannot be produced in the body. They are essential for cell function, help to keep cell membranes flexible and more fluid and are very important for neurotransmitters in the brain. EFAs can reduce blood cholesterol and platelet aggregation. Both omega 3 and 6 have an anti-inflammatory effect due to their ability to convert into anti-inflammatory prostaglandins.

However, omega 6 can also have a pro-inflammatory affect. To maintain the anti-inflammatory effect of EFAs it is necessary to keep the balance of dietary intakes of omega-3 (n-3) and omega-6 (n-6) fats to an approximate ratio of 2:1. High n-6 : n-3 ratios will enhance pro- inflammatory cytokine production. EFA's cannot be made in the body and need to be supplied through diet. Sources of Omega 3 are mainly from oily fish, green leafy veg, pumpkin seeds, hemp seeds, flax seeds and walnuts. Omega 6 is more abundant, found in hemp, pumpkin and sunflower seeds, walnuts, almonds, olives, wheat germ and soya beans.

A diet too high in saturated and trans fats will interfere with EFA function and production of prostaglandins since they compete for the same enzyme.

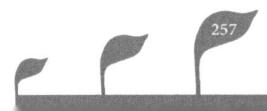

DARK CHOCOLATE NALUA NUT CAKE

SERVES 12 | ⏱ 1 HR | GF DF V

"Dark dense chocolate cake. Start with a sliver... I call this a perfect dish for quality overladening quantity."

A fantastically chocolately, coconutty, refined sugar-free delight. Make sure that you use 70% + dark chocolate for its cocoa solid content rich in polyphenols which are important antioxidants.

The coconut oil, flakes and milk add to the good fat quality of this cake meaning that it is packed with energy. Coconut is high in lauric fatty acids which have proven health benefits particularly providing a great source of energy to the body.

Eggs and walnut provide protein and healthy fats (walnuts are in our top nut choices). The dates and banana provide the sweetness and some good fibre.

Using bananas in cakes are a great way of using up those very ripe bananas. The more ripe the banana the higher the sugar content which you may prefer to sweeten the cake a little more.

INGREDIENTS

125g	Walnuts
150g	Dark chocolate
50g	Coconut flakes
1 tsp	Baking powder
50g	Cocoa powder
Pinch of	Sea salt
5	Medjool dates
2	Bananas
75g	Coconut oil
100ml	Coconut milk
2	Eggs
1 tsp	Vanilla essence
-	
50g	85% Dark chocolate
50ml	Coconut cream
50g	Hazelnuts

EQUIPMENT

Blender
20cm Cake tin, round

METHOD

1. Heat the oven to 180°C.

2. Use a blender to powder 50g (just under half) of the walnuts.

3. Chunkily chop the rest of the walnuts with the dark chocolate.

4. Mix the ground nuts, chopped nuts, coconut flakes, chopped chocolate, baking powder, cocoa powder and salt in a large bowl.

5. Remove the stones from the medjool dates and blend the dates with the bananas.

6. Melt the coconut oil and pour it in the date and banana mixture. Mix in the milk, eggs and vanilla essence.

7. Pour the wet mixture in the bowl with the dry ingredients and mix it all well.

8. Place the batter in the cake dish, best lined with baking parchment.

9. Bake the cake at 180°C for 40-45 minutes. Leave to cool.

10. Heat the chocolate to melt using a pan with a glass dish on top (bain marie) then add the coconut cream and stir. Cover the cake once cooled.

11. Chunkily chop the hazelnuts and decorate the cake.

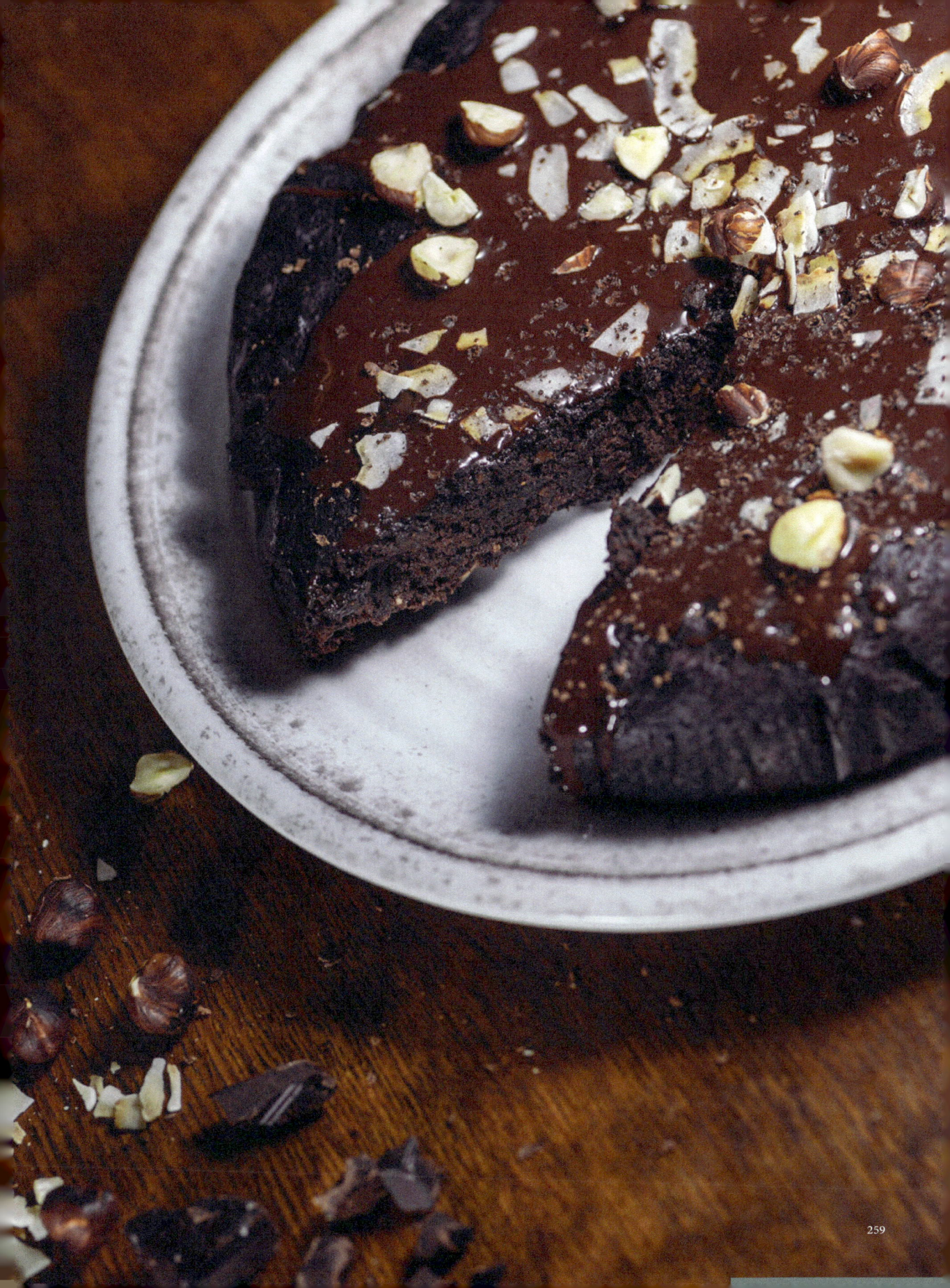

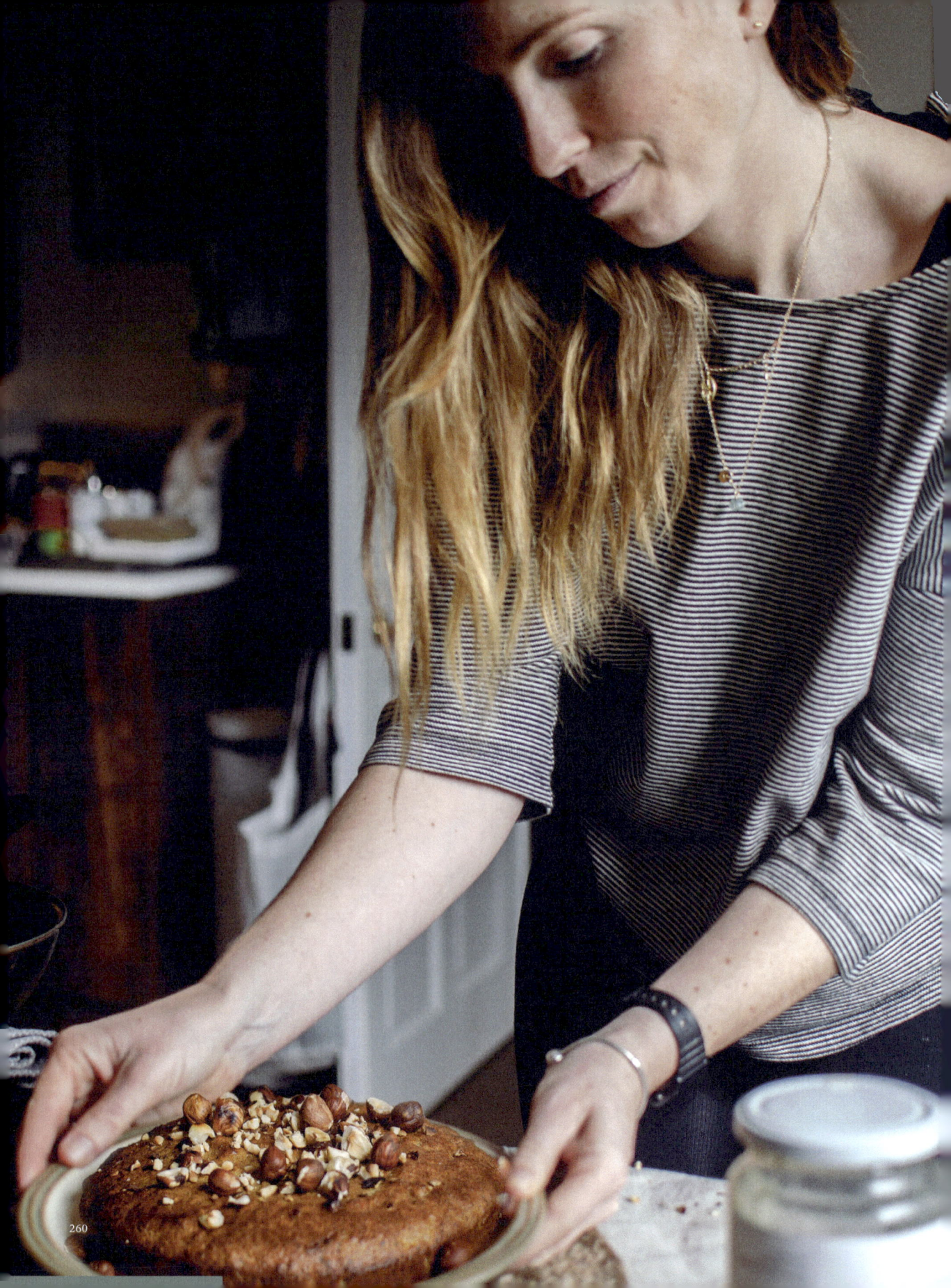

Hazelnut Cake

SERVES 10 | ⏱ 45 MINS | GF DF V

"This is beautifully full through and through with vitamins and protein galore. Fuel for the day! It is the ultimate in healthy cake so you can have your cake and eat it."

Hazelnuts are packed with protein and healthy fats and come under our category of top anticancer foods. They are also high in vitamin E which research has shown to be important for protecting us against many cancers.

The six eggs provides us with some first class protein and just a small amount of spelt flour and honey means these carbs will not spike your blood glucose levels and there is a low amount of gluten. If you are eating dairy enjoy with some yoghurt or pour over some organic double cream.

INGREDIENTS

6	Eggs
250g	Ground hazelnuts
25g	Spelt flour
100ml	Runny honey
20g	Roast hazelnuts

EQUIPMENT

20cm Cake tin, round

METHOD

1. Preheat the oven to 180°C.

2. Seperate the egg whites from the yolks.

3. Add the hazelnuts, spelt flour, 80ml of the honey and egg yolks together in a mixing bowl.

4. Whisk the egg whites and carefully stir into the main cake mix, bursting the lowest amount of bubbles possible.

5. Add to a lined or greased cake tin, and bake for 25 mins.

6. Smash the roast hazelnuts with a pestle and mortar, or loosely chop, and sprinkle upon the cake, drizzle the last of the honey to lightly re-moisten too.

RECIPE

SERVES _____

TIME _____

_____

_____

_____

_____

_____

_____

_____

_____

_____

_____

_____

_____

RECIPE

SERVES _____

TIME _____

_____

_____

_____

_____

_____

_____

_____

_____

_____

_____

_____

_____

RECIPE

SERVES _____

TIME _____

_____

_____

_____

_____

_____

_____

_____

_____

_____

_____

_____

_____

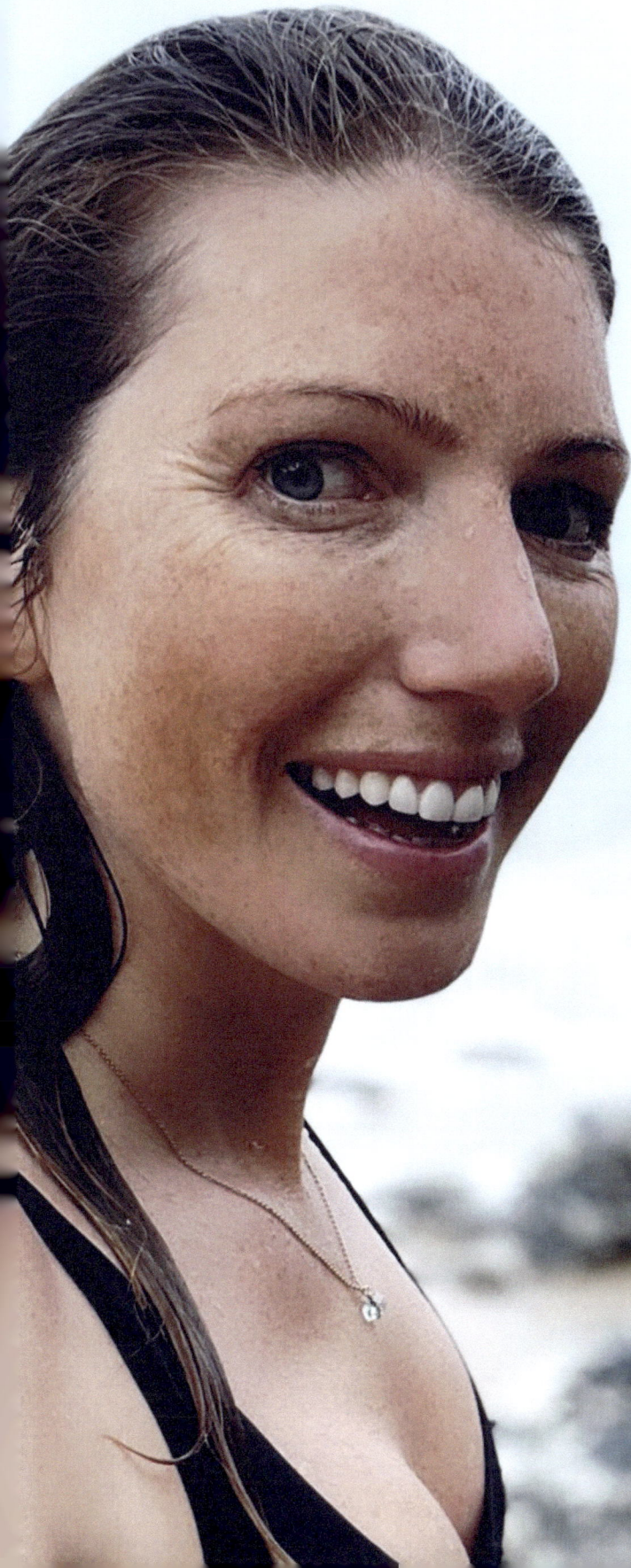

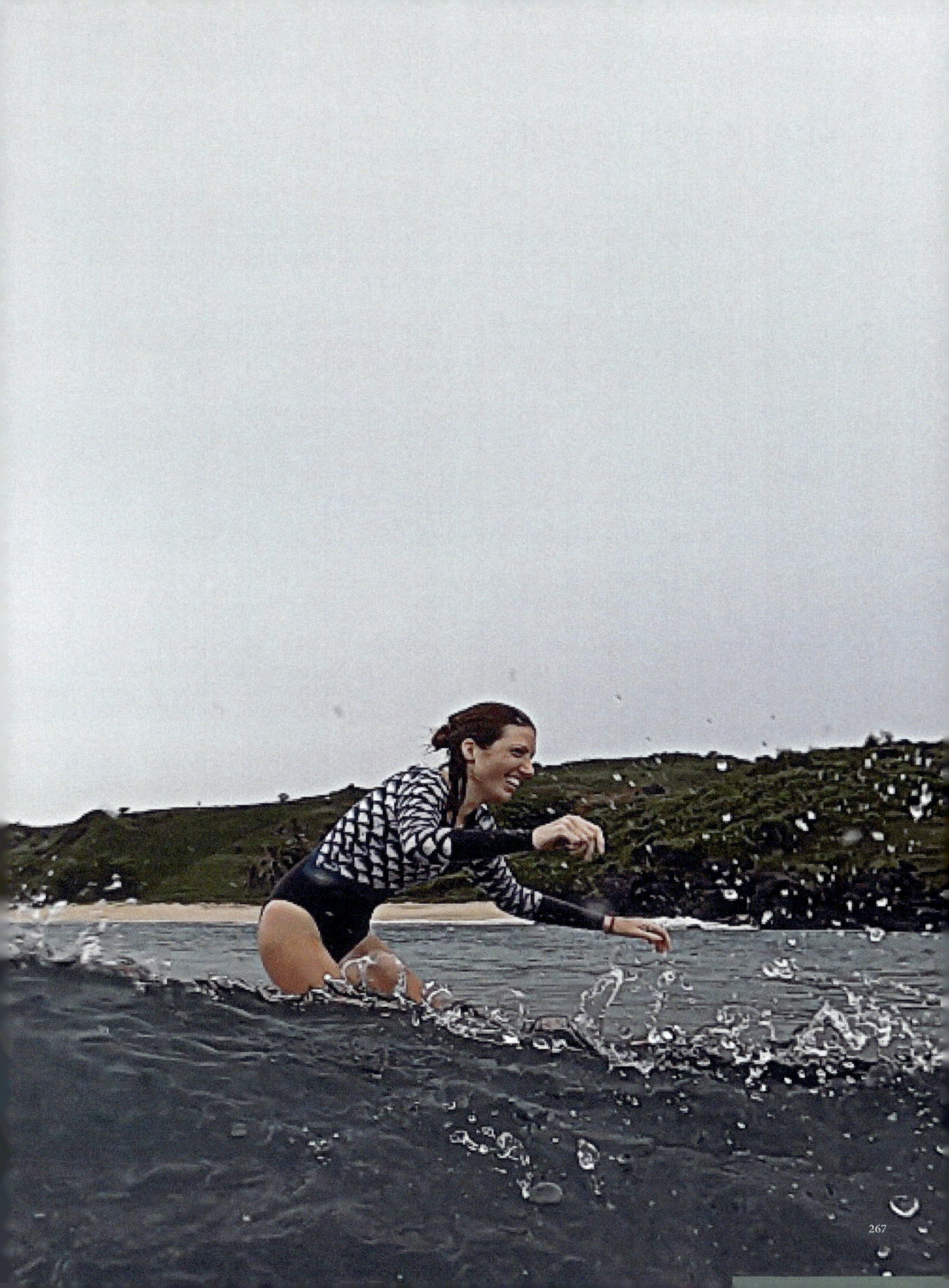

Waves of

Thank You Galore

Catherine Zabilowicz	(Genius) Nutritionist. Catherine has aided the creation of this book hugely. So immense appreciation and thank you. Nutrition Advisor at Maggie's Cancer Caring Centre since graduating with a degree in Nutritional Therapy.
Tim Smit	Founder of both Heligan Gardens and the Eden Project, which are real steps into the natural reality of the worlds nutrition. Seasonal insight on a doorstep of how when and where we can and should find our delicious ingredients.
Riverford Organics	Organic view of life and the importance of its growth to our lives. Beautiful recipes, contributed to the app, sprout in my mind from them and their seasonal local growths.
Dr Jonathan Fenn	NHS qualified doctor, UK based Sports, Exercise and Wellness Doctor. www.DrJonathanFenn.com
Dr Anna de Nazelle	Ahila Health is a holistic health platform centred around the mind, body and medicine connection. Past focus: Rheumatology, Cardiology and Pulmonology. Current focus: Integrative approach to health care and women's health specialist.
Dr Mayoni Gooneratne	Such a beautiful soul, a strong health advisor after her NHS surgery career. She realised the need and time to expand the publics understanding to prevention of health issues, and opened her private healthcare practice, Human Health. It's so important to elevate health issues on ourselves, and enhance the ease on those working for our NHS.
Piers Townley	An amazing man from The Brain Tumour Charity, thank you for your support.
Fran Warde	Fran Warde is my culinary world. Beautiful flavours through her mind and recipes, through the sea, land and air of the world.
Jan Merrills	PG.Dip Psychotherapy & LL.B (Hons) Law. A beautiful woman who understands life influences from the inside and out of your mind. Integrative Psychotherapist and Coach.
Amanda Winwood	The main soul and mind of the clean Made for Life skincare and cancer charity.
Lottie Brook	Pro and geniusly delicioso Chef to start with, very much of a unique soul and a solid pioneer for being so. Thank you for every recipe and moment of your love.
Ben Wigglesworth	Photography galore. He gives such depth to the recipes and the surrounding which falls beautifully in line with his environmental, art and life photography. Have a look at the North Coast Asylum art gallery that he set up with his equally creative, beautiful artist wife, Jo Painter.

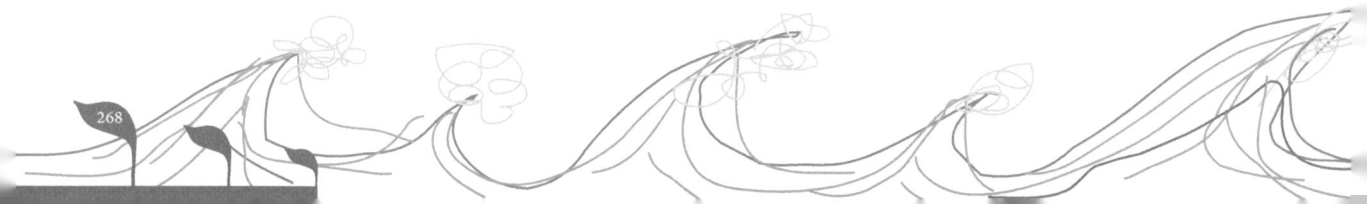

Victoria Cooper	Victoria has been with me through this project as a seed of growth for Wholesome World. Photographer and copywriter, alongside being my alien brain language translator to you lovely readers. Oh and she delightfully is a matching ocean addict. www.bellandbarrel.com
Katy Griffin	Mental health nurse, for the NHS, founder of Thera-Sea, a retreat to open your mind while releasing your body from stress.
Beth Trevethick	A marine and food addict to both souls like Freya the seal and Wholesome ingredient sources and growth. Falmouth University lecturer.
Lettice Rowbotham	Inspiring musician, who has taught me how to appreciate music for health and happiness.
Tor Greaves	Art and sailing addict photographer, who captured our alfresco dining, baking and everything else that occurs in the kitchen, garden and salty waters that she bounces to and from.
Yating Yang	Talented translator, sketcher and artist. Thank you for your heart and never ending time.
Annabelle Inman	Delicious mind and soul. Thank you for your generosity, mind and healthy self.
Ryan Jones	A strong friend, who has been a cushion for me through this change in my life and cookbook creation. An oracle of my music world.
Olivia Cornish	Digital designer, full of techno love, with which she helped to realise the WW cookbook, and moments of its creation.
Kerry Skinner	Giver of flourished local wild flower growth. kerry@rarecreation.co.uk *Find out more:* Rarecreation flower farm, Downhill, St Eval. Cornwall.
Mama & Papa	Just a mountain of love and huge pile of thank yous for your million moments of helping making this book happen.
Family	A delightfully wide group of my Scandi, ginger, blonde, brunette and European semi-freckly family from a wide life ethos.
Laura Hanstein	One of the strongest souls in the world. Amazing from her brain to every other aspect of her being.
Charlie Man	Thank you for all of you. Thank you for supporting me and keeping me happy.
Xanthe Hayes	This woman is my getaway. My meditation space and my positive aura that I have leant on and learnt strength from.
Sarah O'Brien	My London haven and home. A secret sister, united with and attached to forever.

SO much more love and thanks to everyone else who has been part of my Wholesome World. From Falmouth University; Plymouth University; EU digital medicinal authorisation, EPIC; Fred - my digital hero, https://moradigital.co.uk; Kate Brown for her never ending science brain reviews; Chris Snow, sailor of love; James Aiken's coastal filming; Salunke, Will, Millie, Natalie, Sophie Dears yoga, Beautiful Bella and those who have given such big wave of support...

Read More

PUBMED	www. pubmed.ncbi.nlm.nih
Centre for Science in the Public Interest	www.cspinet.org
Anticancer: A New Way of Life	Dr Servan-Schreiber
Headspace	Digital mobile app
Rewire Your Brain: Think Your Way to a Better Life	John B. Arden
The British Dietetic Association Website	www.bda.uk.com
China Study Expanded	Colin Campbell & Thomas Campbell
Whole	Colin Campbell
The Living Well With Cancer Cookbook: An Essential Guide to Nutrition, Lifestyle and Health	Fran Warde & Catherine Zabilowicz
What happened when I open-sourced my brain cancer	Salvatore Iaconesi
My stoke of insight	Jill Bolte
How we're fighting cancer	8 researchers
Type 1 and Type 2 Diabetes Cookbook: Low carb recipes for the whole family	Vickie De Beer & Kath Megaw
Brain Tumour Support	www.braintumoursupport.co.uk

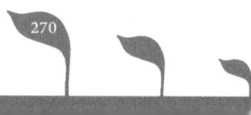

PubMed is a FREE access point which connects you primarily to the MEDLINE database of references and abstracts on life sciences and biomedical topics. It is managed in America; the United States National Library of Medicine at the National Institutes of Health. It is a platform to take your insight to the next level and see what is the most recent insight to medical conditions.

An American company. Research and information on health and nutrition. Main noted options are a resource library & 'news'.

If you read one book, read this one. It's my favourite. While the author was doing research he stepped in to have a brain scan because a participant didn't show up, and he turned out to have a tumour. He did huge amounts of research into all aspects of life which could affect cancer like nutrition, meditation, fitness etc. It's what I'm trying to provide with this app - things additional to medical information that is beneficial to your health and recovery.

A trust-worthy meditation app. I found it really simple to use when I was feeling stressed and needed to calm down. It also provides you with sounds of the wind and waves and things which helps you to fall asleep.

This book explains how you can rewire your thinking to be more positive, which can be really helpful during stressful times. It's really accessibly written and is based on neuroscience.

This webpage was recommended to me for additional information by NHS nutrition experts I saw. It provides really easy to understand and valid advice about nutrition.It clearly states that it is not a substitute for proper medical diagnosis or dietary advice given by a dietitian, and the the importance of getting professional advice.

I love The China Study. It is both easy to understand and scientific; it explores how nutrition and diet can impact on your health and likelihood of getting diseases. It is based on a 20 year study by scientists from the UK, US and China, who looked at the differences in the health of people who eat animal-based or plant-based diets. I massively recommend.

One of the most medically informative books that I read. It gives a comprehensive and well-researched insight in to the benefits of changing your diet. As well as exploring medical knowledge around nutrition, it also gives an honest insight into less established views.

Created through the beautiful cancer charity MAGGIES, by Catherine Zabilowicz, nutritional therapist who researches the impact of diet on health both medically and emotionally, and Fran Warde, a best selling food writer and London cookery school owner. The recipes are simply delicious.

"In this TED Talk, Salvatore, an Italian artist, brain cancer victim, explains how engaged with the world as he worked to understand the medical decisions he was making about his treatment for his brain cancer. Salvatore is artist who went through similar brain cancer to me, and wanted to understand research that helps you to make medical desicions, and implant the understanding into your life.

The woman, Jill Bolte, was a doctor who suffered from a stroke. Her talk is eloquent and unbelievably insightful, giving an intricate and compelling overview of what went wrong. She is so open and relatable as she lets you in to her 'ridiculous' moments."

This is a selection of TED Talks, compiling different viewpoints on cancer, both from scientists and first hand handlers. It's really insightful.

A really lovely insight into the ways that health can be effected by diet. Made by a medical mother for her young son, it is written in an easy and entertaining style to encourage and enthuse people to help themselves, being an active and productive part in maintaining your own health. It focuses on diabetes but a lot of the book can also be beneficial to general health.

Brain Tumour Support is not just for the patients themselves, but also families, carers and loved ones who are dealing with life being imposed by a brain tumour. They have set up one-to-one and group support, as well as online or telephone support and specialist counselling. It's a good door to feeling 'normal' despite the heavy emotional changes cancer imposes.
There is a beautiful amount of insight from the charity and they provide researched information to life changes and benefits that can be found within the government, hospitals and souls who are nearby.

My Beautiful Broken Brain	Lotje Sodderland
Fighting Cancer With Dance	Ananda Shankar Jayant
The Brain Tumour Charity	www.thebraintumourcharity.org
Macmillan	www.macmillan.org.uk
Made for Life	Skincare & Cancer Charity
Tao Te Ching	The Book of the Way	Lao Tzu
How Not To Die: Discover the foods scientifically proven to prevent and reverse disease	Dr Michael Greger
A Scattering	Christopher Reid
One Renegade Cell: The Quest for the Origin of Cancer	Robert Weinberg
Saltwater Buddha: A Surfers Quest to Find Zen on the Sea	Jaimal Yogis
The Private Life of the Brain	Susan Greenfield
The PH Miracle; Balance your diet, reclaim your health	Dr Robert O. Young & Shelley Redford Young
My TherAPPy	NHS
Cancer Research UK	

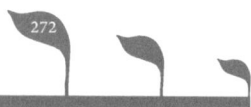

"Film: This is beautiful, stark, honest and firmly planted in reality. Lotje documents how having a stroke changed her life, from soon after she regained consciousness - happy to be alive but very confused. There is often no idea what the outcome will be of going through such brain trauma, and Lotje's problems were similar to the side effects that cancer brought my life. It's amazing to have a full, honest, insight."

A 2009 TED India Talk by a beautiful dancer, Ananda Shankar Jayant, who had breast cancer. Her successful dancing career was attacked by the effects of the cancer and its treatment. It is a beautiful insight from her, that cancer should be seen as a page of your life rather than the whole essence of your life. It's hard to keep cancer from controling your life, but it is unbelievably beautiful if you do manage to have moments, or an entire world, that can mentally override it, throwing cancer into insignificance.

"This is a lovely charity which works from fleet-footed fundraisers, to relentless research scientists. From the brave facing up to a diagnosis, to the health professionals helping them. And from close friends and families to kind strangers and everyone in between. We are a growing movement of people from every walk of life."

"I found Macmillan to be accessible, contactable and there for you. I absurdly slowly became aware of them. When my man was going through cancer, due to his treatment being abroad, we didn't have interaction with the team, but when my health issues arose, they helped me physically and emotionally, helping with my understanding and treatment. There are amazing things to receive from other charities or helpers, who can be more specific to your condition, local to you and be able to cater for your personal needs. But Macmillian is available across the country and able to help with lots of things - mental stress, physical stress, general research and knowledge of other charities that can aid you."

"Made for Life Organics is an ethical and award winning organic skincare range based in Cornwall, UK. It has a simple philosophy - that to be healthy and whole, we simply need to be connected with Nature. The most genuine and lovely skin brand worldwide. Developed by combining a deep knowledge of dermatological science with the strength and purity of botanicals, the formulations have gently evolved and improved with research based on clinical studies, whilst always bearing in mind the rich abundance of nutrients that nature provides us with. Made for Life enables spas to open their doors to people going through cancer. They are Complementary Medical Association accredited and CIBTAC endorsed Cancer Touch Therapy training has changed lives by enabling so many spas. Any profits from training go into the Made for Life Foundation. Made for Life Organics is about a pure and clean way of life which centres on the principles of Mindfulness and kindness. And no animal testing ever."

"A set of poetry which is saying that a calm, quiet life is available for everyone. It focuses on the benefits of meditation and inspiring yourself to relax at any moment. I like the line on page 71: "To know that there are things you cannot know is wisdom.""

This book by Dr Michael Greger focuses on how good nutrition can prevent, as well as assist the teatment of, disease. It's well worth a read and does a great job of translating scientific insight into an accessible book. He also has a website nutritionfacts.org, which promotes itself as being non-commercial and science-based.

I picked up this poetry book while I was waiting for a meeting in the local library. It made me realise that there is a big benefit to being open and writing thoughts down. I see it as a form of meditation and a lovely defocus on stress.

Molecular biologist Robert Weinberg works on treating cancer by destructing cancer stem cells. But his research also explains the construction of cancer and how variations of the disease differ. It is informative and gives simple descriptions and overviews into scientific understanding of cancer.

This memoir explores the author's discovery of meditation. Pushing yourself into a calm space, through different activities which can be translated to that meditation, has benefits for everyone in the world.

I like this book because it's a completely different diet to ones which focus on particular ingredients. But it's very interesting that the health benefits are very similar to the ones that I personally experienced with my own diet choices. Different diets work for different people! It defines a patient as the one who waits, which I found really interesting.

This book explains the brain, personality and mental health from a scientific perspective, explaining complicated medical studies.

This is a good reviewed App list, tested by NHS specialists, for recovery after a stroke or brain injury.

Cancer Research UK is a cancer research and awareness charity in the United Kingdom. It is the world's largest independent cancer research charity, which conducts research into the prevention, diagnosis and treatment of the disease.

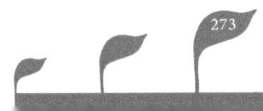

NOTES

Glossary

Acetic Acid	The acid that gives vinegar its characteristic taste.
Adrenaline	Adrenaline, also called epinephrine, is a hormone released by your adrenal glands and some neurons.
Alfafa sprouts	Sprouts are newly grown bud (especially from a germinating seed). Sprouted alfalfa seeds are shown to help lower cholesterol and benefits for blood sugar management.
Ambassador	A brand ambassador is hired by a company in order to bring its products, messaging, and brand image to the community.
Amino Acids	Amino acids are molecules that combine to form proteins. Amino acids and proteins are the building blocks of life.
Antibacterial	Anything that destroys bacteria or suppresses their growth or their ability to reproduce.
Anticancer	Used against or tending to arrest or prevent cancer.
Anti-diabetic	Tending to relieve diabetes: drugs with anti-diabetic properties.
Anti-imflammatory	Reducing inflammation.
Antimicrobial	Destroying or inhibiting the growth of microorganisms and especially pathogenic microorganisms.
Anti-thrombotic	Used against or tending to prevent thrombosis.
Antioxidants	Antioxidants are substances that can prevent or slow damage to cells caused by free radicals, unstable molecules that the body produces as a reaction to environmental and other pressures.
Antispasmodic	(Chiefly of a drug) used to relieve spasm of involuntary muscle.
Antiviral	Medical : acting, effective, or directed against viruses.
Anthocyanins	Any of various soluble glycoside pigments producing blue to red coloring in flowers and plants.
Angiogenesis	Angiogenesis is the process by which new blood vessels form, allowing the delivery of oxygen and nutrients to the body's tissues. It is a vital function, required for growth and development as well as the healing of wounds.
Anxiety	Apprehensive uneasiness or nervousness usually over an impending or anticipated ill : a state of being anxious.
Alimentary	Providing sustenance or nourishment.
Autoimmune Disease	Autoimmune disease happens when the body's natural defense system can't tell the difference between your own cells and foreign cells, causing the body to mistakenly attack normal cells.
Ayurveda	Ayurveda is an ancient Indian system of medicine which began about 5,000 years ago.
Beta Glucans	Beta-glucans are soluble fibers that come from the cell walls of bacteria, fungi, yeasts, and some plants. They might lower the risk for heart disease.
Bioavailability	Bioavailability refers to the extent a substance or drug becomes completely available to its intended biological destination(s).
Biochemical	Biochemistry is the branch of science that explores the chemical processes within and related to living organisms.
Biodiversity	Biodiversity refers to the variety of living species on Earth, including plants, animals, bacteria, and fungi.

Blood Glucose	Blood glucose is a sugar that the bloodstream carries to all cells in the body to supply energy.
Brassica	Commonly known as the mustard family, Brassicaceae contains some 338 genera and more than 3,700 species of flowering plants distributed throughout the world.
Calcium	A mineral most often associated with healthy bones and teeth, although it also plays an important role in blood clotting, helping muscles to contract, and regulating normal heart rhythms and nerve functions.
Capsaicin	Capsaicin is the stuff in chili peppers that makes your mouth feel hot.
Caratenoid	Carotenoids are pigments in plants, algae, and photosynthetic bacteria. These pigments produce the bright yellow, red, and orange colors in plants, vegetables, and fruits. They act as a antioxidant in humans.
Carbohydrates	Carbs are an important part of a balanced diet. Unprocessed carbs contain fiber, vitamins, and minerals.
Carcinogenic	Any substance that causes cancer.
Carminative	Able to relieve flatulence.
Carotenes	Any of four orange-red isomers of an unsaturated hydrocarbon present in many plants (ß-carotene is the orange pigment of carrots) and converted to vitamin A in the liver. Formula: C40 H56
Catechins	Catechins are natural polyphenolic phytochemicals that exist in food and medicinal plants.
CBT	Cognitive behavioural therapy (CBT) is a talking therapy that can help you manage your problems by changing the way you think and behave.
Cells	Cells are the basic building blocks of all living things. The human body is composed of trillions of cells. They provide structure for the body, take in nutrients from food, convert those nutrients into energy, and carry out specialized functions.
Chemotherapy	Chemotherapy is a cancer treatment where medicine is used to kill cancer cells.
Chlorogenic Acid	A polyphenol and the ester of caffeic acid and quinic acid that is found in coffee and black tea, with potential antioxidant and chemopreventive activities.
Cinnamic Acid	Cinnamic acid is commonly used as flavor compound in foods and drinks, and for its aroma in perfumes and cosmetics.
Citric Acid	Citric acid is found naturally in citrus fruits, especially lemons and limes. It's what gives them their tart, sour taste. A manufactured form of citric acid is commonly used as an additive in food, cleaning agents, and nutritional supplements.
Cognative	Relating to, being, or involving conscious intellectual activity (such as thinking, reasoning, or remembering).
Compound	A distinct substance formed by chemical union of two or more ingredients in definite proportion by weight.
Cortisol	Think of cortisol as nature's built-in alarm system. It's your body's main stress hormone. It works with certain parts of your brain to control your mood, motivation, and fear.
Cruciferous	Cruciferous veggies are a diverse group that includes broccoli, cauliflower, cabbage, kale, bok choy, arugula/rocket, Brussels sprouts, collards, watercress and radishes.
Culinary	Of' or 'for' cooking.
Curcumin	A yellow pigment, derived from the rhizome of Curcuma longa, and the main active ingredient of turmeric. It is an antioxidant and has anti-inflammatory properties.
Depression	Depression is more than simply feeling unhappy or fed up for a few days. Most people go through periods of feeling down, but when you're depressed you feel persistently sad for weeks or months, rather than just a few days. nervous system develops, its structure, and what it does.

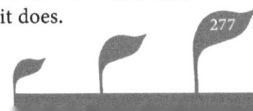

Detoxification	Detoxification or detoxication (detox for short) is the physiological or medicinal removal of toxic substances from a living organism, including the human body, which is mainly carried out by the liver.
Digestion	The process of making food absorbable by mechanically and enzymatically breaking it down into simpler chemical compounds.
Dioxins	Dioxins are environmental pollutants. They belong to the so-called "dirty dozen" - a group of dangerous chemicals known as persistent organic pollutants (POPs).
Distillery	A place where spirits are produced.
DNA	The molecule inside cells that contains the genetic information responsible for the development and function of an organism.
Empty Calories	No nutrients benefits.
Endorphins	Endorphins are chemicals (hormones) your body releases when it feels pain or stress. They're released during pleasurable activities such as exercise, massage, eating and sex too. Endorphins help relieve pain, reduce stress and improve your sense of well-being.
Endocrine	The endocrine system is a complex network of glands and organs. It uses hormones to control and coordinate your body's metabolism, energy level, reproduction, growth and development, and response to injury, stress, and mood.
Enzymes	Enzymes are proteins that help speed up chemical reactions in our bodies.
Epidemic	An epidemic is a disease that affects a large number of people within a community, population, or region.
Essential Healthy Fats	Fat is a type of nutrient, and just like protein and carbohydrates, your body needs some fat for energy, to absorb vitamins, and to protect your heart and brain health.
Ethical Farming	Livestock raised on pasture produce healthier meat, dairy and eggs. Compared to industrially produced meat, pastured foods are lower in fat, calories and cholesterol, and higher in many nutrients.
Fatigue	Fatigue is a term used to describe an overall feeling of tiredness or lack of energy. It isn't the same as simply feeling drowsy or sleepy. When you're fatigued, you have no motivation and no energy.
Ferment (fermented - Fermenting)	Fermentation is the process in which a substance breaks down into a simpler substance.
Fibre	Fiber helps regulate the body's use of sugars, helping to keep hunger and blood sugar in check.
Flavanols	Flavonoids are various compounds found naturally in many fruits and vegetables.
Folate	Folate is the natural form of vitamin B9, water-soluble and naturally found in many foods.
Folic Acid	Folic acid is a form of folate (a B vitamin) that everyone needs.
Free radicals	These are unstable atoms that can damage cells, causing illness and aging.
Fructose	Fructose is a type of sugar known as a monosaccharide.
Gazpacho	A fresh cold soup or broth.
Germinate	To Cause a seed to start growing.
Glucose	Glucose comes from the Greek word for "sweet." It's a type of sugar you get from foods you eat, and your body uses it for energy.
Glut	An excessively abundant supply of something.
Gluten	A general name for the proteins found in wheat.

Glutinous	Like glue in texture; sticky.
Glycaemic Effect	A measure of how much the food affects blood glucose levels. Aim for low glycaemic foods.
GMO	Genetically Modified Organism.
Gut Flora	Flora is the scientific term for a group of plant or bacteria life, typically particular to a certain area.
Haem-iron	Haem (heme) iron is found only in meat, poultry, seafood, and fish, so heme iron is the type of iron that comes from animal proteins in our diet. Non-haem is found in eggs and plants.
Healthy Fats	Monounsaturated and polyunsaturated fats, including omega-3 and omega-6 fatty acids, are both healthful fats. They can aid hormone function, memory, and the absorption of specific nutrients.
Herbicides	Herbicides are chemicals that kill plants or prevent them from growing. Their method of killing plants is as varied as the plants they kill.
Hormones	Hormones are your body's chemical messengers. They travel in your bloodstream to tissues or organs. They work slowly, over time, and affect many different processes.
Hydrogenated Fats	Hydrogenation is a process in which a liquid unsaturated fat is turned into a solid fat by adding hydrogen. During this manufactured partially hydrogenated processing, a type of fat called trans fatis made.
Immune Cells	Immune cells develop from stem cells in the bone marrow and become different types of white blood cells.
Immune System	The immune system is the body's tool for preventing or limiting infection. Without it, the body would be unable to withstand attacks from bacteria, viruses, parasites, and more.
Insulin	A hormone made in the pancreas, which is an organ in your body that helps with digestion.
Insoluble Fibre	Insoluble fibre is the type of fibre that adds bulk to our stools helping to pass solids out more easily.
Intensive Farming	System of cultivation using large amounts of labour and capital relative to land area.
Iodine	An element that is used by the thyroid. Humans cannot produce iodine, so it must be consumed. It is added to some foods and also to salt.
Iron	Iron is a mineral that is naturally present in many foods, added to some food products, and available as a dietary supplement.
Ketogenic	Ketogenic is a term for a low-carb diet. The idea is for you to get more calories from protein and fat and less from carbohydrates. You cut back most on the carbs that are easy to digest, like sugar, soda, pastries, and white bread.
Keytones	Ketones are a type of chemical that your liver produces when it breaks down fats.
Lauric Acid	Lauric Acid is a saturated medium-chain fatty acid with a 12-carbon backbone. Lauric acid is found naturally in various plant and animal fats and oils, and is a major component of coconut oil and palm kernel oil.
Livestock	Animals kept on a farm, such as cows, sheep, chickens, and pigs.
Lycopene	Lycopene is a type of organic pigment called a carotenoid. It is related to beta-carotene and gives some vegetables and fruits (e.g., tomatoes) a red color. Lycopene is a powerful antioxidant that might help protect cells from damage.
Macronutrients	Macronutrients are the nutrients we need in larger quantities that provide us with energy.
Magnese	Manganese is a trace mineral that is present in tiny amounts in the body.
Magnesium	Magnesium is a key factor in making several parts of the body run smoothly: the heart, bones, muscles, nerves, and others.
MCT	Medium chain triglycerides (MCTs) are fats, made in a lab from coconut and palm kernel oils.

Meditation	Meditation can be defined as a set of techniques that are intended to encourage a heightened state of awareness and focused attention.
Microbiome	The microbiome consists of microbes that are both helpful and potentially harmful. Most are symbiotic (where both the human body and microbiota benefit) and some, in smaller numbers, are pathogenic (promoting disease).
Microbiome (Gut)	Your 'gut microbiome' is made up of the trillions of microorganisms and their genetic material that live in your intestinal tract. These microorganisms, mainly comprising bacteria, are involved in functions critical to your health and wellbeing.
Microbiota	The community of micro-organisms themselves.
Microplastic	Tiny plastic particles that result from both commercial product development and the breakdown of larger plastics.
Microorganisms	Bacteria and viruses (more commonly known as germs), fungi or parasites.
Mindfulness	Paying more attention to the present moment – to your own thoughts and feelings, and to the world around you.
Minerals	Minerals are nutrients your body needs in small amounts to work properly and stay healthy.
MRI	Magnetic resonance imaging.
Mylk	Non dairy 'milk'. Oh how legality and allowance changes. It's officially; white liquid like milk but made from nuts or plants rather than produced by an animal.
Nervous System	Your nervous system is your body's command center. Originating from your brain, it controls your movements, thoughts and automatic responses to the world around you.
Neurological Disease	Neurological disorders are medically defined as disorders that affect the brain as well as the nerves found throughout the human body and the spinal cord.
Neuroplascitiy	Neuroplasticity can be viewed as a general umbrella term that refers to the brain's ability to modify, change, and adapt both structure and function throughout life and in response to experience.
Neuroscience	Neuroscience, also known as Neural Science, is the study of how the nervous system develops, its structure, and what it does.
Neurotransmitters	Neurotransmitters are chemical messengers that your body can't function without.
Niacin	Niacin, also known as vitamin B3, is an important nutrient. In fact, every part of your body needs it to function properly.
Oligodendroglioma Cytoma	Oligodendroglioma is a primary central nervous system (CNS) tumor. This means it begins in the brain or spinal cord. This is the type of cancer I, Freyja, dealth with - in the Temporal Lobe.
Omega 3-6-9	Fatty Acids: They all have health benefits, but it's important to get the right balance between them. An imbalance in your diet may contribute to a number of chronic diseases.
Oxidant	An oxidant is a reactant that oxidizes or removes electrons from other reactants during a redox reaction.
Oxidative	"An oxidative chemical reaction adds oxygen to the tissues of the body: it can cause oxidative damage."
Pectin	Pectin is a fiber found in fruits.
Pharmacopeial-grade	The chemical grade of a drug that meets or exceeds the purity, potency, and quality standards and requirements of the United States Pharmacopeia (USP).
Phenolic Acids	Phenolic acids are aromatic secondary plant metabolites, widely spread throughout the plant kingdom.

Phosphorus	Phosphorus is the second most plentiful mineral in your body. The first is calcium. Your body needs phosphorus for many functions, such as filtering waste and repairing tissue and cells.
Phytonutrients	Phytonutrients are natural compounds found in plant foods such as vegetables, fruit, whole grain products and legumes.
Polyphenols	Polyphenols are compounds that we get through certain plant-based foods. They're packed with antioxidants and potential health benefits.
Potassium	Potassium is an essential mineral that is needed by all tissues in the body.
Prebiotic	Prebiotics are a source of food for your gut's healthy bacteria.
Preservatives	Simply, preservatives help prevent the growth of microorganisms, particularly bacteria and fungi, which may cause disease or infection.
Prostagladins	The prostaglandins are a group of lipids made at sites of tissue damage or infection that are involved in dealing with injury and illness.
Protein	Protein is an essential macronutrient, but not all food sources of protein are created equal, and you may not need as much as you think. Learn the basics about protein and shaping your diet with healthy protein foods.
Quercetin	Quercetin is a plant pigment (flavonoid).
Radiotherapy	Radiotherapy is a treatment where radiation is used to kill cancer cells.
Refined Carbohydrates	Processing carbs removes nutrients and results in refined carbs, which people sometimes refer to as empty carbs or empty calories. Refined carbs provide very few vitamins and minerals.
Refined Sugar	Refined sugar comes from sugar cane or sugar beets, which are processed to extract the sugar. It is typically found as sucrose, which is the combination of glucose and fructose.
Replete	Filled or well-supplied with something.
Salubrity / Salubrious	Conducive or favorable to health or well-being.
Saponins	Saponins occur naturally in soybeans, peas, horse chestnut, yams, quinoa and grains.
Sarcoma	A type of cancer that begins in bone or in the soft tissues of the body, including cartilage, fat, muscle, blood vessels, fibrous tissue, or other connective or supportive tissue.
Satiate	To satisfy (a need, a desire, etc.) fully or to excess.
SCOBY	A SCOBY is a cellulose mat that houses the bacteria and yeast cultures that turn sweet tea into kombucha.
Selenium	A mineral found in the soil. Selenium naturally appears in water and some foods. While people only need a very small amount, selenium plays a key role in their metabolism.
Serotonin	Serotonin is a neurotransmitter, and some also consider it a hormone. The body uses it to send messages between nerve cells. It appears to play a role in mood, emotions, appetite, and digestion.
Soluble Fibre	This type of fiber promotes the movement of material through your digestive system and increases stool bulk.
Soluble Nitrogen	A form of fertiliser in which the nitrogen is readily available for uptake by plants, and which provides quick color and growth response.
Stages of Cancer	Number staging systems use the TNM system to divide cancers into stages. Most types of cancer have 4 (IV) stages, numbered from 1 to 4. Interesting when you find our that some cancer types are restrained from the normal I-IV stages. *"Oligodendrogliomas are grouped in two grades based on their characteristics. Grade II & III. Not the general knowledge!"*

Grade II oligodendrogliomas are low grade tumours. This means the tumour cells grow slowly and invade nearby normal tissue. In many cases, they form years before being diagnosed as no symptoms appear.

Grade III oligodendrogliomas are malignant (cancerous). This means they are fast-growing tumours. They are called anaplastic oligodendriogliomas.

Statins	A group of medicines that can help lower the level of low-density lipoprotein (LDL) cholesterol in the blood.
Sterols & Stanols	Plant sterols and stanols are substances naturally found in fruits, vegetables, whole grains, legumes, nuts, and seeds. Research has shown that plant.
Sulphoraphane	Sulforaphane is a natural plant compound found in many cruciferous vegetables. It has been linked to health benefits, such as improved heart health and digestion.
Sulphur	Sulfur is a chemical element that is present in all living tissues. After calcium and phosphorus, it is the third most abundant mineral in the human body.
Temporal Lobe	The temporal lobe is one of the four major lobes of the cerebral cortex. It is the lower lobe of the cortex, sitting close to ear level within the skull.
Thiamine	Thiamine, also known as thiamin or vitamin B1, is one the of B vitamins.
Triglycerides	Triglycerides are a type of fat. They are the most common type of fat in your body. They come from foods, especially butter, oils, and other fats you eat. Your body changes extra calories into triglycerides and stores them in fat cells.
Ursolic acid	Ursolic acid (UA) is a natural triterpene compound found in various fruits and vegetables.
Viruses	A virus is an infectious microbe consisting of a segment of nucleic acid (either DNA or RNA) surrounded by a protein coat.
Vitamins	Vitamins and minerals are nutrients your body needs in small amounts to work properly and stay healthy.
Viability	Ability to work as intended or to succeed.
Wholesome	Good for you, and likely to improve your life either physically, morally, or emotionally.
Wellbeing	The condition of being contented, healthy, or successful; welfare.
Worm Castes	A wonderful worm outlet. As it digests the organic materials it consumes, it refines them. Nutrients, including minerals and trace elements, are reduced to their most usable form. The castings have a neutral pH of 7.0.
Umami	Umami or savoriness, is one of the five basic tastes. It has been described as savory and is characteristic of broths and cooked meats.

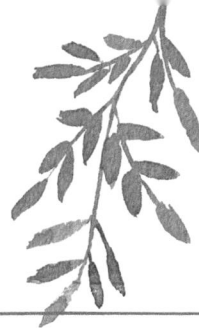

Glossary de la Freyja

Crimble	Christmas.
Delicioso	Delicious.
Et Voila	Voilà is essentially a combination of two words: voir (to see/look) and là (there). So literally speaking, voilà is an instruction.
Galore	In abundance.
Glutinous	Like glue in texture; sticky. "glutinous mud"
Heavenly	Divine, Very good.
Husky	Heavy texture.
Placate	Relaxed, chilled, low effort.
Techno	Vessels... Mobile phones.
Teeny	Small in amount.
Satiation	the act of completely satisfying yourself or a need, especially with food or pleasure.
Sauciness	Sauce, with a good flavour.
Souls	People, humans, you and me...
Slothic	The Oxford dictionary states that Sloth is the noun for 'no effort'. It is the unwillingness to work or make any effort: "The report criticizes the government's sloth in tackling environmental problems."
Sultration	Passionate.
Oodles	High amount of something.
Oral Door	The mouth.
Zinging	Sharp in flavour.
Nutrition Halos	High and beneficial in nutrients.

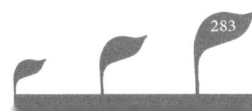

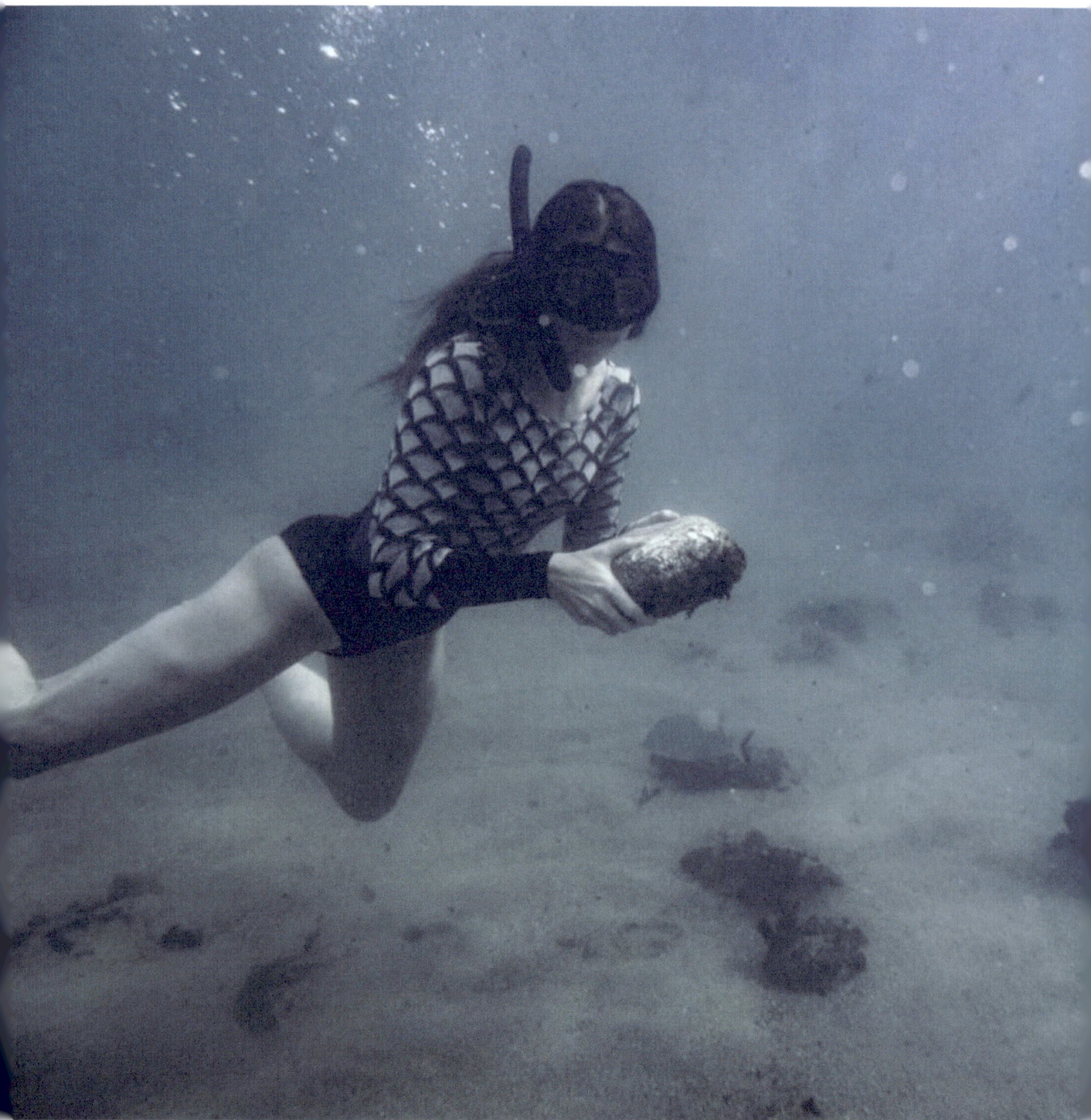

References

p12

1. Burnet NG, Jefferies SJ, Benson RJ, Hunt DP, Treasure FP. Years of life lost (YLL) from cancer is an important measure of population burden--and should be considered when allocating research funds. Br J Cancer. 2005 Jan 31;92(2):241-5. doi: 10.1038/sj.bjc.6602321. PMID: 15655548; PMCID: PMC2361853.
2. The Brain Tumour Charity. Losing Myself: The Reality of Life with a Brain Tumour. 2015. https://www.thebraintumourcharity.org/about-us/our-publications/losing-myself-reality-life-brain-tumour/
3. The Brain Tumour Charity. Barriers to research. 2021. - https://www.thebraintumourcharity.org/about-us/our-research-strategy/barriers-to-research/
4. The Brain Cancer Charity Oligodendroglioma prognosis: https://www.thebraintumourcharity.org/brain-tumour-diagnosis-treatment/types-of-brain-tumour-adult/oligodendroglioma/oligodendroglioma-prognosis/

p17

1. Calder PC. n-3 polyunsaturated fatty acids, inflammation, and inflammatory diseases. Am J Clin Nutr. 2006 Jun;83(6 Suppl):1505S-1519S. doi: 10.1093/ajcn/83.6.1505S. PMID: 16841861.
2. https://neurodigest.co.uk/the-brain-tumour-patient-experience-of-ketogenic-diet-therapy/

p25

1. https://journals.physiology.org/doi/full/10.1152/japplphysiol.01413.2009
2. https://www.ncbi.nlm.nih.gov/pmc/articles/PMC3047226/

p31

1. https://pubmed.ncbi.nlm.nih.gov/20465176/

p33

1. Sharma A, Madaan V, Petty FD. Exercise for mental health. Prim Care Companion J Clin Psychiatry. 2006;8(2):106. doi: 10.4088/pcc.v08n0208a. PMID: 16862239; PMCID: PMC1470658.

p44

1. Donaldson MS. Nutrition and cancer: a review of the evidence for an anti-cancer diet. Nutr J. 2004 Oct 20;3:19. doi: 10.1186/1475-2891-3-19. PMID: 15496224; PMCID: PMC526387.

p60

1. https://www.frontiersin.org/articles/10.3389/fpubh.2016.00057/full
2. Sharma PV, editor. Susrutha Samhitha. (Vol. 1). Varanasi: Chaukhambha Visvabharati (2004). p173
3. https://www.healthline.com/nutrition/black-tea-benefits
4. https://www.healthline.com/nutrition/top-10-evidence-based-health-benefits-of-green-tea#2.-May-improve-brain-function
5. https://www.healthline.com/nutrition/white-tea-benefits#TOC_TITLE_HDR_2
6. https://medium.com/@britishholistic/creating-pukka-herbs-76ca3d7c81bb

p194

1. https://www.webmd.com/diet/organic-beef-good-for-you

Extra Useful Links to the Book Research

1. Donaldson, Michael S., 'Nutrition and cancer: A review of the evidence for an anti-cancer diet', Nutrition Journal, 2004, 3:19
2. World Cancer Research Fund / American Institute for Cancer Research, Food, Nutrition, Physical Activity, and the Prevention of Cancer: A Global Perspective, AIRC, Washington, DC, 2007
3. Key, Timothy, J et al, Diet, nutrition, and cancer risk: what do we know and what is the way forward? BMJ 2020, 368:m511
4. Pelucchi, C, Bosetti, C, Galeone, C, La Vecchia, C. Dietary acrylamide and cancer risk: an updated meta-analysis. Int J Cancer 2015; 136:2912-22
5. Kord-Varkaneh, H, et al, Association between Healthy Eating Index-2015 and Breast cancer Risk: A Case-Control Study. Asian Pac J Cancer Prev, 21 (5), 1363-1367
6. La Vecchia, C, Altieri, A, Tavani, A. Vegetables, fruit, antioxidants and cancer: a review of Italian studies. Eur J Nutr 40: 261-267
7. Borek, C. Dietary antioxidants and human cancer. Integr Cancer Ther. 200 Dec;3(4):333-41

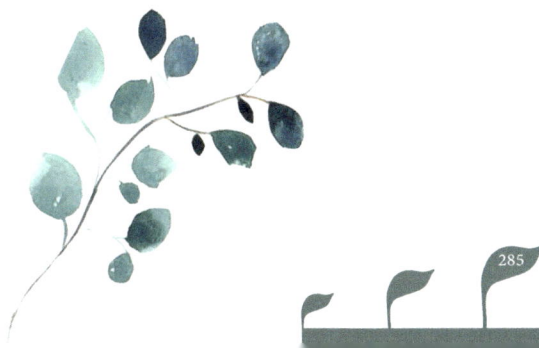

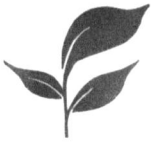

Index: Recipes

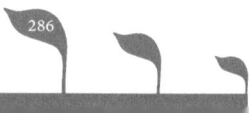

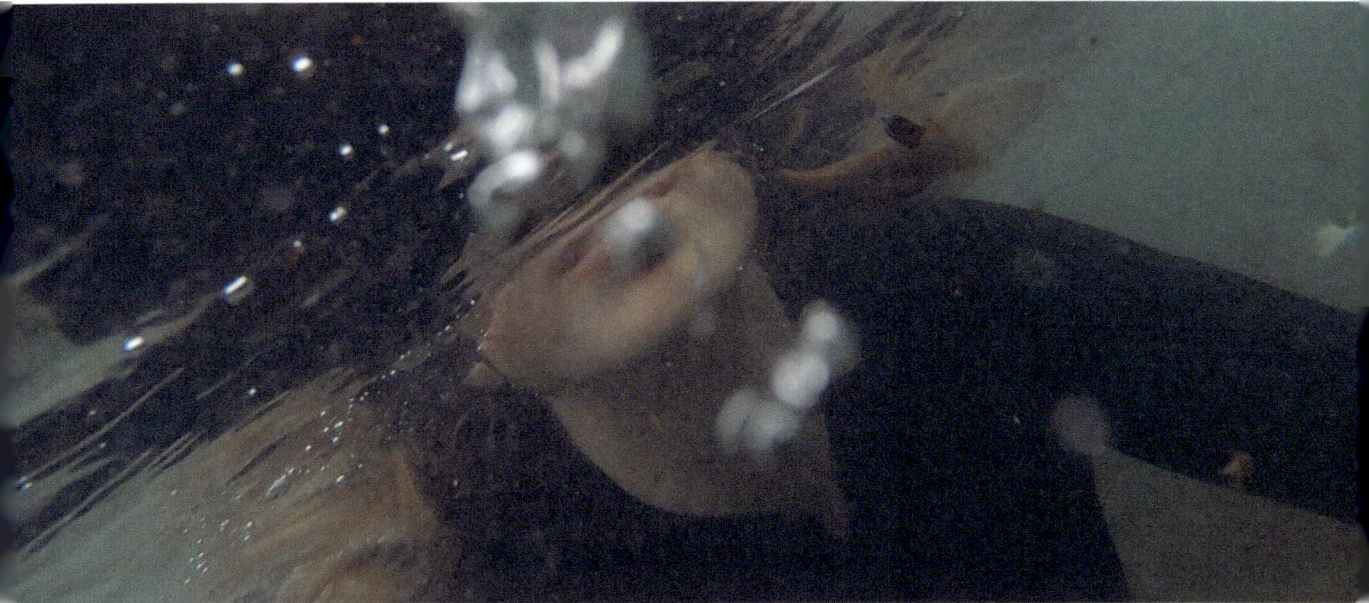

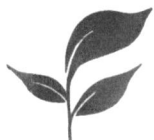

Index: Recipe Ingredients

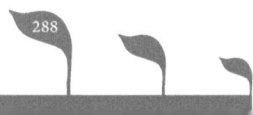

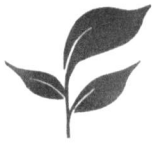

Index: Recipe Ingredients

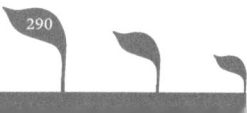

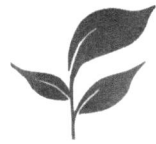

Index: Recipe Ingredients

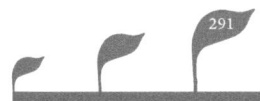

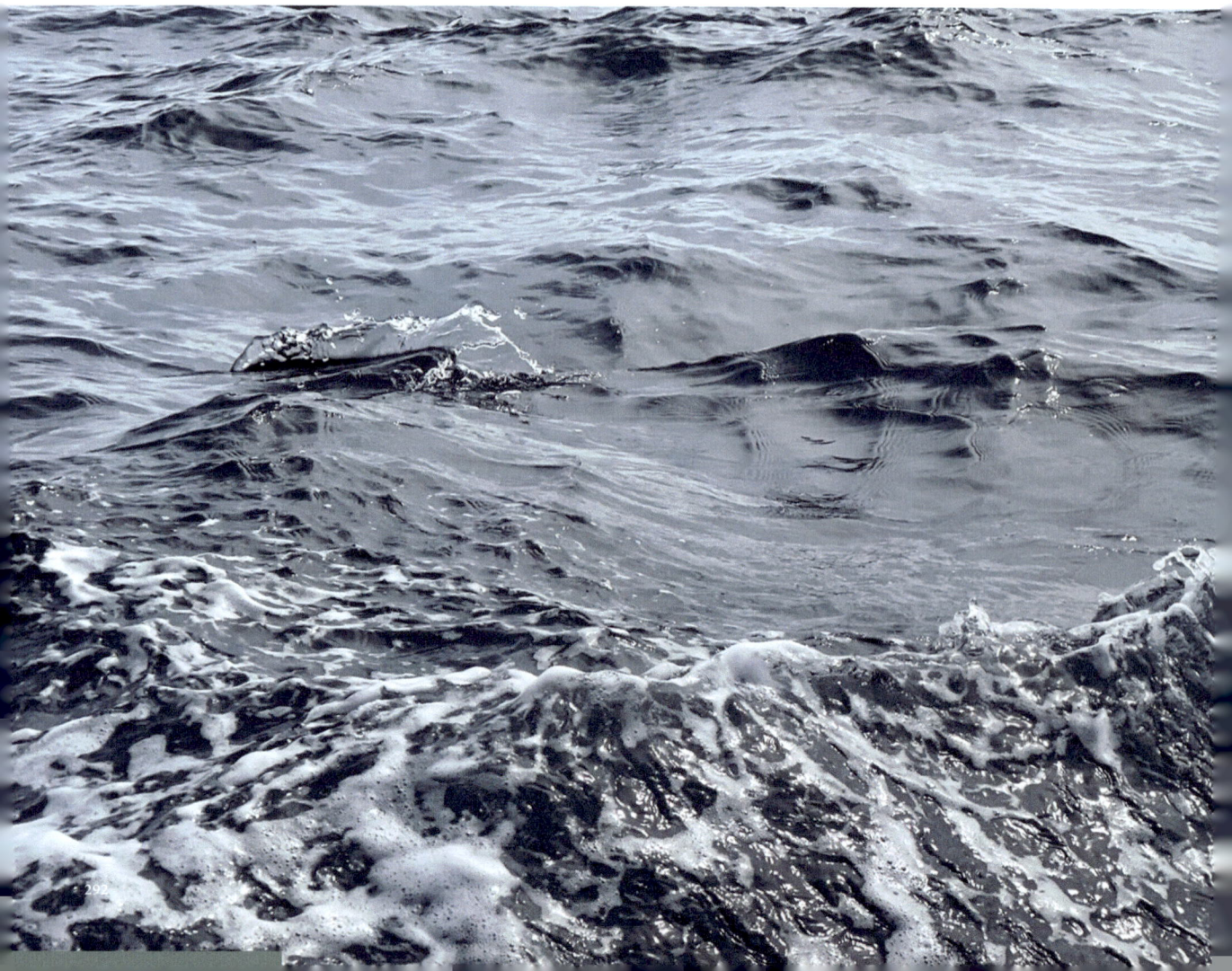

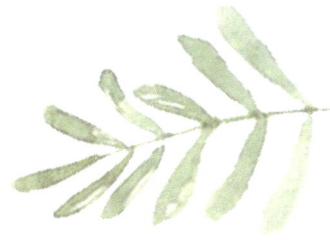

Simply Fusilli - 154

Pear

Ginger, Pear & Apple Smoothie - 75
Maple Pears - 252
Red Cabbage, Pear & Beetroot - 215
Seeded Spelt Pear Bread - 202
Super World Salad - 156

Peas

Pea & Coconut Soup - 12

Peanut Butter

Ribbon Steak, Tenderstem & Asian Slaw - 194

Pea Shoot

Prawn Courgetti Spaghetti - 183

Pine Nuts

Goats Cheese Salad - 169

Plum

Plum & Banana Kombucha Smoothie - 88
Plum Crumble - 254

Pomegranate

Iranian Lamb & Spiced Rice - 192
Super World Salad - 156
Vanilla Sponge Cake - 246

Potatoes

Aubergine & Potato Curry - 144
Celeriac Soup - 124
Coastal Chowder - 132
Fishie Pie - 180

Prawns

Fishie Pie - 180
Prawn Curry - 178

Pumpkin Seeds

Green Soup - 127
Wholesome Crunchy Granola - 98
Super World Salad - 151

Radishes

Coleslaw - 220

Raisins

Wholesome Crunchy Granola - 98

Rapeseed Oil

Coastal Chowder - 132
Wolf's Fish Bowl - 130

Raspberries

Pink Island Smoothie - 73
Vanilla Sponge Cake - 246
Wholesome Kombucha - 86

Red Chard

Prawn Courgetti Spaghetti - 183

Red Grapes

Goats Cheese Salad - 169

Red Pepper

Beef Cacao Stew - 199

Cucumber, Mint & Sumac - 142
Mediterranean Roasted Cod, Fennel & Olive - 173
Super World Salad - 156
Wolf's Fish Bowl - 130
Red Quinoa
Super World Salad - 156
Warm Quinoa Salad - 148

Risotto Rice

Mushroom Risotto - 162

Rhubarb

Rhubarb Panna Cotta - 244

Rocket

Squash & Beetroot Salad - 152

Rosemary

Beef Cacao Stew - 199
My Omelette - 108

Rose Water

Rose & Cardamom Hot Chocolate - 90

Rye Flour

Pecan Pie - 233

Saffron

Wolf's Fish Bowl - 130

Salmon

Coastal Chowder - 132
Spiced Steamed Salmon Parcels - 176
Wolf's Fish Bowl - 130

SCOBY

Wholesome Kombucha - 86

Seabass

Wolf's Fish Bowl - 130

Shallot

Chimchurri - 217
Mushroom Risotto - 162
Walnut & Brazil Nut Salsa - 216

Shrimps

Wolf's Fish Bowl - 130

Sourdough

Mushrooms on Toast with Hazelnuts - 100
Tuna Melt - 110

Soya Sauce

Ribbon Steak, Tenderstem & Asian Slaw - 194

Soya Mylk

Banana Bread - 113
Cacao Carob Smoothie - 80
Rose & Cardamom Hot Chocolate - 92

Spelt Flour

Hazelnut Cake - 260
Seeded Spelt Pear Bread - 202
Spelt Wholegrain Flatbread - 208

Spinach

Aubergine & Potato Curry - 144

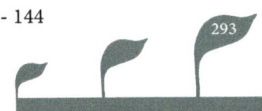

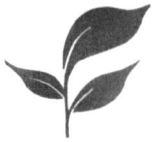

Index: Recipe Ingredients

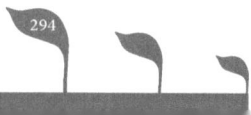

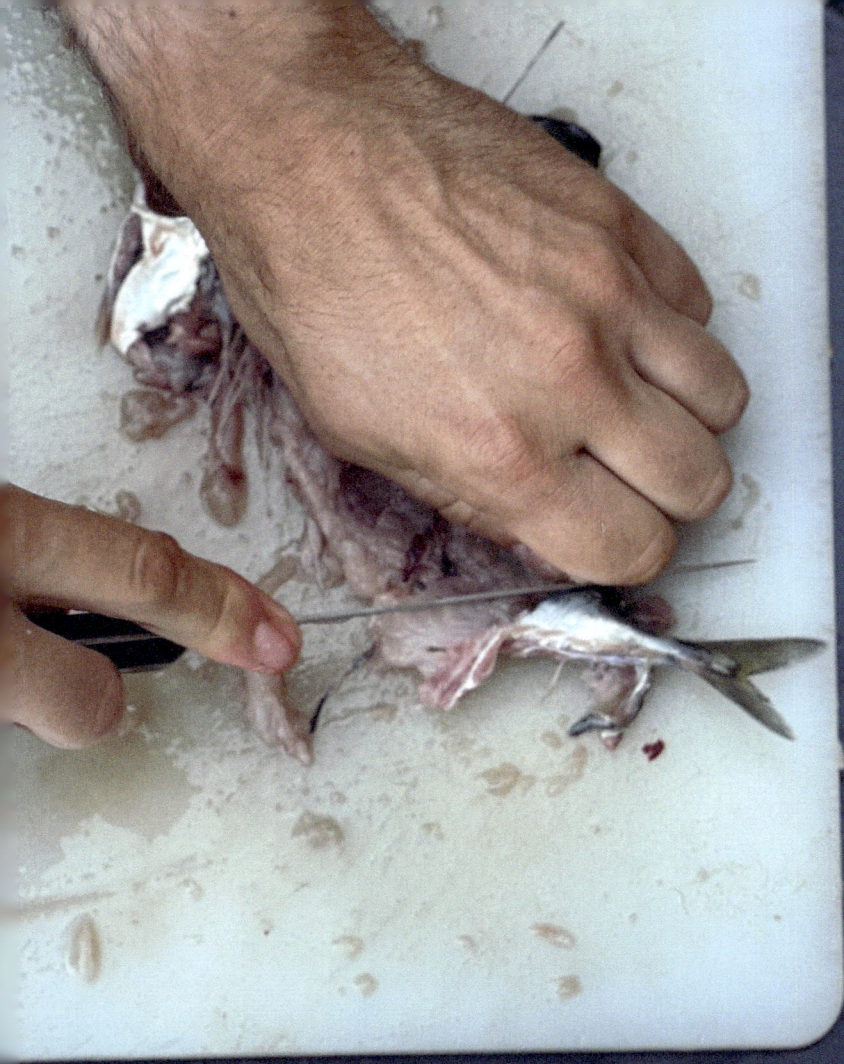
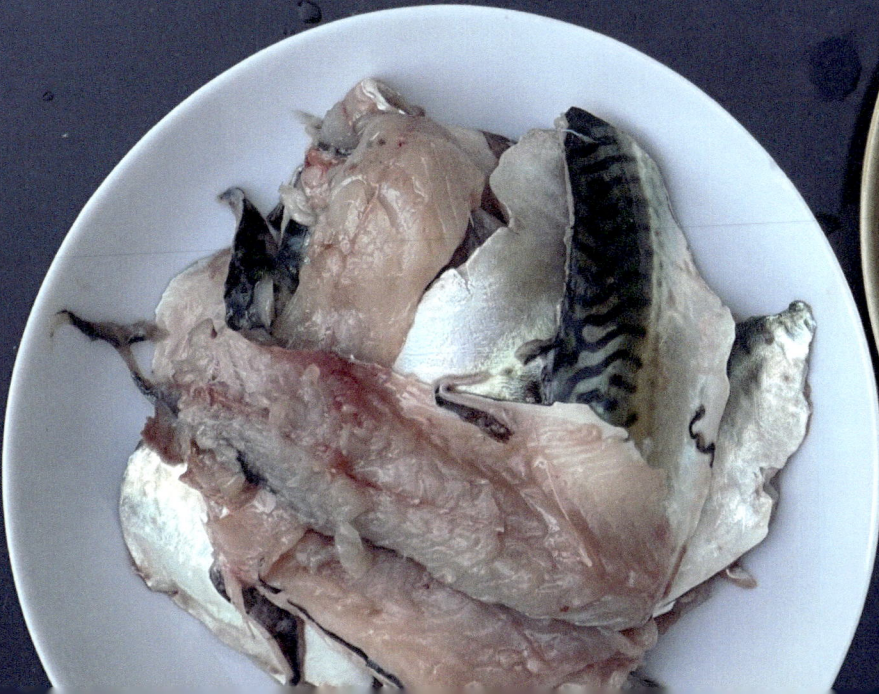
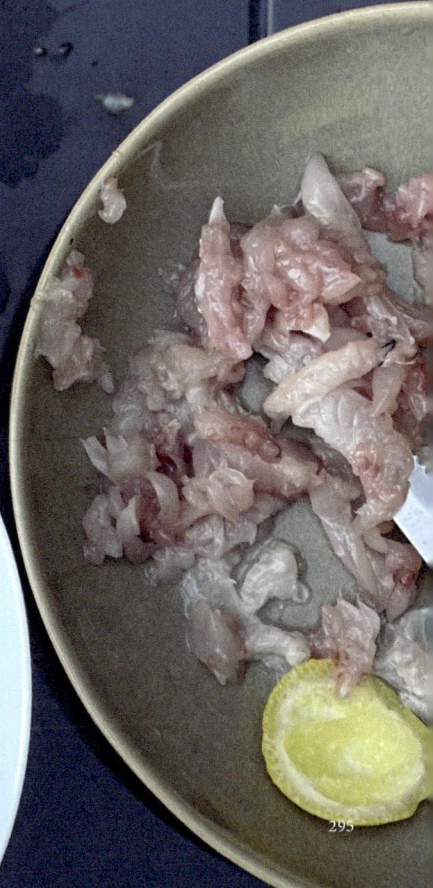

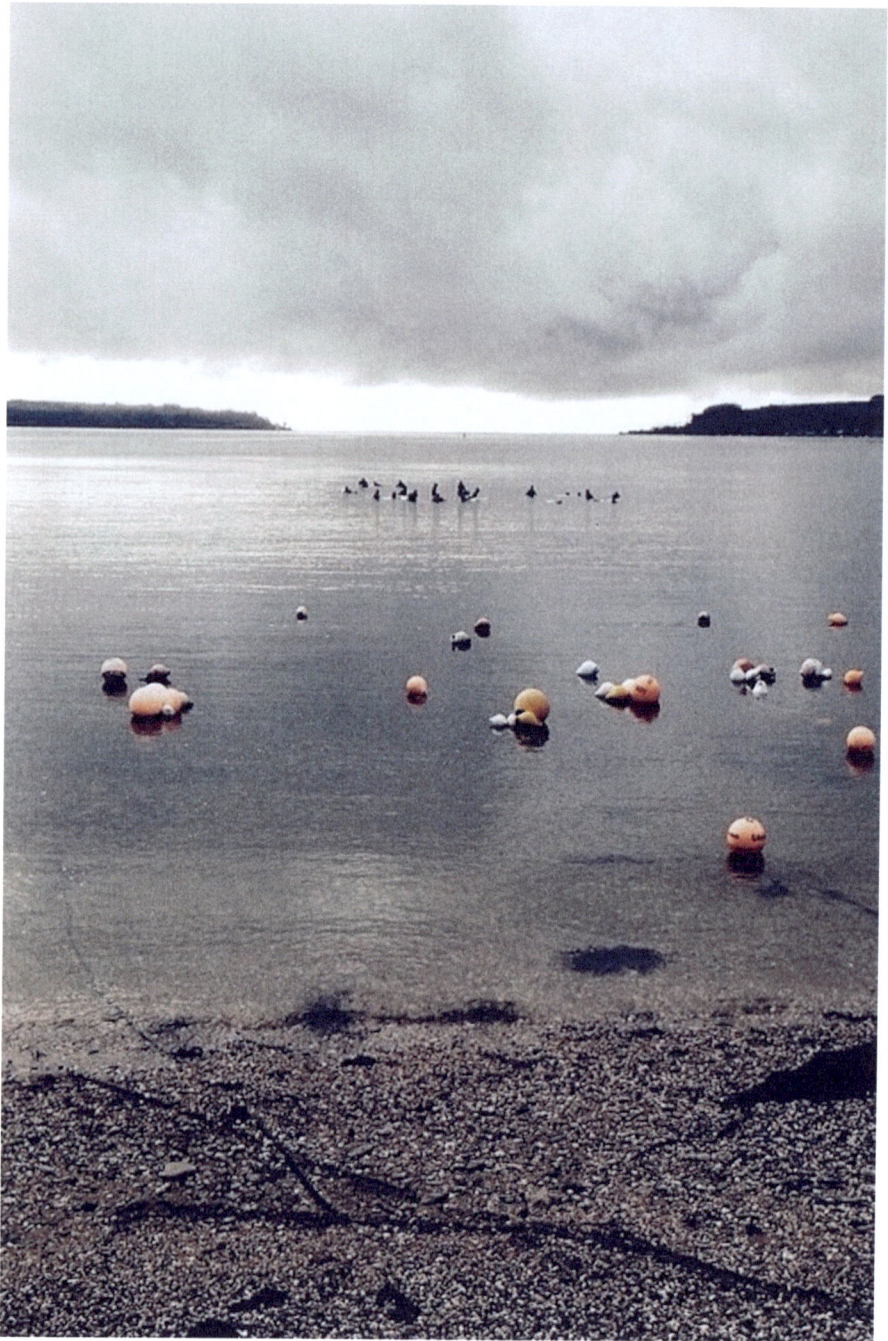